Through the Lens of Humanity

(A Memoir)

Mark E. Anderson

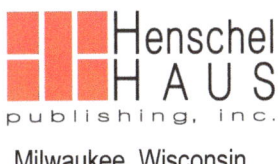

Milwaukee, Wisconsin

Copyright © 2023 by Mark E. Anderson
All rights reserved.

Photographs provided by the author unless otherwise noted.
Maps are public domain licensed via Shutterstock.

Published by HenschelHAUS Publishing, Inc.
www.henschelHAUSbooks, com
Milwaukee, Wisconsin

ISBN: 978159598-977-2
LCCN: 2023946778

Printed in the United States of America.

For my parents

Audie E. Anderson (1923–2014)
Mary Alna Jarman Anderson (1919–2011)

Table of Contents

Foreword i
Introduction i
About This Book v

PART ONE: THE JOURNEYS BEGIN 1
1. Invitation to Miraj 3
2. The Eyes of the Heart 39

PART TWO: BLESSED ARE THE PEACEMAKERS 63
3. "In Thoughts with You…" 65
4. "The Beauty of Holiness" 97
5. "Blessed are the Peacemakers" 121

PART THREE: UNCOMMON JOURNEYS 149
6. Safari! Chronicle of Adventure from South Africa
   to Malawi 151
7. The Mwandi Road 183

PART FOUR: WELCOME TO HELL 219
8. Welcome to Hell 221
9. "Where God Goes to Weep" 245

PART FIVE: ONCE A HOPIE 283
10. "Once a HOPIE, Always a HOPIE" 285

PART SIX: THROUGH THE LENS OF OF HUMANITY 313
11. Through the Lens of Humanity 315

Postscript: *Tempus Fugit* 325
Acknowledgments 327
About the Author 329

FOREWORD

I am delighted and honored to have been asked by Mark Anderson to write the Foreword for his book, *Through the Lens of Humanity*.

I am pleased to see that two major themes of his book are optimism and service. As I read Mark's stories, I was struck not only by his experiences and descriptions of what the world we live in is like, but also the optimism of what the world could be as he recounts his fascinating tales of interactions with Nobel Peace Prize recipients, missionaries, volunteers, and health professionals in service and action, and through his travels to war-torn, impoverished, and desolate areas of the world.

Through the Lens of Humanity allows us to share Mark's conversations with some of the greatest humanitarians and heroes and heroines of peace of the past century. The lives, ideals, and actions of Mother Teresa, Archbishop Desmond Tutu, Dr. Albert Schweitzer, and Dr. Margreitha van der Kreek stand as testament to their courage, compassion and perseverance in the midst of the compelling issues of their day. Hearing directly from them the thoughts, hopes, and aspirations that punctuated their tragedies and successes offers insights I believe can inspire and encourage new generations.

I met Mark while he was serving as Executive Vice President of Wisconsin's premier hospital for children, Children's Hospital of Wisconsin. As Governor of the Great State of Wisconsin, my administration worked closely with Children's to help establish it as one of the top children's hospitals in the country, and ensure Wisconsin's parents and children had access to the best pediatric care available. I'm sure Mark's work and passion at Children's was a precursor to his future involvement with medical missions, volunteerism, and international health education and training organizations.

THROUGH THE LENS OF HUMANITY

Our paths crossed again when I was Secretary of the Department of Health and Human Services (DHHS) in the Bush Administration and Mark was President of the Center for International Health, a consortium of Wisconsin-based academic and health organizations focused on international healthcare. In 2004, with the winddown of hostilities in Afghanistan following the 9/11 attacks in 2001, DHHS through United States Aid for International Development was involved in Kabul, Afghanistan, specifically at Rabia Balkhi Women's Hospital, in efforts to reduce maternal and infant mortality rates which, at the time, were the highest in the world. Mark, the Center for International Health, and a friend and colleague from the University of Wisconsin, Dr. Doug Laube, Chair of the Department of OB-GYN, joined DHHS' efforts to tackle these issues and bring a higher degree of care to Afghanistan's women, infants and children.

Whether it be the war zones of Afghanistan or Sarajevo, or impoverished villages in Africa or Asia, *Through the Lens of Humanity* shares stories of people's lives, the realities of their existence, and the immensity of their struggles. As you read these pages, see and feel the commonality of joys, sorrows, and hopes and aspirations people around the globe have for themselves and their children. The message of *Through the Lens of Humanity* bears witness to the promise of what we can all share: the dignity of humanity.

—The Honorable Tommy G. Thompson

INTRODUCTION

Someone smart once said, "A mind stretched by a new thought can never return to its original dimension." This has certainly been true in my experience. I have found and believe to be true that most defining moments in our lives are serendipitous—they sneak up on us. I have been fortunate throughout my life to have had many such moments and experiences. Moments that have caused seismic shifts in my world view, in my understanding of humanity, in who I believe God to be, moments that have transformed my thinking of how I want to live my life. For me, many of these moments occurred as a consequence of my travels to countries around the world.

Early in my life, I was bitten by the travel bug. In my junior year in high school, I was selected to represent my high school as an exchange student to Barranquilla, Colombia, South America. It was an incredible experience. I stayed in the home of the Faillace family, a Jewish family whose predecessors had fled Germany and immigrated to Colombia to avoid Hitler's persecution prior to the start of the Second World War. Mrs. Faillace was a teacher and taught math and science at the high school I attended. Mr. Faillace owned a shoe factory in Barranquilla that distributed shoes throughout South and Central America. They had three children, two of whom attended high school; their youngest was still in grade school.

Over the seven-week period I was in Colombia, I was the beneficiary of the hospitality not only of the Faillaces, but all the students of the high school I attended in Barranquilla. I was exposed to the Colombian culture, I visited the white, sandy beaches of the resort city of Cartagena, I toured the capital city of Bogota, and I was there for the magical experience of Carnival—the Colombian Mardi Gras! While in Barranquilla, I received a deeply moving letter from my maternal Grandfather Jarman, who had served for decades as a Baptist minister

THROUGH THE LENS OF HUMANITY

in rural Mississippi and Tennessee in the early to mid-1900s. He exhorted me to embrace this experience, to understand the culture of "our southern neighbors," to recognize the "bigger picture" and live with a greater awareness of the whole. In short, to embrace and understand the humanity of others.

As I grew older, my "travel bug" morphed into full-blown wanderlust. As my chosen career in hospital administration advanced, I began to seek opportunities to integrate my healthcare and administrative training with my wanderlust and try to create meaningful ways to assist others in my travels overseas. To that end, over the years, I was able to conceive and plan remarkable journeys and experiences that enabled me to meet and work with fascinating people in exciting and often exotic locales around the world. I volunteered as a short-term medical missionary in hospitals and medical facilities in remote and often desolate areas in Africa, India, Asia, Central Asia, and the Middle East. I travelled to active war zones to deliver medical supplies and develop medical training programs for medical professionals. I met prominent humanitarians like Mother Teresa, Archbishop Desmond Tutu, and Dr. Margrietha van der Kreek, Albert Schweitzer's chief surgeon in Africa, and discussed with them their life's callings. I learned about their hopes and prayers for the future of humanity.

In addition, I worked for world-renowned humanitarian organizations whose missions were educating medical professionals in emerging and developing nations and elevating the standards of care available to all peoples worldwide. Along the way, I met people from all walks and stations of life—peasants, farmers, city dwellers, immigrants, and homeless people. I met victims of war, poverty, disease, and oppression, medical personnel, government officials and heads of state, journalists, translators, clerics, Nobel Peace Prize laureates, senior corporate executives. The list goes on and on.

In his poem *Prelude*, celebrated poet Rudyard Kipling used the biblical imagery of communion and covenant to encourage greater empathy, unity, and community among his various readerships. His verse suggests that as we as individuals move beyond our own sheltered existences and experience life as lived by others, our own consciousness and sense of humanity are expanded.

Introduction

Prelude

I have eaten your bread and salt.
I have drunk your water and wine.
The deaths ye died I have watched beside,
And the lives ye led were mine.

Was there ought that I did not share
In vigil or toil or ease, —
One joy or woe that I did not know,
Dear hearts across the seas?

I have written the tale of our life
For a sheltered people's mirth
In jesting guise - but ye are wise,
And ye know what the jest is worth
   —Rudyard Kipling

Kipling's *Prelude* holds a special place in my own conscience and consciousness. I first came upon the poem shortly after returning from a deeply moving and emotional journey to India in fall 1987. Kipling's poem reflected my experience in India of moving out of my sheltered existence and sharing, at least temporarily, life as experienced by those in a culture completely foreign to me.

I had gone to India as a medical mission volunteer—working for six weeks at Wanless Hospital in Miraj, India, a city about a day's travel by train from Bombay (Mumbai). In Miraj, I was immersed in a completely different culture. The living conditions were harsh, the poverty surrounding the hospital and Miraj was abject and pervasive, the hospital was overwhelmed by the numbers of patients seeking care and handicapped by the lack of state-of-the-art equipment and supplies, and the future facing the vast majority of the population of the region seemed dismal and bleak. It was a profoundly moving and often disturbing experience.

Through the Lens of Humanity

My experiences in India intensely, powerfully, and poignantly pointed out how my life story was so dramatically different from the life stories of so many in Miraj. I was one of those sheltered from the realities of life that Kipling alludes to in Prelude. And yet, despite the cultural differences that separated my life from the realities of life in Miraj, I felt a kinship, a deep sense of fellowship and unity with the patients at Wanless and the people of Miraj.

I've had the opportunity to travel to many parts of the world since my early journey to India. Wherever I've gone, I've been mindful of *Prelude*'s imagery, and this mindfulness has enabled me to experience a deeper, richer, and fuller communion with others abroad as I have *'eaten the bread and salt,' 'drunk the water and wine,'* and *'shared the lives, joys and sorrows'* of so many dear ones across the seas.

My intent for this book is to share tales of the experiences I had with many of the extraordinary people I've met on my journeys over the years. Several of these individuals have been characters on the world stage and have participated in turbulent and world-altering events. Others are unsung heroes living their lives and life realities, often in the midst of the most difficult and harshest circumstance imaginable. My hope is that the spirit, sentiment, and imagery of *Prelude* permeates the stories I share, and that we may all become wise and understand that beyond the tales of our individual lives and our fixed ways of being ourselves and strangers, there is a common humanity that we can all embrace.

ABOUT THIS BOOK

I've organized the stories in **Through the Lens of Humanity** into six parts. In Part One, *The Journeys Begin*, I write of my journeys to India and Malawi in Central Africa—countries and cultures foreign to my own background and upbringing. My awareness and consciousness were broadened and my life irrevocably altered by what I saw, learned, and experienced.

In Part Two, *Blessed are the Peacemakers*, I share my experiences of meeting and spending time with three exceptional humanitarians: Dr. Margrietha van der Kreek, who worked alongside Dr. Albert Schweitzer for years in Africa in Lambarene, Gabon, and Nobel Peace Prize laureates Mother Teresa of Calcutta and Archbishop Desmond Tutu of South Africa. Their wit and wisdom, their descriptions of their own life's journeys and callings, and their perseverance in pursuit of their faith and justice in spite of overwhelming obstacles are inspirational and timeless.

Part Three, *Uncommon Journeys*, describes my adventures in Africa, buying and driving an ambulance from Pretoria, South Africa across Botswana, Zimbabwe, Zambia to a remote mission hospital in Embangweni, Malawi, as well as bungee jumping in Victoria Falls, Zimbabwe. This part includes the story of the village of Mwandi, Zambia, which has forever impacted the lives of hundreds of adult and youth mission volunteers who have visited there.

In Part Four, *Welcome to Hell*, I write of unforgettable journeys to war-torn Sarajevo, Bosnia, and Herzegovina and Kabul, Afghanistan. Made at a time when those cities were considered to be the most dangerous places on earth, these journeys provided medical supplies and humanitarian assistance for the hospitals and clinics in these cities. The faces of our fellow human beings in these cities expressed sadness, weariness, fear, anxiety, anger, despair and so many other tortured emotions. In downtown Sarajevo, "Welcome to Hell" was written on a bullet riddled wall. How does one make one's home in Hell?

Part Five, *Once a HOPIE...* describes my many miles of journeys and experiences while working for Project HOPE, a renowned international charitable organization committed to providing health education and training for health professionals in emerging and developing countries. The moniker "Once a HOPIE, always a HOPIE" is said with pride and reflects a respect and commitment to an organization dedicated to enhancing the health and well-being of all peoples everywhere.

Part Six, *Through the Lens of Humanity*, tells the story of the creation of *Human Reflection: The Photo Symphony*, an artistic endeavor that featured the work of documentary photographer Steve McCurry, best known for capturing people in the midst of their everyday lives, accompanied by original symphonic music composed by a trio of renowned composers. The result was a "symphonic journey through the lens of humanity" that reflected the radiance and sometimes unsettling beauty of life that shines through the joys, sorrows, challenges, limitations, and difficulties that comprise the human condition.

Finally, in Robert Service's poem, *The Wanderlust,* he declares:

> *The Wanderlust has taught me ... it has whispered to my heart*
> *Things all you stay-at-homes will never know....*
> *The Wanderlust will help you understand.....*
> *The Wanderlust has blest me...*
> *I've walked with eyes wide open to the wonders of the world*
> *And I've got to thank the Wanderlust for that....*

The stories in *Through the Lens of Humanity* reflect my wanderlust, my searching for understanding, and the wonders of humankind and of the world. As a dear friend of mine once said, "Sometimes the hand of God just takes you to places you never imagined." I have been taken places I never imagined and I have been "blest" by my wanderlust in all my travels. I hope my stories speak to and inspire others as they explore and pursue their own journeys and quests for understanding.

PART ONE

THE JOURNEYS BEGIN

CHAPTER 1

INVITATION TO MIRAJ

Ever since I was a young boy, I knew I wanted to work in healthcare. Initially, I thought I wanted to be a physician, but by the end of high school, I had determined that I was more interested in the business and operations of healthcare. Specifically, I felt myself drawn to a career in hospital and healthcare administration. After graduating from high school, I pursued an educational track that enabled me to obtain first an undergraduate Business degree in Healthcare Management and then a graduate degree in Hospital and Health Administration from the University of Alabama, Birmingham (UAB). Years later, I added a Master's degree in Theology from McCormick Seminary in Chicago, and a Doctor of Science degree in Administration —Health Science from UAB.

Early in my career, my first administrative positions took place at Children's Hospital of Alabama, University Hospital in Little Rock, Arkansas, and the Children's Hospital of Wisconsin. Throughout these experiences, I retained my interest in traveling abroad, though now my vision had expanded to include using my healthcare background and training to help others in whatever ways I could, wherever and whenever I could in countries around the globe.

In 1986, I was serving as the Executive Vice President of Children's Hospital of Wisconsin and one fall day, I joined two friends for lunch. The two had just recently returned from extended trips abroad; the purpose of the lunch was to discuss the adventures of their respective journeys.

Carol Johnson was an ICU nurse at Children's and I knew her through both the hospital and mutual friends. Carol had just returned from several weeks of volunteer work at a hospital in Bangladesh. She spoke of the poverty of the area and the masses of people living in crowded and squalid conditions. She spoke with tears in her eyes of the children who came to the hospital, most dirty and malnourished, many having never seen a doctor, and the far too many who were beyond medical help. She spoke of the lack of basic medical equipment, medicines and supplies—supplies and medicines which, if they had only been available—could have saved many lives.

A particularly poignant portion of Carol's sharing was her telling of how difficult it was for her to re-adapt to our culture and material possessions once she returned, not only in her personal daily life, but specifically with regard to the plentifulness of resources we had at Children's Hospital. She shared a story of going to the supply room on one of the hospital's floors and being completely overwhelmed at the surplus of supplies she saw at her disposal—items that could have saved so many in Bangladesh. Overcome with emotion, she said she sank to the supply room floor, sobbing uncontrollably. Though haunted by so many depressing images, she shared how she had resolved to do all she could to help others overseas—particularly children—and was contemplating a return trip to Bangladesh.

David Eager was a certified public accountant and the nephew of one of the board members of Children's Hospital. David and I had met at one of the hospital's charitable golf outings. David had just returned from a multi-week journey through India, Pakistan, Thailand, and other Asian countries. David's stories reflected his own serious case of wanderlust—the intrepid traveler willing to go anywhere and see everything. He talked of the mystique of India, of the Taj Mahal, the Ganges River. He spoke of the beauty of Thailand and Pakistan and of the various scenes and states of life in those far away places. His stories were mesmerizing and had the feel of a traveler or journalist of a bygone era sharing impressions of the most exotic and beautiful parts of the world.

As I marveled at their experiences, both Carol and David encouraged me to plan my own journey, answer my own wanderlust, and pursue my own calling to share and experience the lives and culture of others. Carol shared with me the name of the Presbyterian organization that had coordinated her volunteer trip to Bangladesh. I knew I would shortly be pursuing my own call and adventures.

Within days of my lunch meeting, I reached out to the Medical Benevolence Foundation (MBF), a Texas-based not-for-profit organization affiliated with the Presbyterian Church (USA) that had facilitated Carol's volunteer efforts. In a call with MBF staffer Clarence Durham, I indicated I was a hospital administrator interested in volunteering at an overseas mission hospital supported by MBF and the Presbyterian Church. I stated that the summer or fall of 1987 was a workable time for me and that I had availability for a period of approximately four to six weeks. Clarence asked me to send a resume and told me he'd see what he could do. I sent my resume to Clarence and eagerly awaited his response.

A few days later, on November 28th, 1986, I received copies of the communiques that Clarence had forwarded to physicians and hospitals abroad about my interest in volunteering my time. Clarence had forwarded inquiries to hospitals in Kinshasa, Zaire, Africa; Chonju and Kwangju, Korea; and Miraj, India. Clarence's letter to the hospital leaders stated:

> *"He is volunteering his time for a four- or five-week period in the summer or fall, 1987. If you think Mr. Anderson's skills will be useful at your hospital, please respond to me or to Mr. Anderson directly with a copy to me."*

I wondered which, if any, of these hospitals I would hear from. Would it be from Africa, where I had dreamed of going all my life, or mysterious and mystical India, or the Far East and Korea, which I candidly knew the least about?

I got my answer in a letter dated 10 December 1986:

Through the Lens of Humanity

WANLESS HOSPITAL
MIRAJ MEDICAL CENTRE
MIRAJ, Maharashtra (India)

10 December 1986

Mr. Mark Anderson
P.O. Box 2041
Milwaukee, WI 53201
U.S.A.

Dear Mr. Anderson:
We have a copy of your letter to Mr. Clarence Durham of the Presbyterian Medical Mission Fund and his letter to Dr. Paul Jewett of our staff.

We would be very happy to have you come to Miraj as a voluntary consultant in administrative and management skills for 4 - 5 weeks. Any time between July and November of 1987 would be convenient.

I am enclosing our hospital brochure and an information sheet for volunteers. If you have specific questions about the hospital, please do not hesitate to ask.

Yours sincerely,
Cherian Thomas, MD
DIRECTOR

cc: Mr. Clarence Durham

Within days of receiving Dr. Thomas's letter, I received another letter asking if, while I was in India, in addition to consulting at Wanless Hospital in Miraj, would I be willing to consult with Mure Memorial Hospital in Nagpur, India.

As the realization hit that my dream of traveling to a foreign land to try help alleviate the suffering of others was about to become a reality, I turned my thoughts to planning and making this the experience of a lifetime. And, in the unconscious arrogance of ignorance, I had no concept as yet, of how this experience was going to forever alter my life.

INVITATION TO MIRAJ

PLANNING

Armed with an official invitation to travel and consult with a hospital abroad, I needed formal approval for time off from my employer. I had just recently been promoted to Executive Vice President of Children's Hospital, and I wondered if I was pushing my luck to ask for what was in essence a "leave of absence" to go work abroad for four to six weeks.

I met with Children's Hospital's president Jon Vice and was pleasantly surprised with how enthusiastically he approved my request! Not only did he approve my leave, but on several future occasions, he mentioned it publicly to others, challenging them, as he phrased it, "to give back to others, particularly those who aren't as fortunate as ourselves."

Over the Christmas holidays, I began to plan my trip to Miraj. I reviewed all the information that I had received about Miraj from Dr. Thomas' first correspondence. The hospital brochure he'd provided was a folded eight-page document that offered a plethora of information about the hospital and the town of Miraj.

Published in 1986, the brochure noted that Miraj was a town of 110,000 located 275 miles southeast of Bombay. It was an important railway junction and was famous throughout India as a hand-crafted manufacturer of the sitar. Wanless Hospital was opened in 1894 by Dr. William Wanless, a young Canadian Presbyterian medical missionary. The hospital served a 125,000-square-mile rural area with a population of approximately 10 million people. Over the years, the hospital's capacity had grown to 550 beds. The hospital treated more than 100,000 patients annually in its outpatient department and annually admitted over 12,300 patients to the hospital. The entire complex was known as the Miraj Medical Centre, and it had evolved into a regional teaching complex for physicians, nurses, and other health personnel.

On the grounds of the Miraj Medical Centre was the Archie Fletcher Residence for Volunteers, named for Dr. A.G. Fletcher, for many years the Director of the Wanless Hospital. Dr Fletcher, a Presbyterian medical missionary still lived and practiced at the hospital. It was the Fletcher Residence that I'd be calling home during the course of my time in Miraj.

Through the Lens of Humanity

The information sheet for volunteers was several pages of basic information volunteers needed to know and would find useful: visa and passport information, flight information to Bombay and then subsequent train schedules to Miraj, seasonal weather forecasts for the Miraj region, specific items related to Indian culture, etc. I tried to absorb it all and began my planning.

In January 1987, I sent a letter to Dr. Thomas and Clarence at MBF indicating my plans were to travel to Miraj in October of 1987. I immediately received word from Dr. Thomas that October was a wonderful month to be in India and he proceeded to articulate the projects he and staff had identified for me to tackle while in Miraj. We left open the option for me to travel to Nagpur, India, if time permitted during my visit. I felt that Clarence at MBF became my guardian angel, much as Clarence the novice angel became George Bailey's guardian angel in *It's a Wonderful Life*. Clarence (MBF) secured tourist visas for me via contacts at the Indian Embassy, and he sent letters to U.S. personnel in the US embassy in India advising them of the purpose and timing of my trip.

On July 30, 1987, I notified Dr. Thomas of my proposed itinerary. Keeping in mind David Eager's comments about his experiences traveling in this part of the world, I expanded my itinerary to include about ten days of personal travel to various cities *en route* to Miraj. I made every effort to include some of the most mysterious and historic cities in this region of the world as part of my itinerary. My *en-route* destinations included Hong Kong; Kathmandu, Nepal; Varanasi and Agra; India. Then to Bombay and by train to Miraj arriving the evening of October 11, 1987.

By mid-August, I had received Dr. Thomas's agreement with my itinerary dates and a letter as well from Dr. Paul Jewett. Paul and his wife Judy were full-time medical missionaries assigned by the Presbyterian Church (U.S.A.) to Miraj. Originally from Nebraska, Paul was serving as professor and head of the Cardiology Department at Miraj Medical Centre, and Judy was serving in the hospital's Administration Department. Paul requested I bring them some specific medical items in my luggage when I traveled to Miraj, a request I was more than happy to honor if my luggage capacity permitted. Six weeks prior to my departure I had the major portions of my travel schedule planned. I used the remaining weeks before departure to research and become familiar with the countries and cities I was preparing to visit.

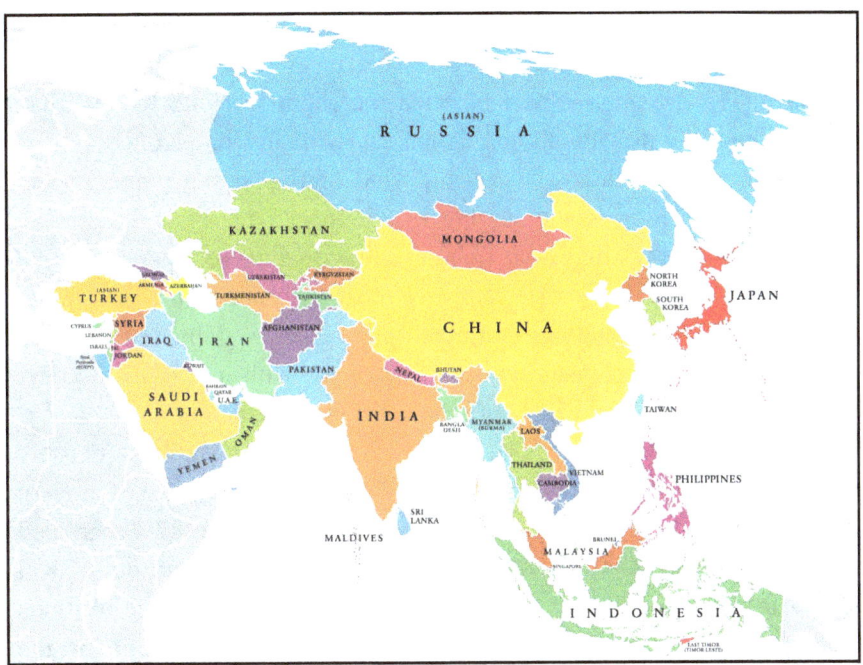

Asia Itinerary Map:
Hong Kong; Kathmandu, Nepal; Varanasi, Agra, Bombay, Miraj, India

Through the Lens of Humanity

The Journey

My departure date of September 30th finally arrived, and I left Milwaukee flying west, first to St. Louis and then onward to Honolulu. Several years earlier, I had house-sat for two weeks for friends in Honolulu while they traveled and camped in the western United States. I had a several hour layover in Honolulu before proceeding on to Hong Kong, so I was able to re-connect with the Dan Rutt family and have an enjoyable dinner with them. They gave me the names of friends of theirs in Hong Kong, so as I boarded the flight to Hong Kong, I had contact names with whom I could connect while in Hong Kong.

The next ten days were a whirlwind of flights and tours. I spent three days in Hong Kong visiting Kowloon and the New Territories, touring Aberdeen Village—a floating village of approximately 30,000 people, Republic Bay—the "gateway" to the South China Sea, Tiger Balm Gardens—containing statutes and dioramas depicting Chinese folklore and Confucianism, and Victoria Peak with its exquisite views of Hong Kong, Victoria Bay, and the surrounding islands.

What a magnificent city Hong Kong is! One of the most densely populated places on earth - the city seemed a curious mixture of modern technology and old traditional Chinese culture. And in 1987, I marveled at our airplane pilots as they navigated our plane into and out of Kai Tak Airport, the international airport of Hong Kong at the time. With its runways jutting out into Victoria Bay and surrounded by mountains, the final approach was technically demanding of pilots as the aircraft flew directly over Chinese junks in Victoria Bay and in a guide path abutted by skyscrapers and mountains! It was a marvelous experience, enjoyed all the more after one safely landed!

Next up was Kathmandu, where I arrived after a brief layover in Bangkok, Thailand. Nepalese soldiers patrolled the airport grounds as we arrived and the airport was abuzz with hundreds of people; Kathmandu airport is the only airport in Nepal, and Kathmandu is the tourist gateway to the Himalayas.

I was struck immediately by the horrid poverty I saw as I traveled from the airport to my hotel. The streets were lined with filthy-looking wooden structures and buildings so dilapidated I was astonished they were even standing. These were the homes and shops of literally thousands of people. A menagerie of animals roamed the streets—dogs, monkeys, cats, cattle—all seemingly on the verge of starvation themselves. Cooking fires were pervasive and smoke and the dust from the streets filled the air. Odors and aromas filled the air—some distinguishable, many not.

In stark contrast to these sour stimuli, were the bright, vibrant colors of the women's saris and the constant noise of hundreds of people on the move. Famed photographer Steve McCurry has described life in this part of the world as "the riot of life carried out on the streets and bazaars." His observation is spot on!

I was the consummate tourist in Kathmandu. My first day, I toured the Hindu temple of Pashupati on the banks of the Bagmati River. Strolling with other tourists along the river's edge, I did see the "riot of life"—a cremation occurring near one of the river ghats (gates), hundreds of animals and humans splashing and bathing in the river, beggars wandering the temple grounds and pleading with tourists for

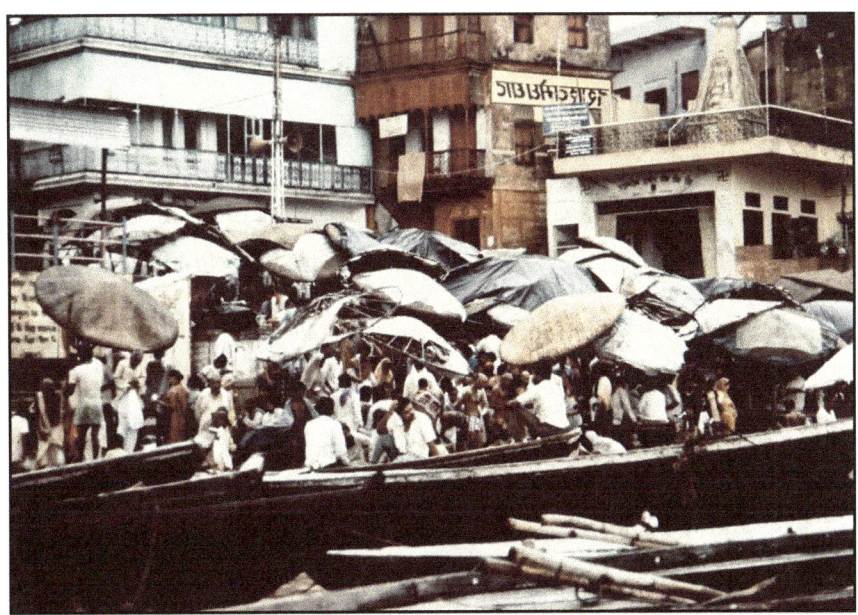

Hindus lining the shores of the Ganges River in Varanasi, India

alms. I toured the Buddhist Stupas of Baudhanath, one of the largest stupas in the world.

My second day in Kathmandu, I traveled to Bhaktapur and Patan, cities which, along with Kathmandu, are known historically as the three royal cities of Kathmandu Valley. These cities possess numerous Hindu and Buddhist temples and are also known for their ornate architecture, stone carvings, and metal statues. I visited the Swayambhunath Stupa, which is said to be over 2,500 years old and is commonly known as the Monkey Temple. It is located several hundred feet up a hillside and affords a wonderful panoramic view of Kathmandu City and the Kathmandu Valley.

My companions as I toured these facilities were a few other tourists and our tour guide, but we were outnumbered by the cattle, monkeys, and beggars, who seemed to match us step for step. I left Kathmandu beginning to grasp just how much the major religions of Buddhism and Hinduism permeated and controlled all of life in this part of the world.

The city of Varanasi was my first "port of call" in India. My first afternoon in Varanasi, I taxied about six miles to Sarnath, one of the holiest places in the world for Buddhists. It is in this area that Buddha delivered his first teachings. Varanasi is also the holiest of the seven sacred cities of Hinduism.

At 5 a.m. on my second morning in Varanasi, I taxied to the *ghats* (gates) on the Ganges River. There, before dawn, I rented a rowboat and guide and we rowed out into the river to observe the literary thousands of Hindus who each morning make their pilgrimage to the Ganges to bathe and worship. Sitting under huge umbrella-like structures that look like mushroom pods were "holy men" who'd bless the pilgrims as they came to the river.

Next we rowed past areas on the shoreline where the cremation *ghats* were located. Each morning at dawn, bodies are carried by family members down the ghats for cremation. Hindus believe that being cremated in the Ganges allows one to attain salvation. The smoke from the pyres provided a dim and murky skyline and filled the air and our lungs with a stinging sensation and pungent odor. The streets were a

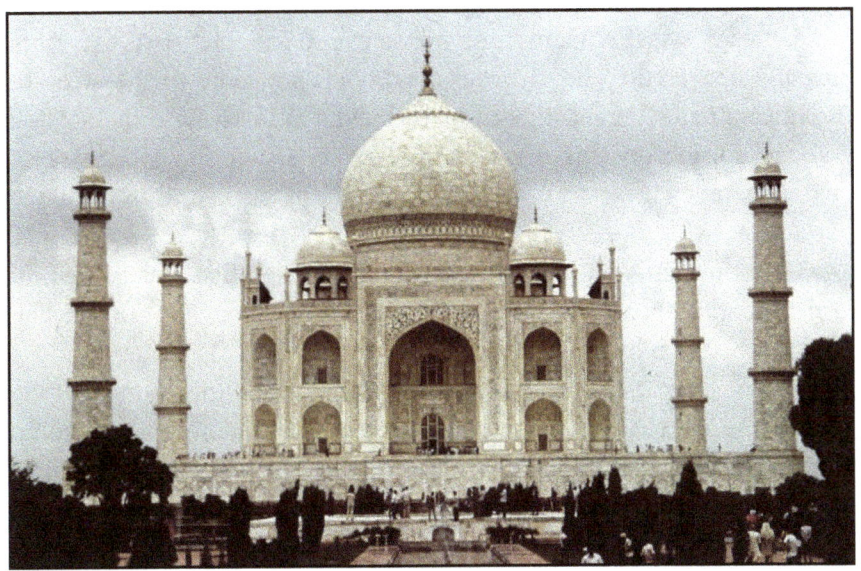

The Taj Mahal in Agra, India

cacophony of sounds. Wailing, the cries of children, barking dogs, honking horns and the noise of thousands of people in motion at dawn all assailed our hearing.

After returning to shore, I walked with a guide through the side streets and bazaars of Varanasi. The city is well known for its silk factories and many shops displayed beautiful and colorful saris, scarves, shawls, silk paintings, carpets, and much more. These products are very inexpensive in Varanasi, but extraordinarily costly outside of India. I left Varanasi much impressed by the vibrancy of the city that I felt my entire time there.

Agra's airport was small and dirty with naked lightbulbs illuminating the large great hall entry room. Taxis and rickshaws were the primary means of transport from the airport to my hotel and the drivers of both were incessant in their pleadings for me to select them as my transport. On the drive to the hotel, I saw all manner of traffic milling through the streets—bicyclists, rickshaws, taxis, cows, pedestrians, water buffalo, and even a few camels.

Poverty was obvious and pervasive, but some parts of Agra actually appeared to be in better condition than some of the areas of Kathmandu and Varanasi that I had visited. On the way to the hotel, a violent rainstorm occurred, muddying the city's streets and side streets, and illustrating how forceful the weather can be in this part of the world.

My time in Agra was spent visiting the magnificent and beautiful Taj Mahal. I spent hours wandering the grounds of the Taj Mahal, taking photographs from all angles, marveling at its beauty and its chameleon-like ability to change its appearance at various times of the day as the marble was reflected in different and shimmering lighting. And I visited the Agra Fort, a red sandstone structure complete with moat and drawbridge in the tradition of the Mogul empire.

Early in the evening of October 10th, I flew to Bombay, arriving late in the evening. I took a taxi to the Advent House, the guest house recommended by Dr. Thomas in Bombay that catered to missionaries, church workers, and volunteers. After some searching for the address with the taxi driver, we finally found my lodgings, and after checking in with Miss Anchees, the aged resident manager of the guest house, I got to bed around midnight. The next morning, October 11th, was my travel day to Miraj!

The Train Ride

After a fitful night's sleep, I arose early, I had been sleeping on a rather uncomfortable roll-away cot in the men's dorm room on the fifth floor of the guest house. I washed up as best I could in the guest house's communal shower facility and made my way to the dining area. Miss Anchees was already up and about and she provided me breakfast and instructed me on how to get to Victoria Train Station for my travel to Miraj. Fortunately, as I was eating, another guest, a Canadian nun in transit, Sister Jocelyn, joined us and indicated that she too was going to the train station that morning. Since she was familiar with the station, she would help me get to the proper train platform. We completed breakfast, gathered our luggage, and shlepped down five flights of stairs

INVITATION TO MIRAJ

(the elevator was out of commission—it appeared this was a common occurrence), and hailed a taxi.

Victoria Station is an enormous, beautiful, old majestic building in the old British colonial tradition. Our driver let Sister Jocelyn and me out as close to the front of the building as he could, and we moved toward the entrance, again shlepping our luggage as we proceeded.

Along the way, we converged on a commotion ahead of us and as we drew near, it was evident that there was an elderly woman's body lying in the road. When we passed, it was obvious that she was deceased and likely had been lying unattended for quite some time. Everyone was moving past her, some actually stepping over her as they moved about their business. Approaching the entrance way, Sister Jocelyn spoke to a police officer about the situation, and he moved toward where the woman lay.

As we moved into the station, I was impressed by the enormity of the building and with the tremendous numbers of people milling about. This train station in India is one of the busiest train stations in the world and it was certainly living up to that billing this particular morning. I had pre-ordered and received my train tickets to Miraj per the suggestion of MBF and Dr. Thomas, so I was able to quickly identify my train platform. Bidding Sister Jocelyn goodbye, I proceeded to the designated track for my train.

My ticket was a second-class ticket entitling me to a train car that was a little more private. I would share the car with others but the space was better suited for longer distance travel; the travel time to Miraj was in excess of 11 hours and the schedule called for us to arrive in Miraj at 9:15 p.m. As the boarding process began, it appeared that there were very few first-class cars, several second-class, with the preponderance of the cars being more general third-class tickets—i.e., cars without much privacy or luggage space. As I watched people boarding, the third-class cars were quickly overflowing. The masses of people streaming into the cars seemingly exceeded the capacity of the cars.

The car that I settled into had storage space over the wooden bench seats, and I nestled my two pieces of luggage and my camera bag, replete with two cameras and film in the area above my head. I was

THROUGH THE LENS OF HUMANITY

sharing the car with about eight other people, what I thought to be two Indian families, parents and children, some of whom were young adults.

As the train pulled out of the station, through the window, I could see the mammoth size of the train station and for the quite a while, I spied parts of Bombay, its skyscraper buildings in the distance. But the real visual was the poverty areas of the city surrounding the station. As

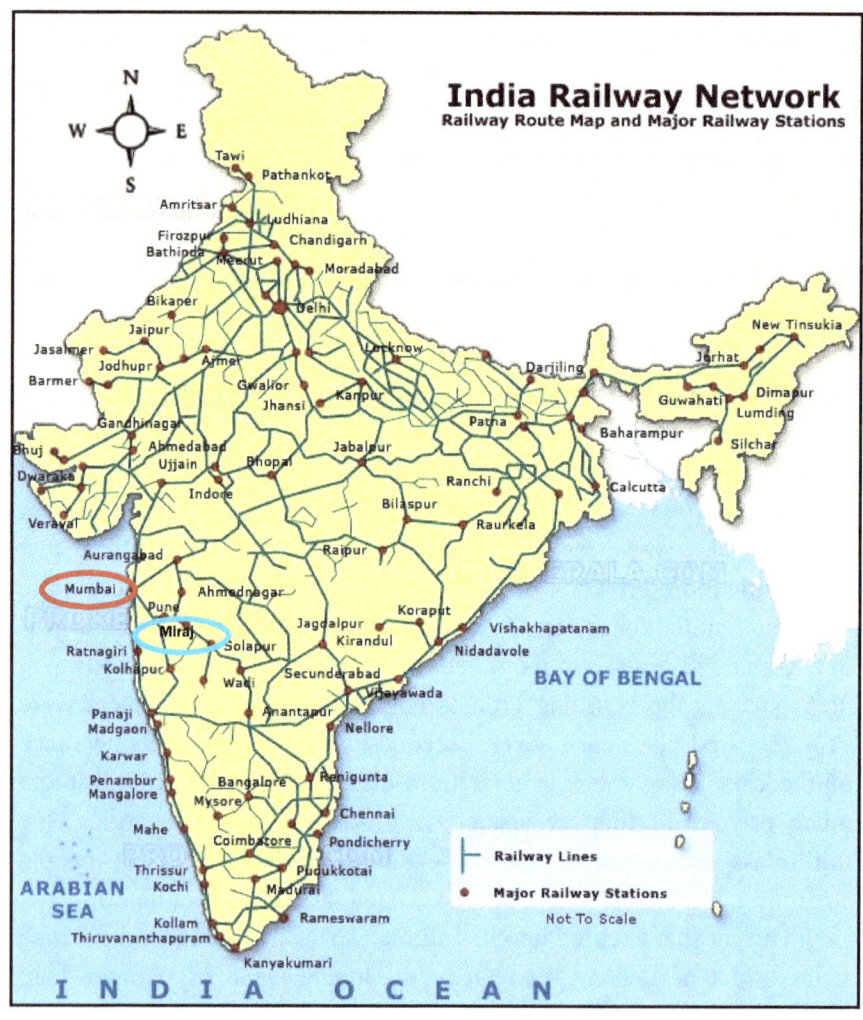

Railway Map of India: From Bombay (red circle) to Miraj (blue circle)

we moved out of the city, I began reading. The other occupants of the car settled in; one family had brought their own food and they started eating a meal. A few people seemed to be dozing.

The benches were un-cushioned, so quite quickly, they became uncomfortable. Gradually, as we traveled along, the car became warmer and warmer. I had brought some water and a sandwich from the guest house, but the soggy sandwich was very unappealing in the heat and it became clear to me that I hadn't brought enough water. During the train's stop in Pune, the largest city between Bombay and Miraj, and about four hours into the trip, several vendors came onto the train and I bought an orange soda. As the day progressed, it got hotter and hotter and in the mid-afternoon at another stop, I bought another soda.

Shortly afterward, I became very sleepy, and as there was room in the storage area, I curled up next to my luggage and tried to rest. Soon I became very groggy and noticed my vision was getting hazy and my peripheral vision was blurred. I tried to sit up but had difficulty getting myself upright. I realized I was dizzy and things were spinning quite a bit, but I was also aware that we had arrived in another station. I looked at my luggage and realized that my camera bag was missing. I started moving things around and the other people in the car noticed my behavior and my searching actions, I asked if anyone had seen my camera bag—I got mostly blank looks but a few shaking of heads no. One man in the car spoke English and I noticed that two of the young men who had been in the car had left. I was told they had just gotten off the train.

Thinking that they must have taken the camera bag, I staggered up and very unsteadily moved toward the car's door and down the steps to the train platform. I suppose my intent was to see if I could spot the two that had left the car, but not seeing them, I thought I should tell someone in authority. I started moving down the platform to see if there was a train office or train official in sight. I felt like things were moving in slow motion—I was unsteadily weaving down the platform, certainly not thinking very clearly, when all of the sudden, I realized the train had started moving in the opposite direction of where I was headed.

I knew I had to get back on the train, otherwise I'd lose the rest of my possessions and be stranded at a train station somewhere in the middle of India. I started stumbling back toward my car, which by this time I was several cars behind, and lurchingly tried to jog back to the train car entrance. At the same time, the train was picking up speed. I got to the car steps and reached for the entrance handle to the train car. I grabbed the handle and got one foot on the first step. But I wasn't able to pull myself up into the car's stairwell and was desperately reaching with my other hand for the handle as the train was rapidly gaining speed. I knew if I let go of the handle, I could fall beneath the train and would likely be killed. I knew time was running out. I either had to somehow pull myself into the stairwell or release the handle and try and push myself away from the train so as not to fall beneath it and be run over.

All of a sudden, I felt hands grasp my arm on the handle and my clothing and pull me into the car stairwell. Two men from my car had seen me and had pulled me in.

"Sir, sir, what are you doing? You could have been killed," said the Indian man who spoke English as we re-entered the train car. The others in the car looked at me with surprise and amazement, and after I caught my breath, I told the Indian man who spoke English and who had helped me, that I thought that the two who had left the car had taken my camera bag and that I was trying to see if I could see them on the platform and report the theft to the police.

He asked me where I was going and I told him Miraj. He indicated that Miraj was still several hours away and I should report the theft there. He told the others in Hindi what had happened and through him, they all expressed sorrow that I had lost my cameras and indicated that they did not know the two young men. They did say that thefts were common on the train. I thanked the two men who had pulled me into the car, and tried to collect myself for the remainder of the train ride.

As the remaining hours of the train trip elapsed, slowly my vision returned to normal and the grogginess subsided. I knew that I had been drugged, probably via the sodas I had purchased, and I knew that I was fortunate not to have injured myself further by leaving the train as I did. As I took stock, I was devastated by the loss of my cameras and all the film that I had already taken—the photos I had taken in Hong Kong,

INVITATION TO MIRAJ

Kathmandu, Varanasi, Agra, all gone. Fortunately, I still had my passport and money—and my life.

> [**Author's Note**: I remember this incident every time I see a train and still shudder when I think what could have happened.]

When we finally got to Miraj, I thanked my train car companions again for helping me. Then, with my remaining luggage, I went into the train station entry lounge and met Mr. Latker from Dr. Cherian Thomas's office who had come to meet me. I explained what had happened on the train, and with his assistance, reported the theft to the railway police at the train station. I knew this was basically a futile effort; I didn't ever expect to see my camera case or its contents again. I felt a little foolish for having allowed myself to be taken advantage of, and I thought, *What a way to begin my four weeks in Miraj!*

Mr. Latker was quite sympathetic, and after reporting the incident, he took me by car to Fletcher Hall in the medical centre. Fletcher Hall is a separate structure with perhaps six large rooms to accommodate volunteers, visiting medical students and medical personnel, and other official guests of the hospital. In addition, it also has a dining area and a small lounge sitting room area for the guests. The lounge area had a TV and a DVD player as well. I was happy to get into my room and get some rest.

MIRAJ

The next morning, though I was still licking my wounds from my train experience from Bombay to Miraj, I was determined not to dwell on this experience and ruin my time in Miraj. I went to the breakfast room and met two young female medical students visiting from the Netherlands, Andrea and Ingeborgh. They were sharing one of the residence rooms and in conversation with them, we determined that their time in Miraj would almost completely coincide with mine. They were in Miraj with permission from the hospital to observe care, but as they were still students, they were not permitted to render care.

THROUGH THE LENS OF HUMANITY

After breakfast, we walked over to the chapel on the Medical Centre campus' grounds. Every morning, chapel services were held primarily for the hospital and medical centre's staff, but also for any patients or patient's families who might want to attend. Chapel services were conducted by the Rev. Agnes Howard, who, in her mid-eighties, was a Scottish force of nature who had been at Miraj for many years—no one I asked seemed to know how many for sure. The entire service only lasted about 20 minutes but with Rev. Agnes in charge, you got your money's worth! Morning chapel after breakfast became a morning staple for the Dutch students and me.

Following chapel, Mr. Latkar took me to Dr. Cherian Thomas's office and there I met Dr. Archie Fletcher and his wife Huldah, who had been missionaries at Miraj for 30 years. Actually, Archie had served as Director of the Wanless Hospital for many years, and had only recently retired and been succeeded by Dr. Thomas. I recognized Huldah as the woman who had played the piano at chapel. The Fletchers had devoted their lives to the mission field, and their eldest son John and his wife were presently serving as Presbyterian medical missionaries in the Congo. Though retired, Archie and Huldah continued to live in Miraj on the medical campus grounds.

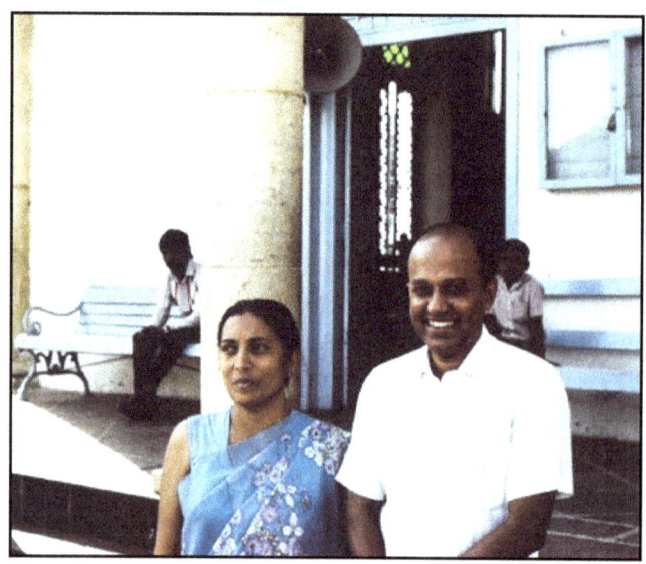

Drs. Cherian and Kalindi Thomas

INVITATION TO MIRAJ

I also met Judy Jewett, who with her husband, Dr. Paul Jewett, were the current Presbyterian missionaries assigned to Miraj. And, in addition to Dr. Cherian Thomas, I also meet his wife, Dr. Kalindi Thomas, who was the Head of the Medical Centre's Community Health Department.

Dr. Thomas and I met briefly and he shared with me his ideas for the various projects they'd like to see me undertake while at the hospital. Basically, we agreed that I'd work to improve efficiencies in the hospital's pharmacy, laboratory, radiology, surgery, and outpatient departments. He asked that I work primarily with Judy Jewett, since she had a background in administration and could help implement my recommendations once I had departed. Once my meeting was complete with Dr. Thomas, Mr. Latkar, who served as Dr. Thomas' administrative assistant, showed me around the hospital.

The tour was educational, fascinating, and depressing. The hospital had approximately 550 beds and a large outpatient department. The hospital operated at almost 100% capacity all the time, as Wanless Hospital was effectively the only major hospital for an area populated by ten million people.

Given its size, I had expected the hospital to be fairly modernized. It was not. It was also quite dirty. The wards and private rooms were poorly lit, and the bed linens looked frayed and stained. In many rooms, the windows were cracked or broken, and the screens covering the verandah and patio areas were blackened by pollution. The nursing stations had very limited supplies and medications. In surgery, I saw soiled bandages being washed and re-washed in order to be reused. Birds flew freely in many areas of the hospital, accessing the building through the open lobby areas and the broken windows. The whole inpatient area was cooled by fans, which meant that most of the year, the fans were mainly simply swirling warm air.

The hospital does not have a dietary department, so if a patient is admitted to the hospital, it is the patient's family who is responsible for providing meals for both the patient and themselves. There are designated areas on the hospital grounds where the families can cook meals, and there are water standpipes where running water is available.

THROUGH THE LENS OF HUMANITY

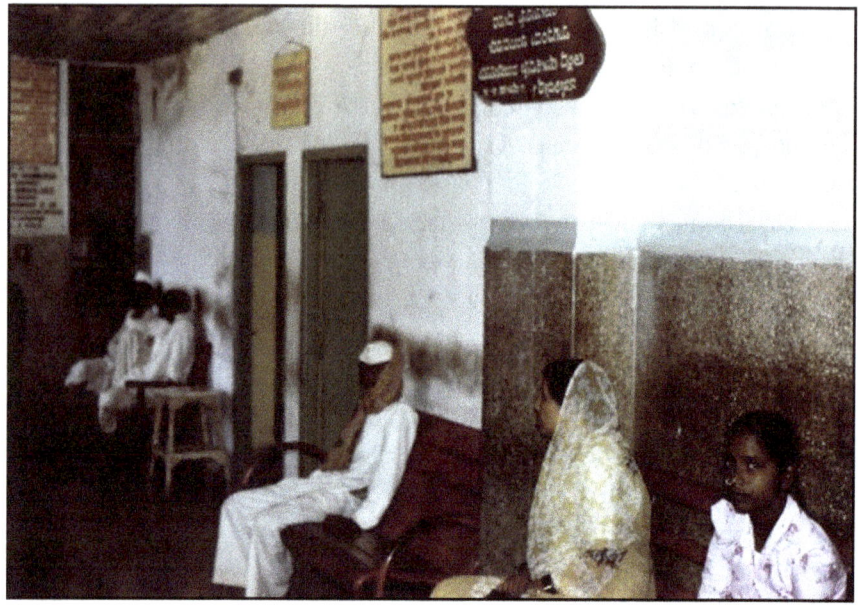

Miraj Hospital Admitting / Waiting Area

Patient's families camp on the hospital grounds. The hospital does have many specialty programs. For example, there is a separate "children's hospital" for pediatric patients, there is a burn unit, ICU and PICU, an orthopedic and prosthesis unit, a chest and cardiology hospital, and a separate leprosy hospital just off the main campus grounds.

After the tour, I met and talked with Mr. Desai, General Superintendent of the hospital, and Judy Jewett about the projects Dr. Thomas and I had discussed and about the hospital in general. After Mr. Desai was called away, I continued to speak with Judy about my impressions of the hospital. Dr. Paul Jewett joined us as he finished his work day at the hospital. End-of-the-day sessions with Paul and Judy became the norm over the course of my time in Miraj, and the Jewetts became close friends and colleagues over the succeeding decades.

My first day ended with dinner at 7:30 in Fletcher Hall with Ingeborgh and Andrea.

Early on my second day, I traveled to the local police district to register as a visiting volunteer. After lunch, Dr. Jewett stopped by Fletcher Hall with a spare camera and several rolls of film and offered

INVITATION TO MIRAJ

them to me for my use while I was at Miraj. I was very appreciative of this gesture, having lost both my cameras in the train theft. I was concerned that I wouldn't have any photos to share of Miraj either. The camera was actually the same model as the one I had lost, so my spirits picked up with Paul's loan of his camera.

Late that evening, Dr. Keith Crowley, a retired pathologist from Australia, arrived for a month volunteer stint. I learned from Dr. Crowley that he had visited Miraj previously—this visit he had come primarily to teach medical students and staff courses in basic and intermediate pathology and to create a meaningful curriculum for future medical students. With Keith's arrival, Fletcher Hall had four volunteer occupants—Keith, Ingeborgh, Andrea, and yours truly.

My daily routine at Miraj emerged pretty quickly. Breakfast at Fletcher Hall, Chapel at 8 a.m., and then I would begin work on my various projects. These basically gave me free run of the hospital and enabled me to interface readily with staff and patients alike. One morning after Chapel, Dr. James Thomas, an Indian cardiovascular surgeon who had trained in Bombay, asked Ingeborgh, Andrea, and me if we'd like to observe an open-heart surgery that he was performing that morning on an eight-year-old girl. Dr. Thomas explained the he was going to correct an atrial septal defect (ASD), saying he felt it'd be

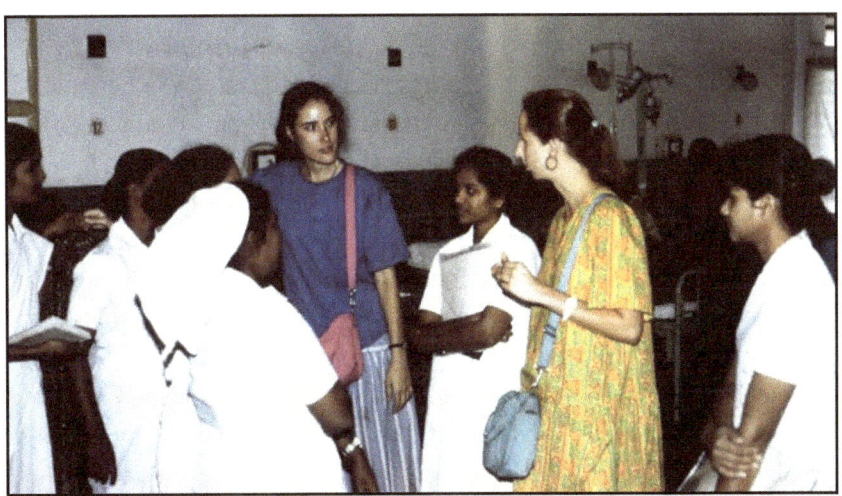

Dutch medical students, Andrea and Ingeborgh

Through the Lens of Humanity

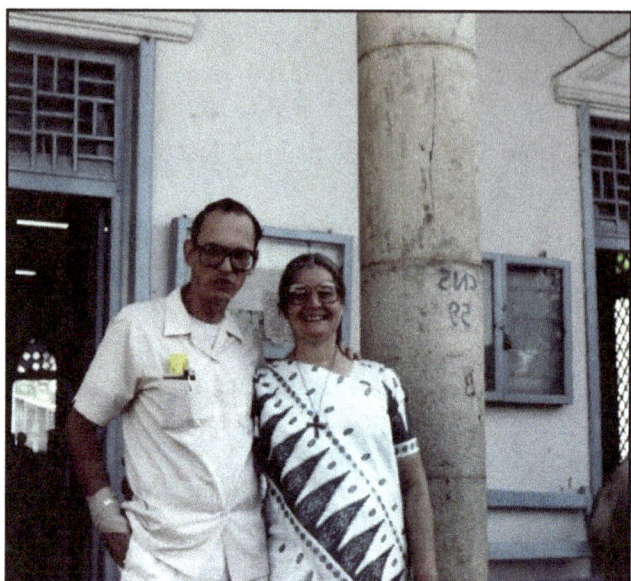

Presbyterian medical missionaries Dr. Paul and Judy Jewett (USA)

a fairly simple case—though he was concerned that the young girl was more the size of a three-year-old child than a normal eight-year-old.

Ingeborg, Andrea, and I, along with a couple of Indian medical students, were in the operating room, and I was surprised at how willing the entire surgical team was to have us observe. As the case progressed, Dr. Thomas periodically commented on what he was doing, but as he was preparing to close and complete the case, it became obvious that he was quite concerned about something. He asked that Dr. Jewett be found and brought into the operating room. After a few moments of quiet discussion between the two physicians, Dr. Thomas indicated that the procedure had not been successful and the patient had died.

Doctors Thomas and Jewett were very distraught. The atmosphere in the operating room was very hushed and subdued. Dr. Jewett departed to speak with the patient's parents. The Indian medical students, Ingeborg, Andrea, and I filed out of the room and spoke quietly among ourselves, wondering what had happened.

Later in the day, I saw Paul and asked what had happened to bring about the girl's death. He said that Dr. Thomas' repair of the child's ASD had caused immediate ventricular failure and the blood was not able to pump properly in the heart, triggering heart failure. At that point, there was nothing more that could be done. Anticipating my next question as to whether or not the young girl might have survived in a setting with better technology and resources, Paul said, "I don't know. I just don't know. But perhaps she could have."

The projects that I was working on allowed me to meet many staff in the hospital. One of these individuals was Mr. Kothari, who had been at the hospital for many years and worked in the pharmacy department. I often chatted with him when I was in the pharmacy doing my fact finding and information gathering for the study that I was doing for Dr. Cherian Thomas. Mr. Kothari was a huge cricket fan and I a huge baseball fan, so we'd often discuss our favorite sports when I was in his area.

One Saturday afternoon Mr. Kothari was working in a part of the hospital where the intravenous drips (IVs) for patients were prepared. Something flammable somehow ignited and Mr. Kothari was critically burned in the resulting explosion and fire. He sustained burns over 80 percent of his body. For days, he hovered between life and death. Mr Kothari was extremely popular among the staff and every morning at Chapel, Rev Agnes gave reports on his status and offered prayers for his recovery. Sadly, 10 days after the explosion, Rev. Agnes announced that Mr. Kothari had passed away the previous evening. Rev. Agnes led the chapel attendees in a moving prayer of remembrance of Mr. Kothari. Mr. Kothari was a Hindu, a Brahmin, and he was cremated later in the day in the Hindu tradition.

Judy told me of the difficulties awaiting Mr. Kothari's widow. She, her young child, and her unborn baby would be cared for by Mr. Kothari's family; the other children would be raised by his brothers. However, the wife would likely be barely tolerated by the family—the children were more important to Mr. Kothari's family. It is strange at times, Judy said, to be a Christian missionary in a land where the basic religion believes in so many gods and there are so many traditions and customs regarding how people will be treated.

During my time in Miraj, my friendship with Paul and Judy Jewett had grown. Often times in the evening, I'd have dinner with Paul and

Judy in their home or at least meet them for afternoon tea in the hospital.

Judy, in addition to being engaged in administrative activities at the hospital, also had taken it upon herself to expand the hospital's medical library. I shared with her that upon my return to the States, I would help collect medical journals ands textbooks for the hospital's library. For several years after my return, I was able to ship medical books and journals to Judy.

The day of Mr. Kothari's death, Judy and I were sitting in the library area of the hospital. She passed me the Bombay newspaper from a couple of days earlier. Two articles caught my attention and resonated deeply with me.

The first was a report that paralleled my experience in Bombay the morning I caught the train for Miraj. Police reported that two people had died in front of the Victoria Station in Bombay. Their bodies were left where they were and were unattended for six hours during the heat of the day due to the inability of the police to access hearses to pick up the corpses.

The second was an article describing an increase of the practice of *sati*—or *suttee*—in rural areas. Sati is a historical Hindu funeral practice whereby a widow sacrifices herself by sitting atop her husband's funeral pyre. While I knew this practice wasn't going to occur with Mr. Kothari's widow, it still gave me pause to know this practice still occurred with such frequency. The article went on to mention the Sati Act, an act passed specifically to criminalize the aiding of the practice of sati. "The uncommon is far too common in India," Judy observed solemnly.

About a mile and a half from Wanless Hospital on the Miraj-to-Sangli Road is the Richardson Leprosy Hospital. Though separated by over a mile, the Richardson Leprosy Hospital is considered part of the Miraj Medical Centre. Comprised of 110 beds, the hospital is newer, cleaner and more modern than the Wanless Hospital. There are about 40 leprosy hospitals in India and Richardson is one of the largest and nicest. In 1985, it was estimated that there were almost 4 million people in India suffering from leprosy. Worldwide, about 35 countries still

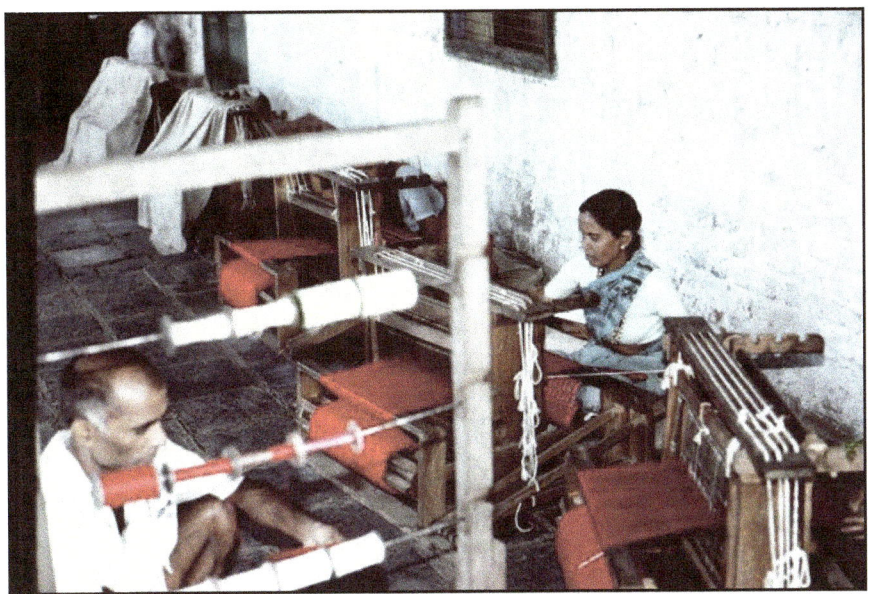

Lepers at the Richardson Leprosy Hospital preparing arts and crafts for sale

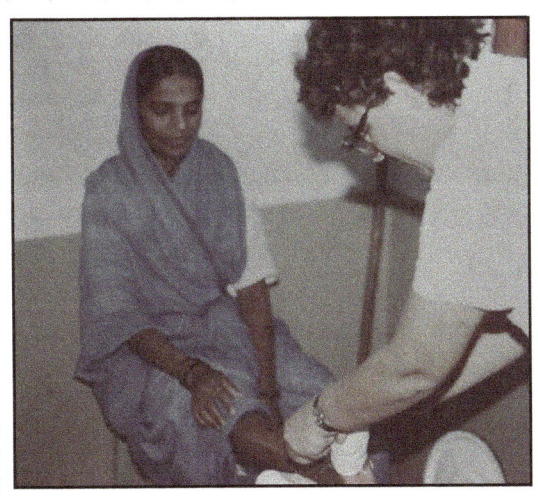

Woman receiving bandage change at Richardson Leprosy Hospital

have significant leprosy populations. At Richardson, both in-patient and outpatient services are provided. Many of the inpatients receive reconstructive surgery in addition to their medical therapies. I was told the disease was not life-threatening among the patients at Richardson, but was more debilitating and deforming. Most of the patients I

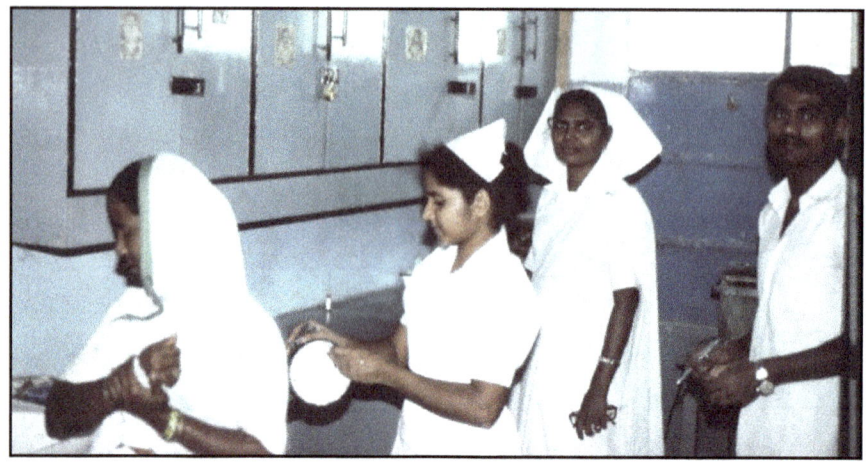
Student nurses and instructors at Miraj Medical Center

saw were women and many were sitting outside the hospital at old-fashioned sewing looms and spinning wheels, making colorful carry bags, towels, table place settings, bookmarks, and other crafts. Sadly, I was told that the hospital's entire 110 beds were almost always full, and I saw numerous patients waiting to be seen in the outpatient clinics.

In addition to visiting the Richardson Leprosy Hospital, several times during my stay, I traveled out into the rural areas surrounding Miraj with the Miraj Hospital's Community Health Department. Led by Dr. Kalindi Thomas, a primary task of the Community Health Department was to assist in setting up medical and community development projects in both rural and urban settings. I accompanied Kalindi and another physician one day to a small village of about 3,000 people approximately 12 miles from Miraj. The village was said to be over 600 years old.

In this village, Kalindi and her staff (Kalindi's department consisted of three physicians, three nurses, and several midwives) had set up a clinic and a nursery, and established ongoing midwifery training courses for women in the village. Recently, because of a drought in the area, water had to be transported into the village due to the community wells having dried up. Children followed us wherever we went in the village, hoping to get into the photos I was taking.

The Eyes of the Heart

I noticed that few homes had electricity, and public latrines were the waste facilities used by the villagers. Several families were eager to show off their stoves, which were fueled by cattle dung and human waste. Kalindi also explained that the villagers would use cattle dung to line the walls and floors in their houses. Once the odor dispersed, the dung served to deflect the heat during the long summer months. The villagers were mostly farmers, growing lentils and peanuts.

The Community Health Department in this village was heavily involved in providing nutritional services to families with children. Kalindi shared with me that most children in rural India were below the normal average weight standards per age group.

In 1987, the estimated population of India was 784 million people, making it the second most populous country in the world, trailing only China. Of this number, over 70 percent live in rural villages. It was estimated that over 60 percent of the total Indian population lived below worldwide poverty-level thresholds. A high population growth rate is a recognized predictor of poverty, illiteracy, and low income. India in 1987 had one of the highest population growth rates in the world.

As Kalindi shared these facts with me, she mentioned that her department was involved in child delivery training. Statistically, she said 80 percent of all Indian births take place in rural settings. Child planning was also a major focus of the Community Health Department. She noted that abortions are provided free in hospitals and birth control is encouraged. Incentives are also provided to encourage women to undergo birth control processes. Kalindi also shared that her department provided women with stainless-steel plates and cups if they would undergo sterilization or have an IUD inserted. She noted that in government hospitals, women were given 100 rupees if they underwent these procedures.

As we returned to Miral from our visit, Kalindi talked about all the things the government and hospitals were doing to impact poverty and improve health. I was impressed by Kalindi's passion that poverty is the number-one issue facing India and that poverty must be eradicated for the people to truly enjoy the fullness of life.

Through the Lens of Humanity

One of the most poignant memories of my time in Miraj came just days before I was to depart. It was the capping service for the nursing students who would be graduating in 1990. Held outside on the hospital's grounds at dusk, the young nurses sat in rows before the stage in their crisp white uniforms and listened to Dr. Thomas issue their charge to care for "the sick, injured, and infirm in the tradition of the dignity and honor of the nursing profession." The service would not have been complete without Rev. Agnes praying for God's blessings on these nurses-to-be—which she did for upwards of 15 minutes. The students then rose and proceeded from the service singing "Onward Christian Soldiers." As they marched out, I couldn't help but wonder what changes these young health professionals would help usher into their country's healthcare system over the course of their careers.

> *We are not divided, all one body we*
> *One in hope and doctrine,*
> *one in charity*
> —From *Onward Christian Soldiers*

Among the most fascinating and enjoyable aspects of the time I spent in Miraj was going to the bazaars in the town of Miraj. On many occasions after a day in the hospital, Dr. Crowley, Ingeborgh, Andrea and I would pay a few rupees to have bicycle-powered rickshaws take us to the bazaars in Miraj. The bazaars were a collection of rows upon rows of wooden or cardboard shacks and stalls where all manner of miscellaneous goods were sold. It seemed as if literally thousands of people were milling around in the bazaars at all times.

There was always a mix of people and animals—chickens, cattle, water buffalo, and monkeys who all seemed to tolerate each other's presence just fine. The odors and aromas were powerful—a mix of flowers, spices, garbage, as well as human and animal waste. Colorful saris, scarves, pajamas, and clothing of all types waved in the warm breeze. There were heaps and mounds of fresh fruits and vegetables—and some not so fresh. Stalls of nuts, seeds, and spices could be spotted in the market. Handicrafts of all types were displayed, and there were special shops for sitars of all sizes and for household products like lamps and vases and bowls. One bargained for everything—there were no set prices.

It seemed too that each time we went to the bazaar, the streets looked different. During Diwali, the Festival of the Lights, firecrackers and paper lanterns and all types of lights sparkled along the walkways. At other times, we observed religious rituals in the streets, weddings and celebrations of births.

Make no mistake about it—the Miraj bazaar was very dirty. Roads and passageways into the bazaar were very poor; rubbish and filth were pervasive. The streets and alleys were full of standing water because of blocked drains, and a putrid odor emanated from the water, which also served to attract mosquitoes and other bugs. Many of the people in the bazaar were in poor health, and personal sanitation was nonexistent for a good many.

Going to the bazaar was a way for us to glimpse the real life of Miraj, to truly immerse ourselves in the culture of the country and the local culture of Miraj. We were welcomed wherever we went—young children often grabbed our hands to pull us toward their families' stalls or shops. We gradually became more adventuresome in buying fruits and vegetables that we took back to Fletcher Hall for washing and then eating. We often drew laughs as we attempted to bargain and barter for the things we wished to purchase.

I believe we all felt that going to the bazaar was a way for us to move out of our comfort zones and into closer fellowship and solidarity with the people of Miraj. In many ways, the bazaar was the bridge between the ancient history of India with the new and emerging history of that amazing nation. For me, the Miraj bazaar was a microcosm of humanity, with all its beauty and its heartache.

Some years after my journey to Miraj, I ran across an observation of daily life in Asia and India by Steve McCurry, the renowned photographer who so eloquently captures the essence of life in India:

> *It is this unbroken continuity with the past and ancient beliefs that still takes me back to Asia, and it's a quality unique in the*

> world. In India in particular, where millions have no homes but the streets, virtually every life event is carried out in public: prayer, eating, sleeping, nursing, crude dentistry, even bodily functions. In the secular West, where nothing is sacred, everything seems hidden; yet in Asia, where nothing is hidden, everything is sacred.

As my time in Miraj drew to a close, it became very important to me that the projects that I worked on positively and meaningfully impacted the experience of patients and families at the hospital. I wanted to ensure that my expertise and time resulted in changes that enabled the hospital's caregivers to render care in more timely or efficient way. I wanted to contribute all that I could toward efforts to raise the standards of care at the hospital and reduce the human suffering that was so prevalent and evident throughout Miraj.

I spent hours with Paul and Judy Jewett and Cherian and Kalindi Thomas discussing ways of getting donations of money, medical books, equipment, and supplies to the hospital. Judy and I developed plans to stay in touch so we could monitor some of the recommendations I had made. We even discussed my returning in 12 to 18 months for another volunteerism tour.

On the night before my departure, Paul and Judy Jewett, Dr. Crowley, Archie and Huldah Fletcher, Cherian and Kalindi Thomas, and I had dinner at the Thomas' house. Dressed in formal Indian attire Kalindi and Cherian hosted a traditional Indian meal that was simply exquisite. We celebrated fellowship and friendship and gave thanks for the blessings we shared together and for the sense of God's presence in our lives that had propelled each of us to work toward eliminating human suffering. That evening I felt we all were aware that in the midst of great suffering, the Indian people we sought to serve had exuded love and generosity towards us even as we strived to serve them. In that moment, I truly knew that the spirit and the beliefs that powers life was inexhaustible.

Twenty-five days after arriving in Miraj, I departed, heading back on the train first to Bombay (no dramatic issues on the train on the way back!), then a flight to Paris for a couple of days vacation, and finally a flight back to Milwaukee. On my way home, I reflected on my various travel experiences and particularly my time in Miraj. I was exhausted and about 15 pounds lighter, but I was gratified to have had all the experiences I had, and content in the knowledge that I had immersed myself, albeit briefly, in a culture far different than mine and that I had contributed towards alleviating the pain and suffering of others.

Once in Milwaukee, it was difficult for me to re-integrate into "Western" daily life. I returned home on a Sunday might and went back to work early Monday morning. Similar to Carol Johnson's experience after returning from Bangladesh, it was disconcerting for me to look around one of the most modern pediatric hospitals in the United States, a variable land of technological and equipment plenty, in comparison to the limited and meager resources at Wanless Hospital. I was haunted by images of Miraj wherever I went—the hospital, the super market, restaurants, malls, public gathering places, etc.

A wise colleague and friend from Children's Hospital was a pediatric psychiatrist, and he commented to me that seeing and experiencing the extreme poverty that I had will almost invariably lead one to comparisons between one's own state of comparative privilege in the world versus others that can give way to feelings of sadness and even guilt. I certainly struggled with feelings like these upon my return home.

These feelings were particularly intense for me when I provided presentations regarding my trip. The photos I had taken in Miraj (with Paul's borrowed camera) were vivid reminders of the overwhelming poverty and suffering of so many in Miraj. I tried always to remember the advice of Judy and Paul when I spoke of my experiences: "Be a good ambassador for those you're speaking about and for. Your job is to spread awareness and to give voice to those who are powerless to speak for themselves."

In early 1988, I wrote an article about my experiences in Miraj to continue to share the story of Miraj Medical Center and the remarkable people who work there, and the thousands who receive care and healing at this venerable institution:

Through the Lens of Humanity

I have eaten your bread and salt.
I have drunk your water and wine.
The deaths ye died I have watched beside
And the lives ye led were mine.
—From "Prelude" by Rudyard Kipling

The article:

"It is stone and it is white. It stands near the outskirts of the quiet, dusty, untidy town of Miraj, India.

Though weathered by time and the elements, this faded four-story building rises majestically from a grove of trees which impart not only shade, but tranquility—and a hint of sadness. Its windows, tall and narrow, are collections of air thickened by dust, soot and haze, which soften the light and make breathing difficult.

Its entrances—massive tunnel-like openings—bid an invitation, while conveying an odd sense of uncertainty. And its grounds are a tapestry of the region—cattle, donkeys and other creatures roam oblivious to the sad, faceless, disinherited bands of people who seemingly wait forever outside the walls of this venerable building.

This is Wanless Hospital. Opened in 1894 by a young Canadian Presbyterian missionary, it traces its roots to a small dispensary that once operated in the Miraj Bazaar.

Over the decades, countless numbers of dedicated physicians, missionaries, nurses and others have journeyed to Miraj. With a vision of tomorrow and God in their hearts, they took up the difficulty task of building a place of healing, teaching and worship. Their memorial is today's Miraj Medical Center, which stands witness to the power of their faith.

Through its doors each day pour the disenfranchised—the poor, the sick and suffering, the repressed and the disposed. Like many other mission hospitals, Wanless is a repository of diseases seldom seen elsewhere. Leprosy, tuberculosis, cholera, and rabies are all too commonplace.

The Eyes of the Heart

And a sense of sadness permeates every corner of this place, a sadness that springs from the fact that many who flock to this place could have been cured if only they had come earlier. It is, for far too many, a place to die.

They converge on Wanless, entire families, from surrounding villages and farms, arriving by crowded trains, by bullock carts and on foot. Many suffer from malnutrition. Often, they are dressed in little more than rags, carrying their few possessions on their backs. These people do not argue the merits of nuclear disarmament, worry about what college their children will attend or wonder whether their car will last another year. Their concern is survival. Will there be enough to eat? Will they be able to clothe themselves and their families? Will they find shelter against the elements? Will they live another day?

When their pilgrimage to Wanless is complete, they camp on the pavement or the bare earth. They cook their meals from meager supplies of food over open fires and bathe at standpipes on the hospital grounds.

And they wait. It is a sight that challenges the very foundations of one's faith, leaving one with a single, persistent question: Is this suffering necessary?

And, they do wait, from dawn to dusk, in dimly lit corridors and cramped rooms spartanly furnished with wooden benches, the air stirred by slowly revolving overhead fans. They wait with a stoic patience to spend a precious few moments with a clinic physician. When a patient is admitted, the family continues its vigil, squatting for days in the hallways of the hospital's wards — the sweat and oil from their bodies staining the walls in mute testimony that they have passed this way.

It occurs to one that these people are either oblivious or all too accustomed to the dirt on the floors and the pervasive stench of disinfectant, urine and feces emanating from the latrines whose doors have long ago been removed and whose drains have been blocked.

Through the Lens of Humanity

They silently accept the crowded patient wards with their seemingly endless rows of beds covered with permanently discolored linens. They accept the unpleasantly warm surgical suites, which are sparsely furnished with metal tables, battered operating lights and rusted shelving. They accept the secondhand medical equipment, fatigued by age and outdated by technology.

Yet, despite the absence of comfortable surroundings and modern facilities taken for granted in the western world, there is a serenity at Wanless—a sense of security that envelopes both patients and staff, which all of the human misery, chaos and technological limitations cannot deny. One is aware that this is a place of heroic accomplishments, where human tragedy is transformed into human potential by care and compassion, courage and determination and, perhaps most all, by love.

Though its emphasis is not evangelical, Wanless is a place which has made enormous contributions to the spiritual life of the region. It is where four major religions—Hindu, Moslem, Buddhist and Christian — share the same hospital ward and are all treated as true brothers and sisters.

It is a place of remarkable men and women, whose source of strength and courage and love is their faith in God and their vocation. And though they live their faith in obscurity, they are bulwarks to a people who have lost much of their own stability.

Caring for one's neighbors is the expression of their faith, and it is the spring from which flows the strength they need to give the extra strength, the extra compassion and the unqualified love to their patients. This strength does as much as their medical skills in relieving the suffering of the sick and injured.

Finally, Wanless is a place of hope. There is an inscription on a Crusader's tomb which reads 'He did the best things in the worst times, and hoped them in the impossible.'

INVITATION TO MIRAJ

So, the worst times lead to thoughts of hope, and where it can be found in seemingly impossible circumstances. At Wanless, hope in the midst of inhuman trials, is manifested through endurance, tolerance, caring, compassion, and, above all, faith—faith that God will provide—that God will succor God's children with divine love.

It is stone and it is white. It is challenge, it is opportunity. It is hope and assurance. It is judgment. And, it is comfort and benediction. It is a microcosm of humanity, with all of its misery and heartache tempered by the invincible strength that comes from the power of love. It is truly God's House, and it belongs right there, where it is, near the outskirts of the quiet, dusty, untidy town of Miraj, India.

What doth the Lord require of thee, but to do justly,
and to love mercy, and to walk humbly with thy God?
—Micah 6:8

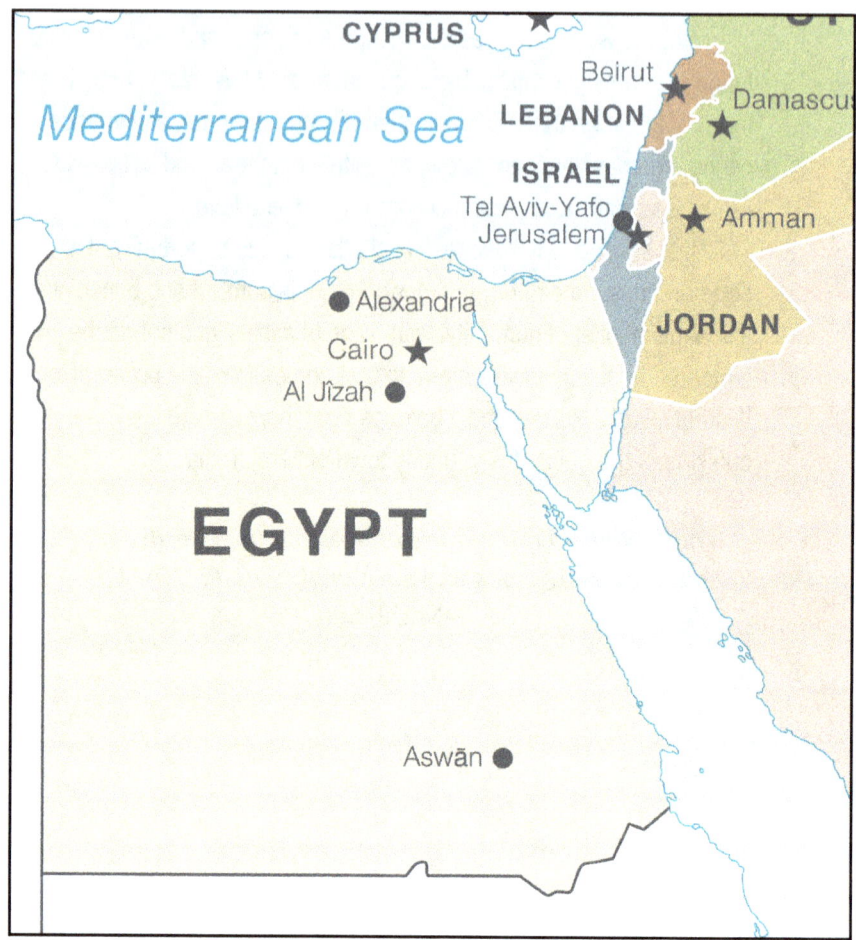

Israel and Egypt destinations: Tel Aviv, Jerusalem, Bethlehem, Israel; Cairo, Egypt

CHAPTER 2

THE EYES OF YOUR HEART

In late summer of 1990, I found myself in Chicago's O'Hare Airport ready to embark on a three-week journey that would take me to Israel, Egypt, followed by the central African countries of Malawi and Zambia. I was scheduled to return to the United States after that.

Thirty months had passed since my return from Miraj. It had been an eventful and trying period for me. Candidly, returning home from India and processing what I had seen and experienced in Miraj had caused me to confront and challenge many of my prevailing notions of place and privilege in the world. I found my emotions often in turmoil as I attempted to re-insert myself into the stream of life that I was accustomed to in Milwaukee. I thought often of those whom I had met in Miraj, and their daily lives and challenges as compared to my own. At the core of my feelings was an illogical guilt regarding my privilege and a sense of impotence to change the social structure. In many ways, though, these feelings also galvanized my desire to raise awareness of the enormous hardships too many in the world face. So it was with a little trepidation that I boarded my flight in Chicago to travel again to several of the world's most impoverished and troubled areas.

I had scheduled the initial portion of my trip to Israel and Egypt because of my long held desire to visit these ancient and historic regions where so much of civilization's religious, cultural, and political history had been born, taken root, and flourished. Not to mention that these two countries have continually dominated the world's headlines and agenda for thousands of years. (See map opposite)

In reality, though, it was the visits to the countries of Malawi and Zambia that comprised the primary intent of my travel. After my journey to Miraj in 1987, Dr. Paul Jewett had recommended to the

Through the Lens of Humanity

Board of the Medical Benevolence Foundation (MBF) that I be invited to become a Foundation Trustee. MBF was the Presbyterian Church USA-supported organization that had helped arrange my trip to Miraj, and also supported Presbyterian medical missionaries like Paul and Judy Jewett. I had joined the MBF Board in 1988, and this trip had evolved out of my attending a MBF board meeting and a desire to visit and see several of the overseas hospitals and projects supported by MBF. My travels to Malawi would include site visits to three MBF-sponsored hospitals—in Nkhoma, Ekwendeni, and Embangweni. This trip would also include re-connecting with Paul and Judy Jewett, who had completed their assignment in Miraj and had relocated to Embangweni as missionaries in residence at the hospital there.

 I am one of those people who enjoys flying and who can sleep easily on planes, so for me, the ten-hour flight from New York to Tel Aviv, following the two hours from Chicago to New York, went quickly and smoothly and without incident. I traveled by small bus from Tel Aviv to Jerusalem and spent several fascinating days there touring the old city: Stephen's Gate, Jaffa Gate, the Mount of Olives, the Dome of the Rock, the Wailing Wall, the Garden of Gethsemane, the Church of the Holy Sepulcher, and of course, the Via Dolorosa, also known as the Stations of the Cross or the "Way of Suffering."

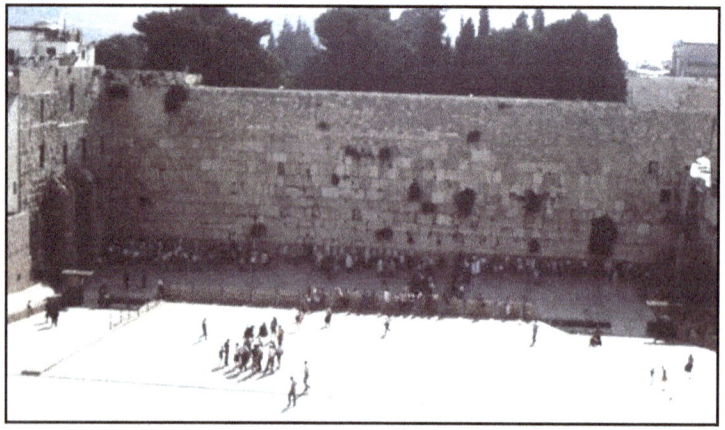

Jerusalem's Wailing Wall

THE EYES OF THE HEART

The day I walked the Via Dolorosa, some excitement occurred at the third Station of the Cross; an elderly man in our tour group collapsed and died, likely from a heart attack. Understandably, his family members were beside themselves with grief—it was a bit traumatic for our little group as well. After the first responders arrived and were aiding the family, we continued somberly along the Via Dolorosa; that day, it yet again had truly been a "way of suffering."

Visiting Jerusalem's sacred sites, I was surprised by the number of merchants hawking their goods to the tourists: postcards, garments, beads, crosses. It struck me as being disrespectful to what had occurred at these sites, and I couldn't help but be reminded of the story of Jesus cleansing the Temple of money changers and merchants.

The final full day I was in Jerusalem, I traveled by bus from Jerusalem to Bethlehem and stopped at the Tomb of Rachel and toured the Church of the Nativity. Rachel was the wife of Jacob, mother of Joseph, and died giving birth to Benjamin. She is revered by Jews, Muslims, and Christians alike and her tomb has been a place of pilgrimage for these three major religions, but especially for Jewish women unable to give birth. Jewish lore maintains that Rachel's tears have special powers, inspiring those visiting her grave to ask her to cry and intercede with God on their behalf. I was touched by the number of

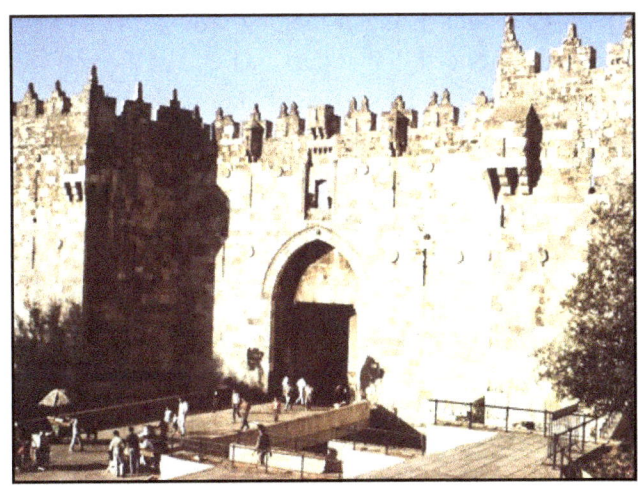

Jaffa Gate, Jerusalem

women, young and old, solemnly touching parts of the tomb structure, many whose own eyes were filled with tears.

The crowd at the Church of the Nativity was sparse the day of my visit and pilgrims roamed the small church and its grounds freely. I was with a small busload of tourists and after about an hour, we departed Bethlehem to return to Jerusalem, but not of course before the tour bus stopped at the obligatory souvenir shop!

The next morning, I took a cab for the approximately 45 minute drive from my hotel to the airport in Tel Aviv. Israel's El Al Airlines is known as the safest airline in the world and Israel's Ben Gurion airport in Tel Aviv is avowed to be the safest airport in the world. As a nation constantly on guard against terrorist attack, Israel has put into place the world's most stringent security measures for its national airline and airport. I had the unnerving and embarrassing experience of finding this to be true.

Per airline instructions to arrive at least three hours early for departing international flights, I reached Ben Gurion airport for my flight to Cairo in accordance with those instructions. Upon arrival, I like others, moved into a large waiting hall to await customs processing for our flight. The hall was very crowded, very warm, and there was no available seating. I ended up standing with my luggage in a central area of the hall. As time passed, I became quite thirsty, and as it was still a long time until the flight, I began looking around the hall for a coffee shop or snack bar. I noticed that at the other end of the hall were several kiosks where soft drinks and food were being sold. While I was wary of leaving my luggage alone, I was becoming increasingly thirsty and I decided that I could walk quickly over to the kiosks, all the while keeping my luggage in sight.

I walked quickly over to the kiosk, keeping an eye on my bags, turned to the kiosk, paid for my selections, turned and walked back to where I had left my bags. They were gone. I glanced around and saw no sign of my luggage. I started walking around the hall to see if anyone had moved them or if I could spot my bags. Nothing. I became more frantic. The bags had been there when I got to the kiosk; in the time it had taken me to turn to the cashier and pay for my drink and snacks, my luggage had vanished. I kept looking around the hall for a few moments and then spotted an Information Center with a uniformed woman sitting at the counter.

She barely looked up as I approached.

"I've lost my luggage. I think my bags might have been stolen."

"What makes you think that?" she said, still seeming to ignore me.

I explained that I had them with me, went just a few feet to get a soda and snacks, and when I returned, they were gone.

She was now looking directly at me—and her glare was laser-like and her voice intense. "You left your luggage alone, Mr. Anderson [I had not told her my name], and we have your luggage. We have removed it to a storage area in the basement."

I stood there, relieved that my luggage was safe, but withering under her gaze and chastisement. After I acknowledged the seriousness of my transgression, the female officer phoned to have my luggage brought out of confinement and delivered to the information counter. After I confirmed this was indeed my baggage and repeatedly apologizing for my lapse, the bags were returned to me. I returned to the waiting hall and attempted to fade into the background as well as I could.

After what seemed an interminable time, my flight was called to begin the customs and clearance processes. With my luggage in tow, I entered the queue for check-in, document review, and personal belongings and baggage searches. As I reached the female security officer whose line I was in, she proceeded to ask me a series of questions—standard questions like why had I come to Israel, where was I going after Cairo, when was I returning to the United States.

As she was searching through my luggage, she asked, "Has your luggage been with you the entire time?"

I responded that it had, except for the time when it had been confiscated by security in the airport waiting lounge. With a trace of a smile and a smirk, she looked at me and said, "That was the correct answer, Mr. Anderson. I have been informed of this issue."

With that, she cleared me through the rest of the customs process. Over the intervening years, as I've gone through the clearance process for countless international and domestic flights, I've smiled to myself as

Through the Lens of Humanity

I remember that episode and give thanks to those security individuals we are indebted too for their commitment to keeping us safe.

After my experience at Ben Guiron, the approximately one-hour flight to Cairo was quick and easy. My time in Egypt was most enjoyable but passed all too quickly. I was awed and mesmerized by the sites: the majestic Sphinx and the pyramids, which I viewed and toured in Giza during the day and then returned for an exquisite dinner and light show at the foot of the pyramids in the evening. I sailed down the Nile at dusk one evening and took a day trip to Luxor and the Valley of the Kings and Queens the next. Though the heat was oppressive, I loved the vibrancy and history of the great ancient city of Cairo.

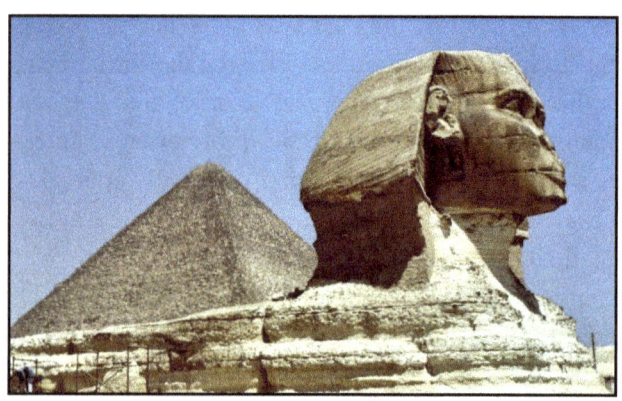

Touring the splendors of ancient Egypt!

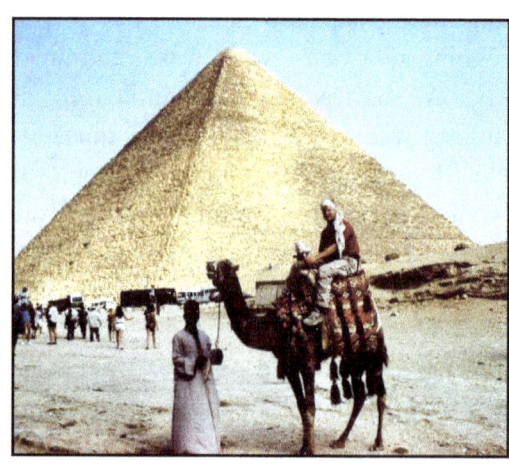

Camel riding at the pyramids!

THE EYES OF THE HEART

Adding some tension and drama during my visit in Cairo, however, was the invasion of Kuwait by Saddam Hussein's Iraqi army. Due to the proximity of Iraq and Kuwait to Egypt and the centuries-old history of conflict, antipathy, and war in the Middle East, the city was abuzz with speculation of what could happen next. Who would be drawn into the conflict and what would be the consequences for the region? Indeed, the day of my departure from Cairo, all departing flights were temporarily delayed due to the influx of Middle Eastern Arab leaders and other international dignitaries for discussions regarding the Iraqi invasion of Kuwait.

My next major port of call was the country of Malawi. My route was through London. Even with the delay out of Cairo, I still had a multiple-hour layover in London. In London I met up with another MBF trustee, Tom Logan of Marion, Illinois. We were both new trustees and had agreed to meet in London and travel together to Malawi.

Traveling with Tom was his teenage son Martin, and the three of us had dinner before boarding the plane. Tom had visited Malawi many times previously; Tom, was an ordained Presbyterian minister but worked in Illinois providing low-income housing. He had created an entity called Marion Medical Missions and his organization was working in Malawian villages helping to dig wells to enable villagers access to a "clean" water supply.

Tom was certainly a fascinating character. He had toured Africa after finishing school and had worked briefly for Albert Schweitzer in Schweitzer's hospital in Lambarene, Equatorial Africa. He had also marched with Martin Luther King in Alabama and Tom himself had been jailed there duing the Freedom March. Tom's mission of digging wells in Malawi coincided with MBF projects at several MBF-sponsored mission hospitals in Malawi. As we ate prior to boarding the aircraft, in addition to trading travel stories and experiences, Tom shared that he had brought equipment and supplies to dig several more wells while he was in Malawi.

Malawi is a small, landlocked, kidney-shaped country located in central Africa. Most of the people of Malawi live in rural areas, in very

THROUGH THE LENS OF HUMANITY

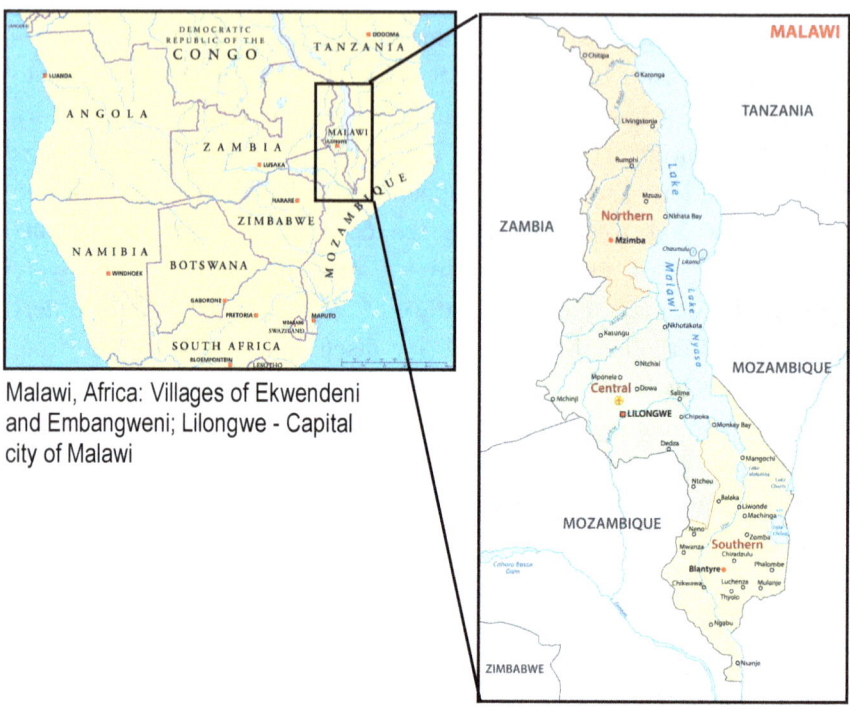

Malawi, Africa: Villages of Ekwendeni and Embangweni; Lilongwe - Capital city of Malawi

traditional villages. Malawi has a rich cultural mix of tribes and its people are described as the warmest, friendliest, and most welcoming in all of Africa, indeed, Malawi is called the "Warm Heart of Africa." Christianity and Islam are the predominant religions in the country.

Lilongwe, Malawi, the capital of Malawi, was our destination. Our flight path took us first from London to Harare, Zimbabwe, and then on to Lilongwe, where we were met by Dr. Jim McGill, a Presbyterian medical missionary. Our itinerary called for us to overnight in Lilongwe and Dr. McGill had arranged for a car and driver to show us around the city. On the way to the hotel, we drove through a large market. I was reminded in many ways of the markets in India—large, open spaces where live animals, as well as fish, were sold or bargained for, as well as fruit, vegetables, pots, pans, and colorful fabrics. The chatter in the markets was interrupted by laughter and singing. The markets seemed to be an enjoyable gathering place, in addition to a place of commerce.

The hotel was adequate, simple with a small lounge and restaurant. It was a nice location to sit and get acquainted with Tom, Martin, and

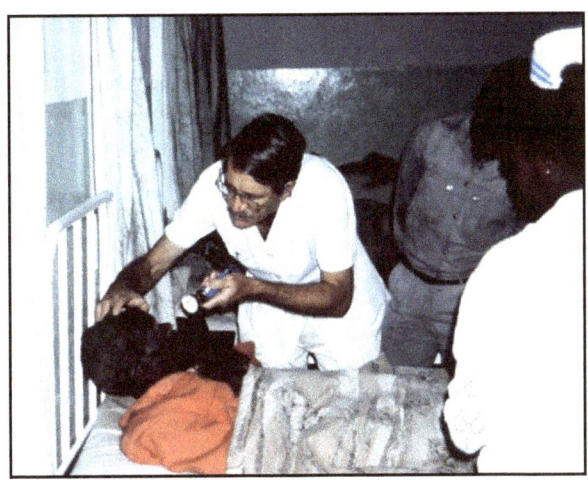

Dr. Chris Blignaut, a South African physician examining an eye patient at Nkhoma Hospital

Dr. McGill. However, due to our travel schedule, we all adjourned early to head to bed.

The drive to Nkhoma the next morning took a little over an hour—the distance was only 60 kilometers. Upon arrival, our driver took us to Dr. Chris Blignaut's house for tea and coffee. Dr. Blignaut was the hospital's eye specialist. He and his wife Julie, a nurse, had been at Nkhoma Hospital for more than three decades. Dr. Blignaut performed hundreds of cataract and eye surgeries annually. Being one of only a handful of eye surgeons in Malawi, Dr. Blignaut was well known by medical personnel throughout the country and patients came to see from all parts. The Blignauts' son Peter was also a general practitioner at the hospital.

We had arrived on a Sunday morning and after tea and coffee, Tom, Martin, and I accompanied the Blignauts to the local church. Several hundred people were in attendance and the highlight of the service was the music. No fewer than six choirs sang *a cappella* during the service; the music was simply beautiful.

At the church, we met Nicholas and Muriel Van Velden, who like Dr. Blignaut and Julie wife, were originally from South Africa and graciously hosted us in their home during our stay in Nkhoma. After the worship service, we adjourned to their home for lunch. Afterwards, Nicholas, a general practitioner himself, gave us a tour of Nkhoma Hospital.

THROUGH THE LENS OF HUMANITY

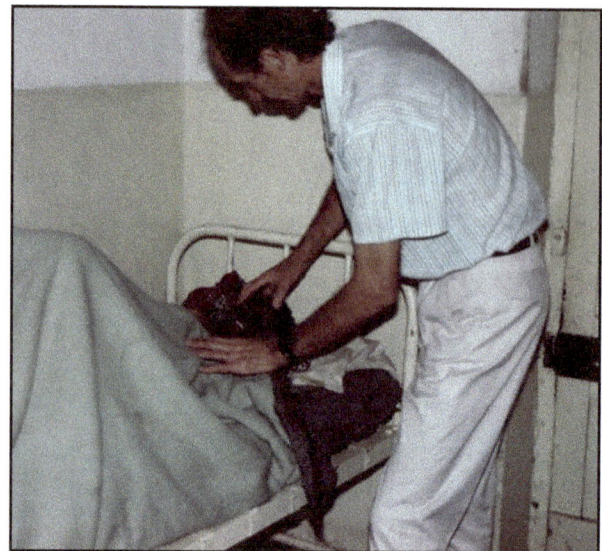

South African physician Dr. Nico Van Velden examining an HIV/AIDS patient.

The hospital was opened in 1915 and had grown from a few mud huts to a hospital of approximately 200 beds spread over a number of single-story brick buildings. The hospital had wards for pediatrics, surgical services, general medicine wards for males and females, tuberculosis rooms, isolation rooms, a maternity ward, a variety of outpatient clinics, and the aforementioned ophthalmology services department run by Dr. Blignaut. The hospital serves thousands of patients from throughout Malawi, many from very rural areas, as well as numerous patients from surrounding countries.

Despite the presence of a "modern" hospital, African traditional medicine is still commonly practiced in the village. Regardless of the influence of Christianity and Islam, there is a continuing adherence to traditional rites and beliefs by many, particularly with respect to medical and health practices.

As we toured, we asked Nico (Nicholas) to describe the types of patients they see. "AIDS, tuberculosis, malaria, infected sores and wounds, malnutrition, leprosy, and of course, the eye patients, including cataracts, all the way to severe eye disease and blindness," he said. "But by far, right now what is increasing the most are AIDS cases, we're seeing two or more new cases every day."

In Africa, he explained, the most common form of AIDS transmission is heterosexual intercourse. The population, he stated, is very, very promiscuous. Ninety-five percent or more of the prostitutes have AIDS, and truck drivers or laborers who travel around Malawi or through neighboring countries seeking work are the most common carriers. Many men, he continued, have several wives in various cities, and through these multi-partner scenarios, many Malawians are infected with AIDS. Significant too is the fact that many people don't get married until after they have children; actually, according to Malawian culture, women become more desirable at the time of childbirth, because of this "proof of fertility." But this practice also promotes multiple partners increasing the spread of AIDS.

Tragically, Nico noted, many Malawians, even when presented with the facts of how the disease is spread and its deadly consequences, are not sufficiently fearful of AIDS to modify their behavior. As a consequence of this burgeoning number of cases, the hospital was unable to house AIDS patients. Rather, the patients were discharged to the care of their families. Most such patients died in their villages rather than the hospital.

Two of the most fascinating people we met in Nkhoma were Corrie Legemate, a primary care nurse form Holland, and Helene Laubsen, a midwife from South Africa. Their jobs included going into the villages to teach sanitation techniques, give inoculations, and provide primary and preventive care services to the villagers. They did this by working with the village "witch doctor." In the rural villages of Malawi, the witch doctor still presides as the primary source of medical care within the village. By working with the witch doctor, Corrie and Helene are able to use the witch doctor's local credibility to provide basic health services to the villagers.

At the time of our visit, Corrie had recently returned from holiday at Lake Malawi, which is one of the largest and prettiest lakes in all of Africa. She related her experience of getting out of the lake after a swim and inadvertently getting between a mother hippo and her infant.

THROUGH THE LENS OF HUMANITY

The hippo charged her, knocking her down and biting her severely on her back and buttocks. Fortunately for Corrie, after the initial attack, the hippo withdrew and Corrie survived the assault, but almost died from her infections. Hippo attacks in Africa are the most common of all animal attacks in Africa, and are almost uniformly deadly. Corrie was indeed lucky to have survived, though she now possesses what will be a life-long limp.

Our final afternoon in Nkhoma, Tom and I took a long walk into some of the surrounding villages. It was wonderful to just walk through the African bush, wandering across scattered fields and dirt roads surrounded by beautiful mountain ranges in the distance. Toward sunset, we strolled into one village where were mobbed by young children who laughed and giggled at us as we talked with them. The children gathered their drums and began playing and dancing for us while the elders offered us water and stew. It was a wonderful and heartfelt display of hospitality.

Tom and I left as it was growing dark; we felt like Pied Pipers because we were followed for a great distance by children singing, dancing, and waving goodbye as we took our leave. Walking back to our lodgings, Tom and I talked about how cheerful and friendly the entire village had been, but especially the children, despite the disturbing and dismal living conditions of the village.

That evening, we enjoyed dinner and the company of the Blignauts and van Veldens and engaged in a lively discussion about David Livingstone and his explorations in Malawi, Zambia, Zimbabwe, and South Africa. We also talked about the political situation between South Africa and Malawi. Indians and Jews from South Africa have established shops in the marketplace and there is growing tension between them and local merchants. There was apparently growing concern that the entrepreneur style of the Indian and Jewish merchants would displace the ability of the local merchants to effectively provide their goods and services as they had in the past. Consequently, restrictions have been imposed to confine the Indian and Jewish merchants to the larger cities and not allow them to infiltrate the rural villages. Doctors

Blignaut and van Velden were concerned that interracial disputes would fester and expand over time.

I turned in, looking forward to our travel the next day to Embangweni and to re-connecting with Paul and Judy Jewett at the Embangweni Mission Hospital.

The drive the next morning to Embangweni took approximately three and a half hours. When we arrived in this small town/village we went first to the home of Dr. Ken and Nancy McGill (Jim's parents) and had lunch along with a volunteer group from California, who had been working in the town of Ekwendeni and had also arrived that morning.

Over lunch, the volunteers described some of their experiences and challenges while in Ekwendeni. The most frightening part of their visit was learning upon arrival that a severe cholera outbreak had occurred the previous year and was still lingering in the village. Adding to their concern was the knowledge that the outbreak had never been officially reported to appropriate authorities, including the World Health Organization (WHO). Dr. McGill noted this was likely the case, and described his own frustrations with local and governmental authorities.

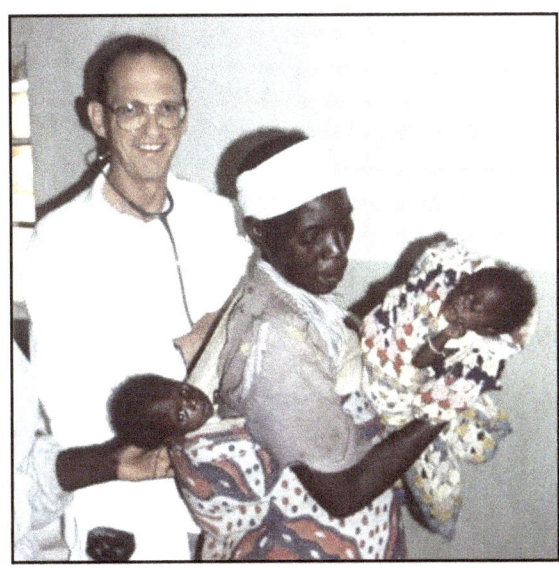

Presbyterian missionary Dr. Paul Jewett with an African mother and babies.

THROUGH THE LENS OF HUMANITY

Dr. McGill explained that most Americans people don't realize that in many countries in Africa, and particularly in Malawi, about 60 percent of the population with AIDS were HIV positive, and probably 90 percent of the police and governmental officials were HIV positive, which meant the nation itself could have severe social turmoil and problems due simply to the vulnerability of senior governmental officials.

"When you go and visit the villages," he continued, "take a look around and you'll see that the main people you see are older adults and young children, so great has been the loss of young adults to AIDS. And so many of the young adults were the parents of the young children you see, who are now either orphans or they're being cared for by their grandparents or other older adults. "It is sobering to think how many of these African countries are on the precipice of disaster," he informed us.

After this sobering discussion, we walked to the Embangweni Hospital and within moments, I bumped into Paul first and shortly thereafter, Judy.

Paul immediately became our tour guide and as we walked through the various sections of the hospital. His words were as chilling as Ken McGill's had been.

In the pediatric ward, he lamented that so many children were admitted with malaria and encephalitis, or were dehydrated and malnourished. Many infants were so malnourished they often died from poor circulation and lack of warmth. Measles was also a greater killer of children. Paul spoke of a woman he had seen the week before who had lost three of her four children to measles. He continued saying that often women who came to the hospital were there delivering their fifth or sixth child, with many of their previous children having died before the age of two or three.

Judy spoke of how compared to the Indian physicians and staff in Miraj, the staff here in Malawi were cheerful, but much more distant than in India.

All of these topics became fodder for our dinner discussions that evening at Paul and Judy's home, with Ken, Nancy, Tom, Martin, and

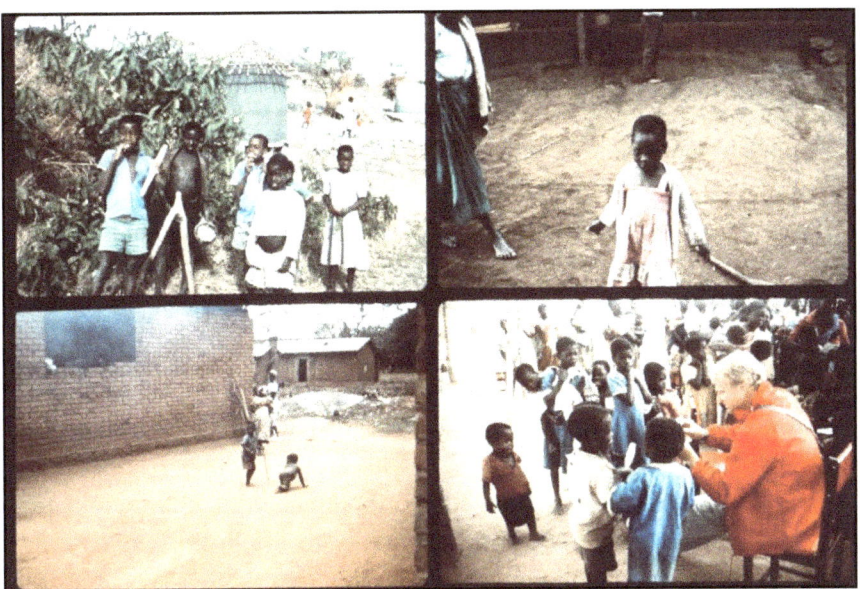

A montage of photographs of the children of Embangweni

myself in attendance. After dinner, Martin excused himself and went to bed, and Tom and I enjoyed being regaled by the stories of Ken and Nancy McGill sharing experiences of decades of medical missionary work in rural Africa, while the Jewetts spoke of their missionary years in Haiti, India, and now Malawi. The stories were remarkable, but not as remarkable as the commitment and passion of the McGills and Jewetts in service of their fellow human beings.

The following day Tom, Martin, and I accompanied nurses from the hospital to a rural village approximately 40 kilometers from the hospital. Once we arrived in the village, the nurses began seeing patients, predominantly women and children. One hundred and thirty-one children were examined, with the infants being weighed and notations made about malnutrition. There were also pre-natal screening checks for expectant others and vaccines were given to both mothers and children for measles, diphtheria, tuberculosis, and smallpox.

Once all the patients had been seen, the nurses gathered all the mothers and children in a group and began teaching about malnutrition and AIDS and other illnesses. What was unique and fascinating is that the nurses taught their material by singing to the women and children, and then having them sing back what they had been taught! Their African voices were beautiful. Everyone all participated, laughing and clapping to the music. It was a truly inspiring sight to see the sense of community achieved by this process.

Another cherished memory of the day was the community lunch that was shared by the entire village. The dishes that had been prepared were traditional Malawian: *chambo,* a fish found in Malawi's lakes; *nsima*, a Malawian loaf or cake made of boiled corn flour; *zitumbuwa*, also known as fried banana; and *kachumbari,* which is made from onions, chili peppers, and tomatoes. Several goats and chickens had also been slaughtered and were part of the feast. The meal was extravagant in terms of the village's available food resources, but the intent of the meal was to be generous in hospitality to the health workers and guests who were visiting the village. During the meal as everyone was eating, the women and children sang and danced and the "Warm Heart of Africa" was in full display.

That evening was my last in Embangweni. The next morning, Paul, Judy, and I were to leave for Lilongwe—they had personal business to do in the city and were dropping me at the airport. My itinerary had me going on to Zambia for several days. Tom and Martin were remaining in Malawi to drill several more wells, so I bid them adieu at dinner that evening at the Jewetts' home.

Paul, Judy, and I left very early the next morning and during our drive, we discussed my visit and what I had seen. Judy also shared that she missed Miraj very much. She didn't feel as integrated into the Embangweni community as yet and she missed the hustle and bustle of Miraj as compared to Embangweni's slower pace. Paul admitted he had some of the same feelings, and as a cardiologist by training, he had "re-engineered" himself to practice more as a primary care and family care physician in Embangweni rather than seeing more complex cardiology patients as he had in Miraj. Regardless, they both said they felt called to Embangweni and were committed to being there for several years.

Three hours after departing Embangweni, we arrived in Lilongwe. Along the way, Paul became concerned about the car engine and immediately upon hitting the outskirts of Lilongwe, we began looking for a service station to check out the car. The car was repaired while we ate lunch. Fortunately, nothing substantial was wrong with the car and we were able to pick it up and continue on to the airport.

As I said goodbye to the Jewetts, I was saddened by the fact that I had only been able to spend such a short time in Malawi. The Jewetts had asked if I could help get them some needed medical supplies and I committed to doing so. I would do my best to return to Embangweni in the near future. As they drove away, I went into the airport and checked in.

I was quite early for my flight and decided to wander through the airport. As I strolled around, I became aware of many people looking and staring at me. I was literally the only white person in the entire airport! I remember thinking to myself how lonely and isolating it felt. In reality, all I saw around me were friendly faces, and the looks and stares seemed to be more from curiosity about my presence than anything else. All the same, I certainly had a greater appreciation of what many racial and ethnic groups must feel in public places in the United States. I began to understand just how intimidating that feeling could be.

Later that day, I landed in Lusaka, Zambia, eager to begin the last portion of my trip.

The next day, I journeyed by car to the Musi-oa-Tunya International Hotel in Livingstone. *Musi-oa-Tunya* is translated from the Lozi tribal language as "The Smoke Which Thunders," referring to what is better known worldwide as Victoria Falls. The Zambezi River forms the border between the countries of Zambia and Zimbabwe, and Victoria Falls is shared by the two countries.

Livingstone was the last stop of my journey and for two days, I relaxed in the city, taking several walking tours of Victoria Falls, which were absolutely stunning with water sprays rising literally hundreds of feet into the air before flowing over a jagged edge of cliffs and plunging several hundred feet down into the Zambezi River. Legend has it that David Livingstone was the first white man to view the falls. Told that

THROUGH THE LENS OF HUMANITY

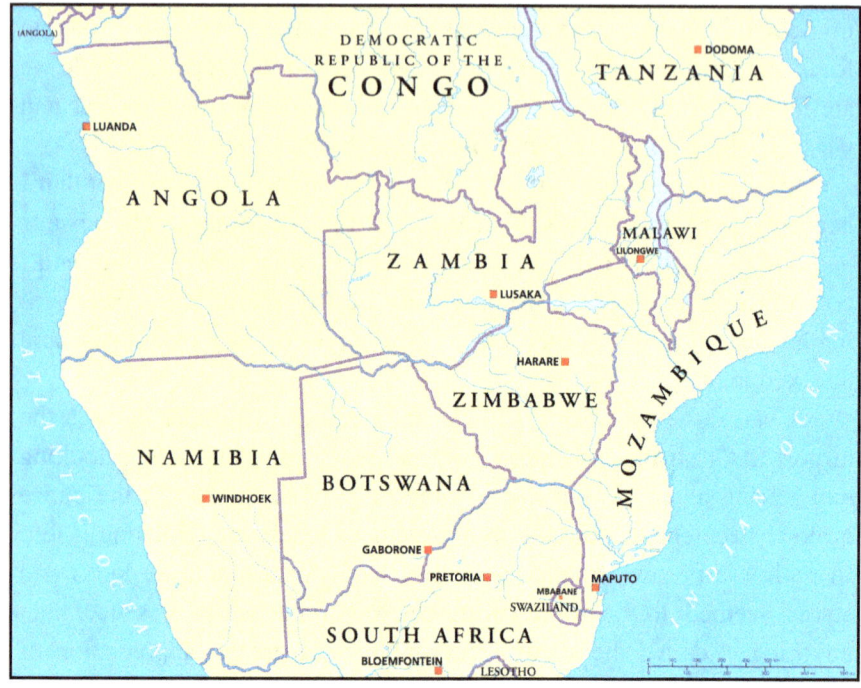

Map of Zambia and Zimbabwe: Destinations: Lusaka, Zambia; Livingstone, Zimbabwe

the natives called it Musi-oa-tunya, he named the magnificent natural wonder Victoria Falls for his queen, Queen Victoria of England.

Spanning the Zambezi River in Livingstone is the Victoria Falls Bridge for both automobile/truck traffic, as well as foot traffic. In the middle of the bridge is the famous Victoria Falls Bungee Jump. I debated with myself for hours as to whether I'd suck up my courage and experience the 350-foot drop from the bridge toward the thundering Zambezi River below as it surges through the Batoka Gorge. I decided to give it a go. So, I paid my $90 for the opportunity to jump off the bridge, and before I had a chance to back out, I was harnessed at my waist and ankles with the bungee rope. The bungee master helped me shuffle to the jumping platform. As I perched on the edge, my fear of heights hit me like a ton of bricks—but then I heard the bungee master calmly speaking the countdown: *5 - 4 - 3 - 2 - 1 - BUNGEE!*

THE EYES OF THE HEART

I closed my eyes and swan-dived off the platform. The adrenaline rush was incredible as for what seemed like an eternity, I hurtled downward toward the Zambezi River. But then I felt a modest tug on my ankles and I began my mid-air bounce when I reached the extension of the bungee rope and for several seconds, I bounced up and down. Slowly I felt myself being winched upward toward the lower spans of the bridge. As I was released from the harness, I was told that if I came back in an hour, for a small price, I could have both a photo and a video of my epic jump, which the attendants assured me was one of the finest they'd ever seen. Dutifully, I showed up in an hour to claim evidence that I had bungee-jumped from the grandest bungee jump in the world!

In addition to touring the Falls, one evening, I took a sunset dinner cruise down the Zambezi River and the sights were stunningly beautiful! The wildlife was resplendent—elephants, hippos, and crocodiles were visible and numerous birds were abundant.

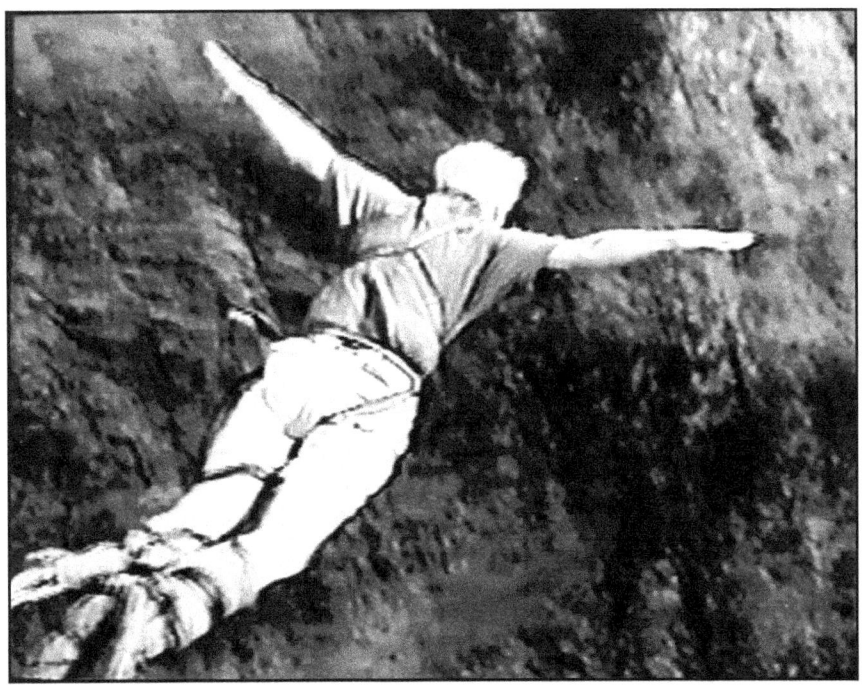

5 - 4 - 3 - 2 - 1 BUNGEE! A 350-foot free-fall adventure off the Victoria Falls Bridge!!

Through the Lens of Humanity

After my two-day sojourn, I returned to Lusaka to catch my flight back to the United States. My driver was getting a little concerned as we got closer to Lusaka. Gas was at a premium due to the conflict in the Middle East between Iraq and Kuwait. Many gas stations along our route were closed and his anxiety transferred to me, but fortunately just after we arrived at the city limits, we found fuel. I breathed a sigh of relief as the driver dropped me at the Lusaka airport.

I returned to Milwaukee, exhausted, but feeling blessed by the experiences I had had. I felt privileged and humbled to have met and seen the work of medical missionaries like Paul and Judy Jewett, Ken and Nancy McGill, Jim and Jody McGill, and Tom and Martin Logan.

I noted earlier that I was deeply affected by my experiences on this trip, as well as on my trip two and a half years earlier to Miraj, India. I have a mixture of feelings that range between sadness and frustration and anger when I see and experience situations where people who are impoverished or who suffer great hardship have little to no control over their situation. What adds to my frustration is I always know that I'm able to board a plane at the end of my visit and return to a life where I'm comfortable and face few of the life challenges confronting so many poor and vulnerable peoples around the globe.

*May the eyes of your heart be enlightened so
that you may know what is the hope to which he has called you.*
—Ephesians 1:18

I believe each of us has a spiritual heart that yearns to be seen, to be illuminated, to be recognized, and to proclaim that we are each entitled to respect and dignity, and to acknowledge this for others as well. My eyes were enlightened on this trip in recognizing that no matter where I found myself, I was connected to a larger whole. I grew beyond my limited sense of self to possess a greater awareness of the whole. And I believe that as we are enlightened to a deeper commitment of respect and dignity for ourself and most importantly others, a greater compassion for all will flourish.

Shortly after returning from my three-week trip, I was asked to write a "mission" piece as part of my church's Stewardship Campaign. The

THE EYES OF THE HEART

Campaign's theme was "Come and See What God Has Done." I chose to reflect on what the "eyes of my heart" had seen in the village of Embangweni, Malawi and in the corridors of the Embangweni Hospital. Below are portions of the piece I wrote entitled, "Having Eyes".

"HAVING EYES"

In Africa, this simple phrase describes an awakening—the physical act of being able to open one's eyes and see the world.

We read in the book of Job, "*I was the eyes to the blind.*" The Apostle Paul expands on this theme in the Book of Ephesians, telling us to "have eyes" in a spiritual sense. He prays that "*the eyes of your heart may be enlightened so that you may know ...*"

Not long ago, I visited several mission sites in Malawi, Africa, as part of a medical missions contingent. I saw with my own eyes how you, through your generosity, have enabled Christianity to be a vital life-saving, life-giving force in one of the world's most deprived regions.

I invite you to join me, to open your heart, to "Have Eyes" and to come and see what God has done in Embangweni, Malawi.

The little town of Embangweni is little more than a collection of mud-cake brick buildings with corrugated iron roofs. It lies closely sheltered by a large hill in the bush country of northern Malawi. Surrounded by small villages, Embangweni is accessible only by dusty, rutted trails that pass for roads. It is one of many, lonely, isolated towns that dot the vast expanse of the African continent.

Living conditions are primitive. There is no disguising the fact that most Malawians live in dirt and filth, yet they do so with a quiet dignity.

As you walk through Embangweni, you pass the small clusters of brick and wooden buildings. You notice the ground between these buildings is a raw, un-landscaped, dusty terrain cluttered by dead leaves, twigs, rocks, and animal excrement. It bears little resemblance to what you left behind in the United States.

All of the activities that normally occur between birth and death in these African towns—gathering firewood, hunting flood, fetching water, cooking with soot-blackened utensils, unceremonious eating, desultory working, resting, mending, babysitting, marriage, play, joy and grief—occur in Embangweni with complete candor.

You notice that most garbage, but not all, is burned. Your nose alerts you to the presence of poorly concealed latrines. You are struck by the prevalence of pregnancy.

But despite the sometimes cruel and always harsh conditions, the Malawin family retains its ancient pattern and strength. Families are bound together by tribes. In turn, the tribes protect the families against the enemies that menace their lives. Family love is not expressed in words, as is our practice, but in the solidarity with which the family unit meets the struggles of life. Joy, too, is present in laughter and play. And when disaster strikes, the reaction of the Malawian family is expressed by the enigma of silence.

Disaster, the visitor learns, is commonplace among Malawians. The rigors of life, ravages of disease, high infant mortality and many natural hazards claim the weak and the unfortunate. The remaining distillate—the rugged survivors—is in many ways hard and hardy. They possess resilience in depth.

Just beyond Embangweni lies the mission hospital. Perhaps the words "mission hospital" convey too much. The 'hospital" is, in actuality, a cluster of sturdy brick buildings. Stepping inside, the visitor sees the various "wards," examination activities, laboratory and X-ray facilities, and the surgical rooms.

Within the hospital walls, life is lived in a simple manner. Plumbing is quite basic. Electricity, which is generated by solar panels, is rationed for the X-ray machine and other equipment. Water is stored in tanks, distilled and filtered frequently.

The Eyes of the Heart

Although the equipment and patient areas are reasonably clean, the average healthcare professional and layman would worry about "quality" and "appearance." Where are the marble floors, indirect lighting, color coordinated walls and drapes, state-of-the-art equipment and personal computers? However, this haven of mercy cannot be held up to comparisons for no rival health facilities exist in this area.

Outside the hospital buildings, groups of Malawian women and children sit, almost like statues, as if waiting indefinitely were an integral part of their lives. But this is a hospital where no one ever asks, "Are you insured?" Here, all in need are treated without question. Patients who can afford the care do pay a minimal fee - in the local currency or with produce, a chicken, eggs or a goat.

The average Embangweni Hospital patient usually presents one immediate problem and many chronic illnesses. Malaria, intestinal parasites, dysentery, malnutrition, tuberculosis, and AIDS are but a few of the ailments routinely discovered upon preliminary examination.

However, the staff's spiritual courage is brought into shining relief by the bitter irony that comes in knowing that the cured will depart only to return, reinfected by the environmental conditions which affect the area.

Jesus was prodigious in seeing, with the eyes of his head and his heart, the moral and ethical truths which have proved enduring, timeless. At Embangweni Hospital, it is apparent that the hospital and its staff spiritually "Have Eyes" and are living instruments of Christ's dynamic truth. Through its ministry to the physically and spiritually sick, this hospital and staff stand as a symbol of mercy, compassion and love. It is a safe haven of respect for the worth of the poor, the humble and the destitute. It is a hospital where the common denominator among the staff is a disinterest in wealth and a love of service. They give of themselves—totally—not alone to a people, but to the river of life. Through their efforts, they have created a treasured hospital, which neither moth nor rust can corrupt. Perhaps the ultimate impact of Embangweni Hospital is directed in a preventive way at the chronic ills of the world, the suppurating, ever-running sores of world society. At Embangweni Hospital to "Have Eyes" is to illuminate the promise of divinity within humanity.

Part Two

Blessed are the Peacemakers

CHAPTER 3
"In Thoughts With You..."

One of the most famous humanitarians ever to receive the Nobel Peace Prize was Dr. Albert Schweitzer. What is astonishing in examining Schweitzer's life story is the depth and spectrum of his life and career. Born in 1875 in Alsace, a territory that alternately came under French and German sovereignty, Schweitzer possessed one of the most powerful and wide-ranging intellects the world has ever known. His interests spanned philosophy, music, theology, and medicine. His academic studies led to pastoral as well as theological faculty posts in Strasbourg. His theological writings on the origins of Christianity drew wide acclaim and critique. He was a celebrated organist and organ builder and his interpretation of the life and music of Johann Sebastian Bach made him one of the leading classical musical figures of his time.

But in Schweitzer's own words, one morning the thought came to him that he should not just accept the good fortune that had come to him in his academic and musical pursuits. Instead, he wrote friends he had decided he could not just devote himself to scholarship and the arts, he must also devote himself to serving humanity. To this end, and despite the protestations of friends and family, he took up the study of medicine and once his studies were complete, he became a medical missionary. In 1913, working with the Paris Missionary Society, he left for Africa and established a hospital in Lambarene, a small village in what was then French Equatorial Africa. For the next 50-plus years, he treated thousands of Africans suffering from leprosy, yellow fever, dysentery, malaria, sleeping sickness, and many other maladies and diseases, all the while continuing to write and express himself via his scholarly writings.

THROUGH THE LENS OF HUMANITY

In 1952, Schwietzer was awarded the Nobel Peace Prize. He used his Nobel Prize stipend to renovate and expand the hospital and to construct a leper colony to house and care for the many afflicted by this disease.

I came to know of the life of Schweitzer at Lambarene Hospital through a book written by Norman Cousins, who at the time was himself an award-winning author, political journalist, and editor of the *Saturday Review Magazine*. The book, *Dr. Schweitzer of Lambarene*, published in 1960, chronicles a visit to Lambarene by Norman Cousins in 1957 to meet and interview Dr. Schweitzer and to gain insight, as Cousins said, "… into one of the towering figures of the twentieth century." Cousins' book of observations, discussions, and encounters with Schweitzer while in Lambarene provided an intimate view into the life, work, purpose, and spirit of Dr. Schweitzer. Additionally, the book also offers profiles of many of the staff surrounding Schweitzer—the young doctors and nurses at his hospital—why they came to Lambarene, the difficulties they faced in their daily work, and how they responded to the persona of Schweitzer.

Similar to Cousins, I too had long admired Schweitzer, indeed I had read several of Schweitzer's books, as well as narratives and books about Schweitzer's life. And yet, while I read Cousins' book with eager anticipation regarding my interest in Schweitzer, it was Cousins' comments and observations about a young staff member, Dr. Margrietha van der Kreek, that captured my attention. Dr. van der Kreek was the chief surgeon at Lambarene Hospital and was affectionately known to everyone as "La Doctoresse."

Describing her "as a lovely young woman of about thirty from the Netherlands," Cousins offered this portrait and description of Dr. Margrietha:

> …. I looked over at Dr. Margrietha … She was busy filling out some prescriptions. I could readily understand why Clara (Clara Urquhart, a nurse colleague of Margrietha's at Lambarene) had called her one of the most beautiful young women in the world…

"IN THOUGHTS WITH YOU..."

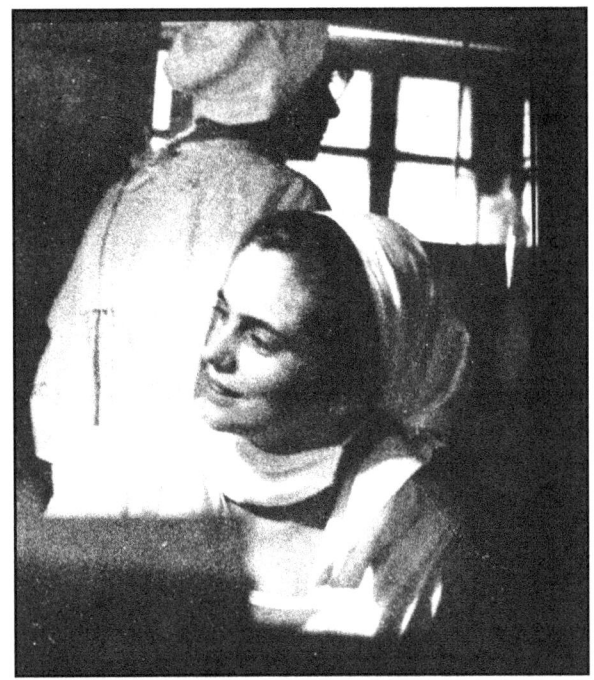

Dr. Margrietha van der Kreek, "La Doctoresse."

From *Dr. Schweitzer of Lambarene* by Norman Cousins, Photograph by Clara Urquhart

> Light-colored hair was combed straight back and held in place by a simple ribbon. She wore no lipstick or other make-up. Yet she possessed an unmistakable quality of classic loveliness both of feature and expression. I wondered about this attractive creature - how she happened to go into medicine and surgery, why she came to Lambarene. Here was the raw material from which legends were fashioned.

And then there was this moving and powerful observation of an encounter Cousins witnessed between "La Doctoresse" and a young African mother and her child:

> A young African mother, her face heavy with apprehension, carried in a five- or six-year old girl and set her down next to La Doctoresse. The child was wide-eyed and fearful. She clung to her mother's faded skirt with both hands....The mother said the child had a persistent fever.

> Kneeling and speaking softly, La Doctoresse took her stethoscope and applied it to the child's chest. Then very deftly, she put a tongue depressor in the child's mouth .... La Doctoresse reached behind her and took a little wooden doll from one of the drawers in her desk. She made small clucking sounds as she held the doll alluringly in front of the little girl. While the child scrutinized the doll, La Doctoresse lifted the child's dress and examined the lower part of her body ... La Doctoresse told the mother the child had malaria but that it could be brought under control.
>
> I could see that the woman had something to say to La Doctoresse but was choked up. The heavy apprehension in her face was gone; now there was measureless relief and gratitude ... I could tell the woman was struggling for a correct way to make known her feelings. Then she reached out and lightly touched Dr. Margrietha's arm. It was a simple gesture but profound in intent. Dr. Margrietha responded with the smile not of a doctor but of one woman communicating with another in a universal language....

I was fascinated and intrigued by Cousins' vignettes and references to Dr. van der Kreek. As I had begun traveling overseas more and more as a medical missions volunteer, I had become increasingly interested in the sense of "call" certain individuals possessed toward living their lives in service to others. Of particular interest to me were stories of individuals who made great personal sacrifices in support of their own sense of "call." So, as I read Cousins' accounts of Dr. Margrietha, aka La Doctoresse, I wanted to meet her and talk with her about her time with Schweitzer.

I shared Cousins' questions about her: Why in the world had she gone to Lambarene to work with Schweitzer? What was her "call" to service? What had happened to her and her career after Schweitzer's death in 1965? Trouble was, I didn't know if Margrietha was still alive or where she lived. After all, Cousins' book had been published over 30

"In Thoughts with You..."

years earlier. The only hard information I possessed about Dr. van der Kreek was what I had read in Cousins' book.

At the time I was reading Cousin's book—early 1991—I was an administrative officer at the Children's Hospital of Wisconsin. A good friend and colleague of mine was Leigh Morris, the hospital's Director of Communications. I shared with Leigh my interest in trying to track down Margrietha van der Kreek and my frustration about not knowing how to find out more about her, whether she was still alive, where she lived, was she still practicing medicine, what had happened to her in the intervening 30 years since Cousin's book had been published.

Leigh took an interest in Margrietha's story and my desire to track her down. Prior to joining the hospital, Leigh had been an investigative reporter for *Chicago Today* newspaper. Leigh told me he'd take a stab finding out what he could about Margrietha and see if his past contacts and resources could help turn up anything about Margrietha.

I was stunned, excited, and appreciative when Leigh showed up in my office a few days later with an address for Margrietha van der Kreek and her husband, Guy Barthelemy. Frankly, Leigh's investigative skills not withstanding, I had had little hope that he'd have much success in tracking her down. I thought too much time had elapsed and despite the fact that she had been prominently mentioned in Cousin's book, I had doubted Leigh would find any current information about her. But Leigh performed his "investigative magic" and it turned out that she was alive and well and living, at least based upon Leigh's information, in Tourves, France.

So, now what? I had her address, or at least what I suspected to be her current address. Now what was I going to do with it?

Well, following the old adage "nothing ventured, nothing gained," I set about composing a letter to her explaining who I was, how I had learned about her, and my eagerness to talk with her, and understand what possessed her to go work for Schweitzer at a remote hospital in Africa.

I developed several versions of a letter, all trying to persuade someone I didn't know, and who didn't know me from Adam's house cat, why she should speak to me about her personal life and life's journeys. After much editing, I finally settled on the following version:

June 20, 1991
Mme. Dr. M. Barthelemy van der Kreek
Villages sans Frontiers
B.P. 18
83170 Tourves, France

Dear Dr. van der Kreek,

Your work as a surgeon in Africa has for many years held my fascination and admiration. A spiritual belief of mine is that each of us are "called" by our creator to fulfill certain missions during our lives. From my knowledge of your work and experiences in Africa, I sense you too share this feeling, and have lived your live in faithfulness to your "call."

I am writing requesting to speak with you, as one who has met the challenges and struggles inherent in responding to their "call". My hope is to shed greater light on the issue of people's "calls" to service by interviewing individuals from various walks of life about their concept of their life's "call", and then writing profiles of these people's feelings and experiences. By focusing on people who are well known, my hope is that others will become responsive to their own "calls.".

I realize, however, you might wish to not be publicly profiled, if that is the case I ask simply for the opportunity to spend some time with you on an informal, personal basis—I strongly believe the opportunity to discuss your life and values will be one of enlightenment and growth for me as I pursue my own life's goals.

"In Thoughts with You..."

I plan to travel to India this Fall (probably August or September) to do some volunteer work in a Presbyterian Mission Hospital and plan to spend some time in France on my return journey to the United States. Will you please write me at either of the enclosed addresses letting me know if I might speak with you while in France? If you are agreeable, I can make specific arrangements as to the dates I can travel to Tourves.

I hope to hear positively from you, and thank you for your consideration.

Sincerely,
Mark E. Anderson
Executive Vice President
Children's Hospital of Wisconsin

P.S. As a bit of my own personal profile, I am currently a hospital administrator at Children's Hospital of Wisconsin, USA. I have been a Volunteer-in-Mission for the Presbyterian Church at the Miraj Medical Center in Miraj, India in 1987 and at several Presbyterian Mission hospitals in Malawi, Africa in 1990. In the fall of this year, I plan to enter a Presbyterian seminary with the intent of combining theological studies with my healthcare background and ultimately devoting myself to missionary activities in third-world countries.

I finished and mailed this version of the letter on June 20, 1991—my 36th birthday. However, instead of sending the letter through normal mail channels, I decided to mail it in a way that would catch her attention and indicate that this letter was not normal correspondence. I purchased the largest letter envelope that Federal Express carried and sent the letter to her via express mail. And then I settled down to wait and see what, if any response I would receive.

Through the Lens of Humanity

I didn't have long to wait. On Wednesday, July 10th, I received Margrietha's reply by Priority Mail. And what an incredible and remarkable response it was!

> Tourves
> 28.6.91
>
> Dear Mr. Anderson,
> Thank you for your letter of 21 June 1991 which I received yesterday. You want to exchange about my call—in French "vocation"—in Dutch, "roeping."
> Somewhere it reminds me the expression of Ghandi who said I want my windows and doors to be open—in that way the spirit can enter my house from all over the world.
> Today there is a strong wind here—a MISTRAL which blows away all the clouds. For my open door it makes a lot of noise but I like it—the branches of an oak dance up and down. The blue sky behind is marvelous. It is warm—24 C.
> It is a pity you plan only in the return of India to come to France. I would have proposed to come now to talk together … I have also worked in India and have still a great attachment for that country (Very good friends are writing to me regularly and that is an exception in India).
> In uniting your and my experiences somewhere a creative power could develop to serve mankind. Schweitzer would say the power of an ideal can work like a drop of water. You cannot see how strong it is, but the moment it falls in the split of a rock it freezes…the rock will explode.
> Perhaps we need here the coming of someone like you. Now and not after some months! We started a project here 4 years ago - 100 acres of land with ruins on it, with a group of volunteers we rebuilt the most of the ruins and started a biological vegetable garden. Actually the danger for our project is that it will fall to pieces.

"In Thoughts with You..."

> Some of the founders ask the money back and the property will be sold. Marvelous big oak trees of 300 years old, with a view of the mountains. The spirit of pioneers you can feel at every corner. Is it a hasard you write just now? I do not know and wait for your answer. Be welcome and see in your heart what says your call.
>
> In thoughts with you,
> Greet Barthelemy van der Kreek
>
> Biological vegetable garden with fraises de bois (wild strawberries) and framboises (raspberries) wait to offer you a fresh meal of fruits ....

Quite frankly, I had been concerned whether Margrietha would reply at all. While I clearly wanted to connect and speak with Margrietha, I believed it was only remotely possible that she would respond to my request. So I was astonished and ecstatic at her reply. Not only had she responded immediately and positively to my request, but her response also had a poetic allure to it, and, it seemed to me, an innate understanding and prescience about the very topics I wished to discuss with her and an importance of our getting together. Come now, she suggests, so that we may talk together! And her words, "In uniting your and my experiences somewhere a creative power could develop to serve mankind..." Was this perhaps an invitation to work together in the project that she and her husband had founded?

A particularly endearing part of Margrietha's letter was her closing salutation, 'In thoughts with you.' I remember how I was struck by the use of this phrase the first time I read Margrietha's letter. It radiated an immediate sense of togetherness, transparency, encouragement even - a warm feeling of intimate comfort between friends.

Margrietha had included her phone number in France within her letter, and several days later, on a Saturday morning, I placed a call to the number in France.

"*Oui?*" answered a woman's voice on the phone.

THROUGH THE LENS OF HUMANITY

"Good morning," I said, "I'm looking for Dr. Margrietha van der Kreek. This is Mark Anderson calling from the United States."

After a brief pause, "Ahhhh, yes" came the reply in English. "You are the letter writer, you are the *chercheur*—the searcher. You wish to come talk to me in France." Even now I can hear the hint of amusement and lightness in her voice as she responded.

"Yes," I said chuckling at her comment, "I am the letter writer and the searcher!"

And so began the process of planning my trip to France and India. Margrietha reiterated again in our phone conversation how important she felt my coming to France first was, and then afterwards to India.

And thus began too a 25-year friendship and connection with one of the most remarkable and incredible people I have ever met.

* * *

After another call and letter with Margrietha (she had by now instructed me to call her "Greet," a shortened version of Margrietha), the framework for my journey to France and India was in place. My itinerary spanned the dates of August 8th through August 16th in France, visiting Greet and her family on their 100-acre commune in Touvres, and August 17th through August 30th in India, with time spent in Varanasi, Agra, and Delhi, culminating with five days volunteering with Mother Teresa and the Missionaries of Charity in Calcutta.

On August 8, 1991, my flight to France left at 5:10 pm out of O'Hare Field in Chicago. I would first fly to Orly airport in Paris, then take a connecting flight to Toulon, where I would be picked up by Guy Barthelemy, Greet's husband. After that, we would drive from Toulon to Touvres.

During my flights, I noticed that the closer and closer I got to Touvres and to meeting Greet, the more and more excited—and anxious—I was getting. Though we had now communicated several times, I still really didn't know what to expect. What would Dr. Margrietha van der Kreek really be like? What did she expect of me?

"IN THOUGHTS WITH YOU..."

Guy Barthelemy picked me up at the Toulon; he was standing in the arrival area of the airport, waving a sign with my name on it. He was accompanied by a young woman, Fuku Davuout, a family friend of the Barthelemys who was visiting with them for the summer.

We ran a quick errand in Toulon and then were on the road to *Villages sans Frontiers*, the commune for the disadvantaged and mentally handicapped that Greet and Guy had established. Both Guy and Fuku spoke English, Fuku better than Guy, but Guy was hard of hearing so our conversation on the trip to the commune was limited.

After about an hour's drive, we turned up a winding, rock-strewn lane that led to the commune. The commune, the ruins that Greet had first referred to in her letter, sat upon a hill at the end of the lane. The structure itself appeared to be several connected buildings. I was reminded of an old farmhouse. The buildings were a rambling mixture of stone and wood surrounded by trees that stretched beyond the buildings and up a hillside. The buildings were situated on a large expanse of land—we were clearly out in the countryside. No other residences or buildings were to be seen.

As we pulled up into the open area in front of the buildings, Greet walked out to welcome us. Though her hair had grayed, she still had it pulled into a bun similar to the photos I had seen of her in the Cousins' book. Though over three decades had elapsed since those photos were taken, as Cousins had observed years earlier, Greet still possessed 'an unmistakable quality of classic loveliness, both of feature and expression.' We greeted each other warmly, both I think a little amused and bemused at the circumstances that had brought us together.

Greet quickly introduced her daughter, Maria, and her granddaughter, Irina, who had also stepped out of the main building. They all spoke English to me, but it was clear they were multi-lingual. When addressing one another, they spoke French.

I collected my couple of pieces of luggage and knapsack out of the car, and followed Greet to my guest room. We walked around the corner of the main building and up a staircase to a second-level bedroom. Along the way, Greet explained that she and Guy had done most of the remodeling of the buildings themselves. There were many guest rooms for "travelers and friends who were always coming and going."

My room had a bed, a table, a couple of chairs, and a small closet. Greet had placed a vase of lovely flowers on the table. She said Schweitzer always liked rooms to have fresh flowers—it was the first of many references to Schweitzer during my visit.

Shortly after my arrival, Greet guided me to a favorite place of hers, a little clearing a short distance up the hill from the farmhouse and buildings where a bench, table, and chairs had been arranged beneath a sprawling and beautiful oak tree: the 300 year old oak tree that Greet had mentioned in her letter. A late afternoon breeze rustled in the trees as the sun set and we began to get acquainted. Greet mentioned that she and Guy had been on the property for several years and that they had worked very hard renovating the buildings and grounds. For them, this was a special place. They loved the location, their family lived on the grounds, Guy was a professional writer and the beauty and quietness of the area suited his work style and manner. Greet shared all this in English that was a little halting and interspersed with the occasional French or Dutch phrase. She was direct and I sensed, like me, a little curious about how our upcoming conversations would go.

I told Greet a little about myself, about my work and family, where I lived and thanked her for agreeing to talk with me. She started laughing, saying she was quite surprised when she got such a long letter from a stranger in America asking to come speak to her. She added that she was very happy to get the letter. As we had communicated further, she had been excited about my visit and was eager to talk of "the things of my interest." She was curious to learn more about how I had learned of her.

I had brought with me, as gifts for Greet, two books: *Dr. Schweitzer of Lambarene* by Norman Cousins, and *The Words of Albert Schweitzer* as selected by Norman Cousins. Both books had photographs of Greet inside. I explained to her that I learned of her as I read the Lambarene book, and I had become enthralled with her story as I read of her and saw the pictures of her in Cousins' book. I asked her if she had ever seen the book. "*Oui*," she said. She had read it years ago and thought she might even have a copy, but she didn't know where it was.

When I gave her both books, Greet took them and opened the book about Schweitzer in Lambarene. I had paper-clipped many of the pages where she was mentioned and pictured. Greet grew silent and sat back in her chair. After a few moments, she started smiling and giggling a little as memories flooded her mind. The years seemed to fade from her face, and behold, "*La Doctoresse*" of Lambarene sat quietly reminiscing .

After a few moments, I asked Greet if it would be okay to record our conversations with a small recorder. Again she laughed and said that would be fine; she remembered Norman Cousins also recording conversations during his visit to Lambarene so long ago.

For the next week, I was the guest of the Barthelemys at a quaint, remote, and beautiful location in South France. I ate meals with them, ran errands with Guy and Greet to local French villages and towns, and even went with them, Maria, her husband Pascal, and their daughter

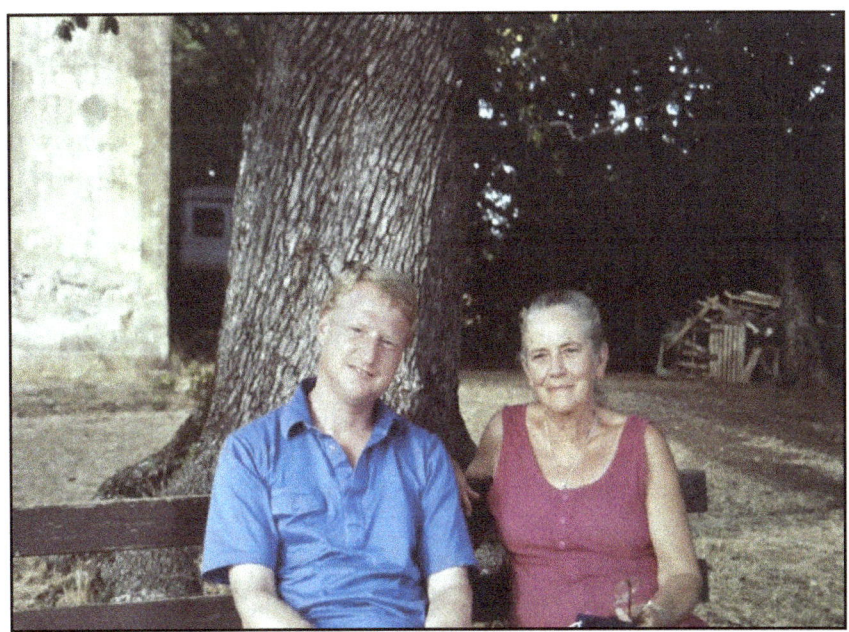

The author and "Greet" under the 300-year-old oak tree.

THROUGH THE LENS OF HUMANITY

Irina on a family outing to a beach near Marseilles. But it was my time with Greet over the next several days under this beautiful old oak tree that created one of the most meaningful memories and experiences of my life.

Every day for the next week, often after breakfast or after running errands to the local village, or helping with the chores around the commune, Greet and I would adjourn to the clearing under the grand old oak tree and talk for hours. She did permit me to record our conversations, which was wonderful, allowing us to chat without my having to worry about capturing our conversations through note-taking, but more importantly, enabling me to recollect her precise words and her voice for the future.

I had shared with Greet some of the areas I wanted to ask her about, and our discussions usually started with a specific question which she would address. Often, though, we'd spin off into other areas as our conversations got underway. Greet was always very open and frequently answered my questions, and then ask me a similar question.

Since I had told Greet that I had learned of her by reading Cousins' book about Schweitzer, my initial interest was how she how met Schweitzer and had gone to Lambarene. And so our conversations began! (The following conversations were recorded with permission.)

"When I first read of you," I said, "I was fascinated by why you might want to go to Africa. And as I read more about you, I recall you made a comment that you went because you felt you heard voices which called you there?"

Greet replied with a chuckle. "When you say voices, that is not exactly the truth. I did not actually hear voices, but it is hard to explain it. Psychiatrists, when they hear people say they hear voices, they say '*hum*,' this person is rather suspect, perhaps not normal."

"But you ask why did I go, I say I heard the voice of my heart, and my guideline for my life from the beginning and has always been the same, to be where I am needed."

"And how did you know that you were needed in Africa," I asked.

"Well, there were first steps that foretold the journey," she said. "There was first someone who said to me, 'Ah, do you know about

"In Thoughts with You..."

Albert Schweitzer. And I said, 'No, I don't know. Is that the fellow with the mustache who did something remarkable? I was studying to be a doctor and one day, a student gave me a photo of African villagers and they said Schweitzer is doing great things in the middle of these people.

"When I finished my degree as a doctor I went to the World Health Organization and asked if they needed me in Indonesia or in the World Health Organization and they say doctors who just got their degree, we do nothing with them, no experience they are useless. Ahhh....

"So I looked in the medical newspaper that every doctor in Holland reads and I found an announcement that a surgeon in a small town needs an assistant. So I went there. I got the job and I stayed there for one and a half years.

"After that time, I make a small holiday trip and one of the student's parents told me that Schweitzer was now in Europe. I was in the town where he was, and people asked if I would like to meet him. And I said 'why not?'

"So I went and I met Schweitzer and we talked about my working in Africa and he asked me two questions. "Can you sleep well?" and "Do you have a sense of humor?" I laughed and I said I have a sense of humor and I sleep very well wherever I am."

"Those are interesting job interview questions," I said.

"Ah, yes, but that was Schweitzer," Greet said. "It is something in a tropical country to have a sense of humor even if everything breaks down around you and you can laugh about it, eh? In Africa, about three quarters of the time if you plan to do something, it comes out differently or not at all. You need a sense of humor. It is necessary to do the work. The second thing to be able to sleep is very necessary and if you have to work very hard, you must be able to in between sleep properly. And happily, I have almost all of my life been able to sleep properly. And when you sleep, you wash away the poison that could just accumulate."

"When was this that you met Schweitzer. What was the date?" I inquired.

"So that meeting with Schweitzer was in July of 1954, and he told me if I need you, we will write you. At the end of 1954, one of nurses of Schweitzer wrote me asking me for a *curriculum vitae*, and I sent it. And then in the beginning of January of 1955, I received a letter from Schweitzer himself, a small letter telling me I was needed."

"In Holland that day was the birthday of my father and Schweitzer asked for a telegram saying yes or no. And I sent a telegram *oui*, yes. And the next day, I told my parents. And my parents, ah, my father he was silent then, he was not happy about it. He was like that. But my mother, she understood. She said, 'But you who are so sensitive and will see everything, how will it be possible for you to go to a place where it must be very difficult. How will you fare in that circumstance?'

I said, "I don't know, but we will see."

Greet paused at this point in the story and I could tell she was reliving these memories and feeling quite a bit of emotion. After a moment, she continued.

"But what was also really typical for my mother, she put in my luggage and I found it when I arrived there—two small papers. And on the small papers was written the beginning of a hymn that I learned when I was 7 years old in the center for rehabilitation where my aunt was the head director. [*Greet had shared with me when she was seven she contracted diphtheria and for five days was on the cusp of death. Her rehabilitation time is what she is referring to here.*] "We were always singing this hymn what the future would bring us." [*Based upon what Greet told me, the hymn she is referring to is: Abide Among Us with Thy Grace by Joshua Stegmann, written in 1630.*] "It is curious when I sing this, I feel emotion coming up. This is the same hymn we also sang at my marriage in the church. The other paper said keep both of my hands together as in prayer. My mother has sent these two things in my luggage. It was very beautiful."

Again, Greet paused for a moment and sat very still. She looked at me and said, "I see you have emotion as well." I said I had had a similar experience and told her that when I went to India in 1987, my mother had sent me a very moving, encouraging, and intimate note and that I was remembering that as she spoke. We sat for a moment and then again she moved ahead.

"In Thoughts with You…"

"You must realize that if you go in an unknown continent, this was not only another country, it was another continent. I went first to France, to Paris. I was four days alone in Paris and then I took a plane and went to Africa and everything is different. You went to India, you went to Africa and you were also older. I was 27 years old at that time. But it was a good thing to have taken this step. I knew my step was the right one. It was a right and straight step and inside my soul, I knew it was straight and right what I did."

I spoke then. "You mentioned yesterday you felt divinely guided in your decision?"

"Yes, I felt guided. I told you yesterday, when I was a child seven or eight years old, I blushed when I pronounced the word God, so even today I am shy to talk … to use the word God. I prefer always to say Divine, or Supreme Spirit. Of course, I believe it is the same, but I prefer to say another word than God."

"Because you have so much respect for that which for you is God?" I asked.

"Yes, That is it. There are some things in your life, I am sure you have the same thought—for certain things, you do not need to pronounce words for it. Something so very—essential, very true—there are no words.

She continued. "You asked me yesterday if I was afraid when I went. No I was not afraid, not afraid at all. I felt guided. This was my way to go and I knew it in my soul."

"And so, you were on your way to Lambarene?" I asked.

"Yes, I flew in a small plane into the airport of Lambarene. As I was gathering my things—I remember I couldn't find my red umbrella," Greet said, laughing.

"There was Emma from the hospital looking for the new *doctoresse*. She was standing there in a white dress and white helmet and I was looking for my red umbrella! But she gathered me up and took me in a truck to the ferry to go to the island of Lambarene.

"We got into the canoes, several of us, including some lepers, and we started toward the hospital. After about three quarters of an hour, Emma said, 'There you can see the hospital.' I saw nothing but a lot of palm trees and a small house in between. I kept searching for something that looked like a hospital, and as we got nearer and nearer, I saw buildings, long buildings, but nothing in my imagination that looked like a hospital. And we got closer and Emma said, 'See all the people coming to welcome you.' And I saw people coming from the left and right and they came all to the landing. There was at least one hundred, maybe even two hundred people. And then ah, there he is coming, Dr. Schweitzer. With Schweitzer, there was a group of about 10 people. Schweitzer was in a big white helmet and he was the first who gave me his hand.

"And I looked around and saw people with big bandages and crutches. And I walked up toward the buildings with Schweitzer and some Dutch people and he brought me to my room. My room was in a building, the name was Sansouci. It was all painted white. There were no windows. There were mosquito nets, there was a bed and a table and a chair and a small corner desk and that was all. It looked a bit poor. But I think as I remember now, with the time in between, the essential was there and there was a very big tree next to my room and big fruit and later on, I understood the value of this tree. Trees like this feed many people. But the first night I was there, the fruits were falling on the roof and I thought there were bombs going off, but they were just the fruits of this tree. I also heard other noises that first night, rats running above the platform of the ceiling."

"What an incredible story," I said. "So once you got to Lambarene, you stayed there for five and a half years? Did you ever doubt that you were in the wrong place or have feelings of 'what did I do,' or 'why am I here'?"

She looked at me wide-eyed. "Yes, I was in that place for five and a half years. I didn't have a doubt. I felt this was the way to go. There was especially in the first months a feeling of loneliness. There was nobody among the people who were there that I felt really attracted to. Even the first night, everything was strange. I even cried a bit. But then I heard the rain falling on the roof and I felt the drops of my tears and they are mixing with the rain and I think at least the rain is the same as in my own country. I think as I looked at the sky I saw the moon and

"In Thoughts with You..."

the next day the sun and it was at least something I knew. But everything else was strange. But there was not any doubts that I was on the right way.

"I wanted to be where I was needed, but in the beginning I felt I was not very useful. In the beginning I remember I dreamt every night, every night I dreamt for my world in Holland, but slowly, slowly it changed and then I changed. Then one day, I started to get a real connection with Schweitzer. Schweitzer was a shy character; he would never impose or question people. In an interview with an American lady named Marion Rogers, I stated my admiration for Schweitzer and what he did in Lambarene."

"I never said this directly to him, but through this interview he knew that I admired what he did. And from that moment, he began to show his affection for me. He laid his hand on my shoulder or he brought me a small booklet or later on he even asked me to check his blood pressure and then slowly, there was a fine relationship where he slowly started to talk even at the table. After the community meals, he even started talking to me about the first Christians."

Greet paused again and became very reflective. She continued, but I could tell she was again having a difficult time controlling her emotions.

"Due perhaps to this..." Again she paused. "One day, I asked him to baptize me and I wanted also to have other relationships with my patients. Not only to be their doctor, but also as he did that in his work, I wanted also to be able to preach. And how can you preach if you are not baptized," I thought.

"And so one day, he baptized me in my room and I had the small box my mother painted [*Greet's mother was an artist*], I had to go and put some water in it and he baptized me. It was a very special moment and he gave me a small bible what was his bible from 1890 or something like that, as a memory of this baptismal day of 2nd of August 1957."

"And then one day after three and a half years about the time I go for my holiday, and I said goodbye to Schweitzer. Schweitzer said goodbye also and give me a kiss on my cheek but he didn't ask me to

THROUGH THE LENS OF HUMANITY

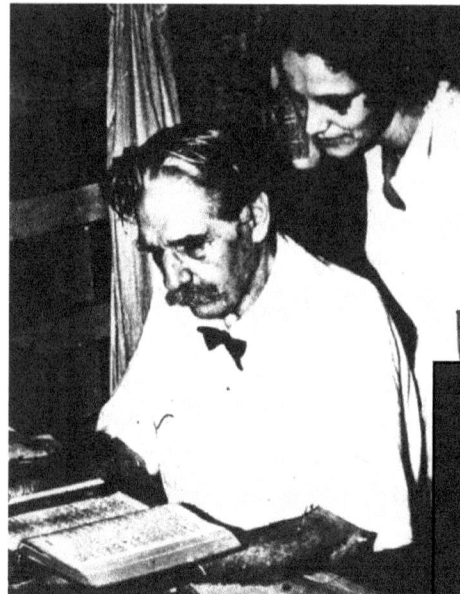

Dr. Schweitzer and Dr. van der Kreek in Lambarene - mid 1950s
From:*Dr. Schweitzer of Lambarene*
by Norman Cousins
Photographs: Clara Urquhart

come back, which was typical of Schweitzer. Schweitzer was fine in his relationship with people in not obligating them. So that was their free choice. And I said, 'I am not sure I will come back'. He said nothing. He give me this kiss and I went."

"But after seven months in Europe, talking about him and giving some conferences and so on regarding the work in Lambarene, I compared my life in Holland with what I did in Lambarene and I chose to go back to Lambarene. And I was there one and a half more years."

"In Thoughts with You..."

"And then you decided to, after your year and a half or so, to leave again," I said.

Greet started smiling and laughing, "Yes, but that was because there was a charming French fellow who came on my road."

"And who is still on your road," I responded.

"Yes, he is still on my road. That was also difficult for Schweitzer, but he never kept people back. He understood that people had to go on their way. Both Guy and I had grown very close to Schweitzer, but it was not his way to hold people back."

"So after you left Lambarene, you married Guy Barthelemy, who also had been at Lambarene for a number of years?"

"Yes, we married on September 24th, 1960. It was very difficult for Guy and me to leave Lambarene—we had grown close to Schweitzer and to others—we had been there for long time—and Guy, he knew Schweitzer a longer time than I."

"What other special memories of Schweitzer at Lambarene do you have?" I asked.

"Schweitzer was a shy fellow as I told you, but he was also a considerate fellow, but he was very private. I learned from my parents, that after I had come to Lambarene, he wrote a handwritten letter to my parents thanking them for letting me come to Lambarene. Schweitzer, he never told this to me. I found out from my parents. It was very special to me that he did that. So many kindnesses he did for others that no one knows, that he just did."

"May I tell you a true story about Schweitzer that I know from a friend of mine?" I asked.

"Yes," she answered, looking at me quizzically as if 'how did I know someone else who knew Schweitzer after all these years.'

"A friend of mine named Tom Logan graduated from high school in the early 1960s. Instead of going away to college right away, Tom decided that he'd travel through Africa for a number of months. Tom started out his travels in South Africa and gradually worked his way up through Africa. After he'd been in Africa several months, Tom arrived in Lambarene, and started working unloading the boats that came in and out of the town. He did this for about two months. Tom knew who

Schweitzer was, had seen him around, but had had very little contact with him.

"Then one day, Schweitzer asked Tom to come see him at his cabin. Schweitzer wanted to know what Tom's plans were and Tom told Schweitzer he planned to go to the Congo next. Schweitzer told Tom he should go home, the Congo is far too dangerous. Tom insisted that he was going to go as planned. Schweitzer told Tom he'd need money to keep going and asked him if he had sufficient funds. Tom answered he had some money and didn't need any. Schweitzer kept telling Tom the Congo and other parts of Africa were very dangerous and he should go home, but Tom kept insisting he was going to continue on his travels in Africa. So Schweitzer wrote a handwritten letter telling Tom to use the letter if he got into trouble. The letter explained that Schweitzer wanted to be contacted if Tom needed any kind of help. Schweitzer also gave Tom a couple of books that he had written.

"Soon after Tom left Lambarene, he looked at the books Schweitzer had given him. He discovered that Schweitzer had put a $100 bill in the one of the books in the event that Tom needed money. This was Tom's experience of Schweitzer."

"When Tom told me this story, the books Schweitzer had given him were *Out of My Life and Thought*, and *The Story of My Pelican*. Tom also told me that he still had the letter that Schweitzer had written —it is framed and hanging in his office."

Greet nodded and smiled, "Ah yes, that was Schweitzer's way," she said. "I am not surprised. Schweitzer, he was concerned about everyone. But you might not always know it," she chuckled.

Then she said, "You asked me about other memories of Schweitzer. At Lambarene, the staff were all aware of Schweitzer's gift of music. He often played the piano at night. The piano, he could not keep it tuned because of the tropic heat, but still he played. We also often saw him studying music even when he did not play. He played for staff birthdays, but mostly he played hymns. Many times while he played, there was singing by the staff of what he was playing. But we knew he was a remarkable musician. I loved listening at night after meals to him.

"In Thoughts with You..."

Many nights too, he would sit and read his Bible. Sometimes he would read out loud, but many times he would sit and read silently. Sometimes he'd pray after the playing and singing of hymns, mostly it was the 'Our Father'.

"Schweitzer loved animals. He had many animals—he liked cats, he had many cats. But he had other animals. He even wrote a book about his pelican," she laughed. "He told me this one day. I was surprised he would write a book about a pelican, but he loved all types of animals.

"With Schweitzer, I think of so many things. I think that life as you live it, makes you become aware of things. Life is something that goes above us, eh? It is not me who is developing awareness—I learn that from above. Life makes me aware that certain things are important and others aren't and that is how I think it is so natural that you have felt it in this week that you are with us that every time whenever we talk about important things the name of Schweitzer is connected to that.

Greet went on. "I remember many things that Schweitzer said, and his thoughts were very fundamental and his thoughts were very up to date. Schweitzer used to say and I know it was what he believed in his life, 'The real civilization starts there where you start to limit your needs and not like in our actual society where we want to have more and more from everything.' This thought I think is important in giving service to others. If you think of this and then you come to the point of having people around you who need you, you have no time anymore for yourself."

As Schweitzer said, 'If you want to give service to people, do not expect they will take away any stone from your path. On the contrary, they will put more stones on it. But he said also it is important to overcome obstacles. Have the tough skin of an old hippopotamus, but also the tender heart of a young antelope'. This is what Schweitzer did in his life and why today he still inspires people."

"And so how did it go when you told Dr. Schweitzer that you and Guy were going to get married?" I asked, drawing the conversation back to when she was about to depart Lambarene. "Did he approve?"

"Ah," he said, "This is a very good fellow. He is a very good fellow."

"So Schweitzer saw you off when you left the second time?"

"Yes, he never tried to keep people back. That was very beautiful in Schweitzer. He never kept people. He received, he was happy when they were there. The connection with him was very deep and wonderful when we left and when we told him that we wanted to make an Albert Schweitzer's village in France, he wrote us a beautiful letter, he was always fantastic in his encouragement of us."

Greet became reflective and said, "It was very difficult when he died, not to have any more possibility to write him and to get an answer. It was very difficult for Guy to hear he died, Guy and Schweitzer had a very close relationship. It was difficult time for me, Schweitzer died on September 4, 1965. My mother she died on September 13th of that same year."

As had been our practice during my visit, when Greet and I talked, we sat beside the 300-year-old oak tree that she truly loved. This day, it was late afternoon and she noticed that her daughter Maria was approaching. It was a good stopping point for the day, I knew Greet had grown a little melancholy as she spoke about Schweitzer's and her mother's deaths. After dinner that night, she told me she was going to look more at the books I had brought her, as well as search for some photos she had of her time in Lambarene.

The next morning, Greet was in a very excited and animated mood. After breakfast, as we adjourned to the clearing and the old oak tree, Greet's eyes grew moist as she shared with me that she had searched and found among her things the prayer that her mother had included within her luggage as Greet traveled to Lambarene. This treasure from her mother was handwritten on a small sheet of paper. The page was torn a little around the edges and the writing was faded by age. On another small sheet of paper, Greet had translated it into English for me:

> "Just a little bit of a dazzling ray of God's grace in response to your love for HIM cancels all your ignorance, all your difficulties, setbacks, drawbacks, all your childish games in just one moment."

"In Thoughts with You..."

"What a wonderful gift from your mother," I said. "And how meaningful it must have been for you when you found it when you arrived in Lambarene."

"Yes. My mother taught me two small prayers - this one and the *Our Father,* but it is this one that I pray when I want to have a direct connection."

"Were your mother and father very religious? Did you grow up in a very religious environment?"

"My mother and father, both in their own way, they were religious. They were believers but they didn't go to church."

She thought for a minute and then said, " I was seven years old and I got diphtheria and they gave me some serum and I was almost dead. Five days between life and death and I was so sick my mother was sitting next to my bed praying and singing hymns. I was sent to a convalescence home for six months where my aunt was director, and my mother was there praying and there was singing of hymns.

"But they didn't go to church, and when I was 11 years and needed a contact with religion, I went to different churches alone, and the only one where they didn't make me sit in a chair in front of everybody was the Baptist one, and so I kept going there for a while. So I did my religious education more myself.

"My father was from a Catholic family but I believe my mother was more deeper religiously. I went to Catholic church some and I know in the Catholic church, liturgy and things like that are important, and you need to kneel at the right time and make your cross in a certain way but I was not good at that.

"I think," she said in a teasing way and with a twinkle in her eye, "that there is too much fondness for a bit of theater."

She laughed and asked me, "Do Presbyterians have a fondness for theater?"

"A little bit," I said. "But Presbyterians mostly have a fondness for meetings of any kind," I said laughing.

"Ah, yes." Greet said amused. "Of course, those things are important, but I didn't want to be pressed into a certain way. I wanted to be able to choose my way myself—and that is why it was so important and moving to me to be baptized by Schweitzer."

As my time with Greet and her family on their farm began to wind down, we began to discuss her life with Guy and her family post-Lambarene and post-Schweitzer. Dr. Schweitzer continued to have an impact on her and Guy's lives—they corresponded frequently with him until his death in 1965, and Schweitzer also assisted in providing some funding for projects they established in France. Greet describes the challenges, opportunities, and joys in following along the path of Schweitzer:

"On the 24th of September, 1960, Guy and I got married in Holland. I had a dream to do something in the style and spirit of Schweitzer. Guy and I decided to look first to do something in France. We found on a map a village called Paunat in the Dorbogne region. It was Guy's idea that we develop the ruins in this place to do something where we could help people. And in this place, we started with 24 hectares of property and buildings, some in ruins and some in rather good shape. In honor of Schweitzer, we created the Albert Schweitzer Village.

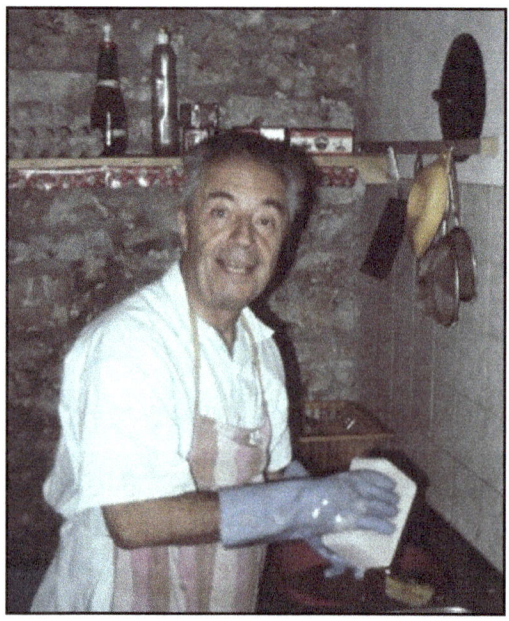

Guy Barthelemy at Tourves, France

"In Thoughts with You..."

"We saw in the beginning abandoned children, and later on refugees, and then also other people who needed our help. In 1967, we had been doing this seven years and it had grown so quickly that we felt overwhelmed, and we felt it became too much.

"We left Paunat in 1967 and we went to India. We were invited by the Indian government; they had heard of our previous work. But we only stayed in India for about five weeks and then returned to France. As we were deciding what our next course would be, I had a friend in Holland who said to me 'I have a place for you in Holland, you can come and practice as a plastic surgeon or as a psychiatrist.' And though I was not trained as a psychiatrist, I received more training and I became a psychiatrist at The Hague in Holland. My daughter Maria went with me and we lived in Holland eight years, with Guy coming to visit every three to four weeks.

"As a psychiatrist, I felt as I told you before—it was there that I was needed, and I saw all the misery I believe people can have. I saw the drunks, and the drug addicts and the people who were suicidal and the completely mad and dangerous people. In Lambarene I had seen the physically pained people with their diseases, but in Holland, I saw all the misery and suffering people can have in their minds and spirit. It was painful to see such misery and suffering, but beautiful to help them and see them help themselves.

"After eight years of working in Holland as a psychiatrist, Guy he says it is time for me to leave Holland and for us to start a new place, and I realized Guy was right and I left and we went back to India for four years. I liked India very much. Guy and I had gone on several visits to India for almost 20 years and I could have settled in India, but Guy, he was not really very happy there and after four years, we returned to France.

"And now we are here, and I wait, I wait and see where, as you say, my call brings me, and wherever people need me."

Greet became very reflective as she said, "I have been privileged in comparison with most people in the world. I am a privileged person but if you have this privilege, you have to pay for it. Schweitzer said that also, if you have learned and if you have had privilege, you have to pay for it towards those who have not had the chance that you have - but too many people don't do it.

"We are all connected together. It is true and sometimes an invisible door is opened and we can see part of the soul of the other and it is a wonderful privilege if you can get more connected to the other. But if I think, for example, of my parents who died. What is the essence of them is still alive in me? But I come again to the seeds of the thoughts of Schweitzer. There are people alive throughout the world and their spirits clamor for a chance to expand their spirits too and have a greater spiritual privilege."

"Do you think the thoughts of Schweitzer are still flourishing?" I asked.

"The thoughts of Schweitzer, oh, it is forgotten most of the time so perhaps it is up to you and up to us to let the world see they are not dead. It did not disappear in us, in Guy and me. It is still alive and I know that my daughter is teaching her little daughter things she learns from us. But perhaps the way we do it is too hidden and perhaps it is not for nothing you are here today and perhaps in connection to you, then you could represent the way in which the thoughts of Schweitzer will come again up to the surface. Not in certain ways people do with famous people that they brush off every day the old clothes or the old books or hats.

"No, his thoughts were fundamental and his thoughts were very up to date. We can practice them today and it can be the power of the steam in a motor and it can be like he says, 'the drop of water, you cannot see the strength in it, but the moment it freezes, it can come into a split of a rock and it can break open a rock. That is what you call the strength of an idea and it is then born in the thought of somebody who is ripened and then it can do fantastic things'

"I believe today the thoughts of Schweitzer and the service of Schweitzer are still important, but as time passes, people do not remember Schweitzer as I believe he should be remembered. Guy and I, and my family, we try and keep the thoughts of Schweitzer alive—and now there is you as well," she said, smiling.

"In Thoughts with You..."

As I recall Greet's words about the life and spirit of Schweitzer and the impact that he had on her life, I am reminded of the lyric that expresses the life of the soul as *'a presence of the dead in the dreams of the living.'*

And I'm reminded too, of a quote of Schweitzer's: "You may think it strange that I have spoken so much about death and not a word about immortality, the word one generally uses to dispel one's fears...No one has ever come back from the other world. I can't console you, but one thing I can tell you, as long as my ideas are alive, I will be alive.'

* * *

On the morning I was to leave Greet, Guy, and their family, Greet and I met one last time beneath the 300-year-old oak tree. She brought two small packages for me. The first was a small bottle of oils and perfume she asked me to give to Mother Teresa in India. Greet was absolutely certain that I would be able to see and speak with Mother Teresa once I reached Calcutta. She predicted that Mother Teresa would be very much like Schweitzer—"when she is with you, her entire presence will be with you," but when she feels she is needed by others more than you, she will go to them.'

The other item was the book, *The Words of Albert Schweitzer*, selected by Norman Cousins, one of the books that I had given her when I first arrived. When I looked a little surprised that she was giving it back, she said, "I have gone through this book of Schweitzer's words and made some small notes for you. You have asked me how I connect with the Divine. I have written that in the book."

Amazed and touched, I opened the book and looked through it. One of the chapters of the book is entitled "Reverence for Life" and features quotes of Schweitzer's philosophy on this topic. Opposite the title page of the chapter was a photograph of Greet in Lambarene wearing a pith helmet, bending over a tiny baby who had been placed in a pith helmet. On the chapter's title page, Greet had written:

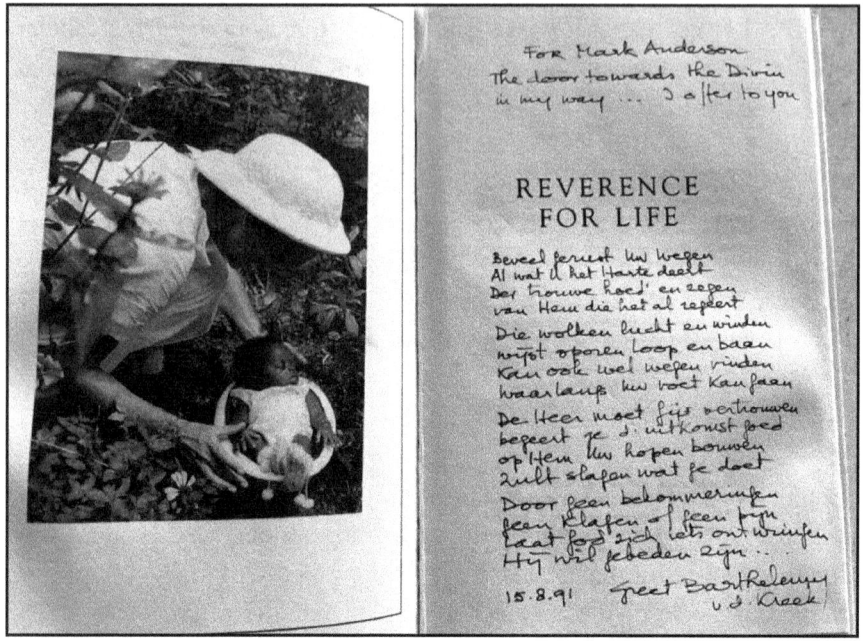

Greet's "Way to the Divine"
Inscribed by Greet in the book *The Words of Albert Schweitzer*
Photograph by Clara Urquhart
(Greet and infant in pith helmets)

For Mark Anderson
The door towards the Divine in my way ... I offer to you.

The chapter's title was "Reverence for Life," which was one of Schweitzer's ethical standards regarding maintaining and enhancing all life. Beneath the subtitle, Greet had written her comments in Dutch. When I looked up at Greet, she laughed, smiled and said, Ah, I didn't want to make it too easy for you!

I was deeply moved by Greet's "gift"—the translation of her comments follows:

"In Thoughts with You..."

Do not fear to entrust
All that your heart desires
To the faithful care and blessing
of Him who governs all.

Those clouds, air and winds
show ethereal courses, trails and paths
They also can reveal ways
along which your feet may pass.

You must trust in the Lord
if you wish for a good outcome
Build your hopes on Him
and you will succeed in all you do.

You cannot force your wants
from God
through sorrows, complaints or pain
He desires your prayers ....

—Greet Barthelemy v.d. Kreek
August 15, 1991

Throughout my conversations with Greet, the spirit of Schweitzer seemed to be present in our midst. As I reflect back on my visit and conversations with her, it seems apropos that the words of Schweitzer I think provide a glimpse of the spiritual ties that have bound Greet to Schweitzer and her life and calling beyond Lambarene. Dr. Schweitzer wrote:

> "I always think that we all live spiritually by what others have given us in the significant hours of our life. If we had before us those who have been a blessing to us and could tells us how it came about, they would be amazed to learn what passed over from their lives into ours."

Through the Lens of Humanity

I think Dr. Schweitzer would be amazed and pleased to learn what passed over from his life into Margrietha's (Greet's) life, and how her life nourished others to go forward and to be in that place where you are needed.

In thoughts with you. Dr. Margrietha Barthelemy van der Kreek died in 2016. Indeed, hers was a life well-lived—in service to others and to the One she called the Divine.

[Author's Note: Greet's daughter Maria and her husband Pascal continue to honor the memory of her parents, Greet and Guy. They maintain an organization, Villages Sans Frontieres, and a website of the same name that describes the mission activities they support around the world including Greet and Guy's beloved France and India. I offered Maria my chapter on her mother and asked if she had comments she'd like to share. I received the following reply:

I do remember your visit to my parent's farm so many years ago.
I read with emotion your passages about my mother and have two small things to add. Actually my mother's first name was Margrietha (in Dutch, which is equivalent to Margaret in English). Further in the little anecdote my mother often told: During her first interview with Dr. Schweitzer, before agreeing for her to come to the hospital in Gabon, he asked her if she slept well (so if she slept well) and if she had a sense of humor. It was only after her positive responses that he agreed for here to come to Lamborene. I think I have nothing else to add to your pages which put my mother in the spotlight.
Thank you for honoring her memory.

Maria

CHAPTER 4
"THE BEAUTY OF HOLINESS"

"People like Mother Teresa of Calcutta do not have biographies," prominent British journalist and television commentator Malcolm Muggeridge once observed. "They live their lives in the present. Questions about the past are passed off as irrelevant."

Many credit Muggeridge as providing the first major exposure of Mother Teresa and her work to the world. Muggeridge first encountered Mother Teresa while filming a documentary of her work in Calcutta in 1969 [to which she only reluctantly agreed ... but permitted as long, she said, that it would help others love God more]. Inspired by his interviews with Mother Teresa, Muggeridge released the documentary, entitled *Something Beautiful for God*, and published a book of the same name in 1971. Muggeridge's story of this tiny, quiet nun tirelessly dedicated to the poor and destitute among us captivated the hearts of millions throughout the world.

Those familiar with Malcolm Muggeridge also know the impact that his relationship with Mother Teresa had upon him—a skeptic was swayed, and an agnostic deeply invested in the intellectual influences of his day shed his doubts and his spirit was inspired by the work of an ordinary Albanian woman doing extraordinary things in the service of the poor. Muggeridge himself credits Mother Teresa with influencing his eventual reception into the Catholic Church in 1982.

In his 1988 book, *Confessions of a Twentieth-Century Pilgrim*, Muggeridge offers a poignant, yet powerful and moving description of Mother Teresa:

THROUGH THE LENS OF HUMANITY

> When I first set eyes on her, ... I at once realized that I was in the presence of someone of unique quality. This was not due to her appearance, which is homely and unassuming, so that words like "charm" or "charisma" do not apply. Nor to her shrewdness and quick understanding, though these are very marked; nor even to her manifest piety and true humility and ready laughter. There is phrase in one of the Psalms that always, for me, evokes her presence: 'the beauty of holiness' - that special beauty, amounting to a kind of pervasive luminosity generated by a life dedicated wholly to loving God and His creation. This, I imagine, is what the haloes in medieval paintings of saints were intended to convey.

My own meeting with Mother Teresa took place in May of 1991 when I initiated efforts to travel to Calcutta and work as a volunteer in Mother Teresa's Missionaries of Charity, a Roman Catholic religious congregation she had established in Calcutta in 1950. By 1991, Mother Teresa was a major international personality. Prestigious magazines, newspapers and television programs had featured her and her work. This tiny woman with her well-creased face and familiar white and blue sari was one of the most recognizable personalities in the world. She had won the Nobel Peace Prize in 1979 for her work "undertaken in the struggle to overcome poverty and distress, which also constitutes a threat to peace" primarily for her efforts among the poor in Calcutta, but also for work that was being conducted at mission sites she had established in various parts of the world. Mother Teresa had recently toured several cities in the United States, including Milwaukee, Wisconsin, the city in which I resided at the time, where she had been honored by Marquette University for her humanitarian work among the poor and disenfranchised.

I had long been intrigued by Mother Teresa's life and commitment to helping others, particularly those suffering in such utter poverty. As with Dr. Margrietha van der Kreek, I had a desire to speak with her and ask her what was the nature of her "call to service" and what compelled her to follow the path she had chosen.

"The Beauty of Holiness"

In early May 1991, I composed a short letter expressing my desire to travel to Calcutta and volunteer with the Missionaries of Charity. In my letter, I expressed my hope that I would have the opportunity to meet and speak with Mother Teresa while there. My original intent for this trip was to travel to India and volunteer with the Missionaries of Charity, return to cities I had first visited in my 1987 journey work at the Miraj Medical Center in Miraj, India, and then travel to France to meet Dr. Margrietha van der Kreek, an associate of Dr. Albert Schweitzer at Schweitzer's hospital in Lambarene, Gabon in central Africa.

Shortly after I sent my letter of volunteer inquiry to the Missionaries of Charity, I received the following reply:

> Missionaries of Charity
> 54A Lower Circular Road
> Calcutta 700016
> India
>
> May 24, 1991
>
> Dear Mark Anderson,
>
> Thank you for your letter. You are welcome to share in our humble works of love for the poor. Come with a heart to love and hands to serve Jesus in the crippled, the abandoned, the sick and dying in anyone of our centres.
>
> I enclose for your information a list of accommodations. On arrival you may put up at one of these as they do not make reservations. You can meet Sr. M. Priscilla or Sr. M. Josma at the above address after your arrival in the city for Registration between 8.00-9.00 a.m. or 5.00-6.00 p.m. daily except Thursday and Sunday. Regarding your visa you can come on a tourist visa and of course you would be expected to tour. Mother is out of India at present. If you want to come when she is in

Calcutta, you may call her on Telephone 033/297115 before you come, to make sure she will be here.

God loves you. He will reward your generous desire to serve Him in His little ones—the poor.

God bless you
Sr. M. Frederick MC
For Mother Teresa MC

With this letter in hand, I immediately began exploring possible dates to travel to India.

I was employed at the time as Executive Vice President of Children's Hospital of Wisconsin in Milwaukee and I received enthusiastic support for my plans to travel to India and France from Jon Vice, President and Chief Executive Officer of Children's Hospital. Jon understood my wanderlust and had previously supported my six weeks of volunteerism in India in 1987 when I worked as a volunteer and consultant at Miraj Mission Hospital in Miraj, India.

Thinking that India was to be the first leg of an incredible trip that would hopefully include visits to India to volunteer with Mother Teresa's organization and to France to meet with Dr. Margrietha van der Kreek, former chief surgeon for Dr. Albert Schweitzer, I turned my attention toward contacting Dr. van der Kreek to inquire about visiting and meeting with her. I immediately received a resoundingly affirmative response from Dr. van der Kreek with her added instructive—that I should come and see her first!

I was amazed. Incredibly, with relative ease, I had been able to arrange meetings with these two remarkable women. Once I heard from Dr. van der Kreek, I began to outline my travel plans. Per Dr. van der Kreek's request, I would plan to go to France first, and then on to India. I contacted Dr. van der Kreek and established potential dates for visiting her. Next, I needed to determine whether the range of dates I had discussed with Dr. van der Kreek would include dates that would permit me to volunteer with Mother Teresa at a time when she would be in residence at the Mother House in Calcutta.

Following Sr. Frederick's directive, I decided to call the Mother House in Calcutta and see if I could somehow determine if Mother Teresa would be there the dates I was contemplating being in Calcutta. Allowing for the time difference between Milwaukee and Calcutta (approximately 10 hours), one July night around midnight, I called the Mother House in India using the number provided by Sr. Frederick. The phone was answered right away; the answerer indicated that I had reached the Missionaries of Charity and identified herself as Sister Josma. I explained to Sr. Josma who I was and that I was calling because I was interested in coming as a volunteer. Sr. Josma was quite welcoming in her response.

I then mentioned to Sr. Josma the specific dates that I hoped to be in Calcutta and then I asked the question I was anxious to ask, "Do you know if Mother Teresa will be in Calcutta on those dates?"

"I don't know," Sr. Josma responded in a lilting Indian accent, "but if you permit me a moment, I'll go and ask her."

Oh, okay, I thought, absolutely amazed that Mother Teresa was this accessible. I heard Sr. Josma put down the phone. Then there was silence for perhaps a full minute. I was beginning to get concerned about the connection having been severed when finally I heard the phone being picked up again.

"Hello?", said Sr. Josma. "Mother says she will be here. She says you are welcome to come."

And with that, I began finalizing my travel arrangements to visit France and India in August, 1991.

* * *

I arrived in Calcutta on Friday, August 23, 1991, after spending an incredible week with Dr. Margrietha van der Kreek—"Greet" as she preferred to be called—at her home in France. With my head filled with Greet's stories of working alongside the great theologian, humanitarian, and Nobel Peace Prize laureate, Dr. Albert Schweitzer, I journeyed from France to Varanasi and Agra, India, retracing the steps of a journey I made in 1987 to volunteer at Miraj Mission Hospital in Miraj, India.

My meeting and discussions with Greet about her experiences and work with Schweitzer and her own life's call to service of others had stirred my soul. I found myself eager and anxious to resume my spiritual journey in Calcutta with Mother Teresa and the Missionaries of Charity.

When I landed in Calcutta, I didn't have any prior hotel reservations, so again I followed the suggestion made in Sr. Frederick's letter, I immediately took the airport shuttle to Sudder Street, the area where Sr. Frederick had indicated there were options for accommodations. Before arriving in India, I had looked into the Lytton Hotel, which is where I headed first.

I was really pleased to book a room at the Lytton for the week at a cost of 600 rupees per night (approximately $24 at that time). Once ensconced in my room at the Lytton, I called Sr. Frederick and indicated that I had arrived in Calcutta and had secured lodgings. She suggested I come right away to the Mother House and register as a volunteer. In addition, she confirmed that Mother Teresa was in Calcutta and would be here throughout the upcoming week! Needless to say I was delighted with this news.

On the way to Sudder Street from the airport, I began to see and experience the extremes of this amazing city. Calcutta is a city rich with history—it is the former capital of British India, which was evident in some of the architecture of historic buildings and other magnificent memorials and structures. In addition to the images of an urban power center, I also saw a city where a deep, enduring poverty had settled into the very marrow of the city. I saw dirty, crowded, and noisy streets with thousands of pavement dwellers, street children and scavengers struggling to grind out a living in the midst of overwhelming poverty. I saw flimsy lean-tos and cardboard and burlap hovels that are homes to literally tens of thousands of people who dwell in Calcutta's vast slums. Grime and pollution are pervasive along the streets, and there is no way

"The Beauty of Holiness"

to tally an accurate number of people who live either on the street or cling precariously to rudimentary and barely livable indoor space.

Sudder Street was a little better than some of the areas we passed through, and the Lytton Hotel seemed to be one of the nicer hotels on the street. I was thankful for a room in a hotel that had functioning air-conditioning and what appeared to be a nice restaurant.

After stowing my luggage in my room, I caught a cab outside the front of the hotel to go to the Mother House of the Missionaries of Charity. However, it quickly became clear the cabbie either didn't know where the Mother House was or hadn't understood where I wanted to go, so I made him return to the hotel and I took another cab.

Unfortunately my experience with the second cab wasn't much better. We first ended up at an orphanage run by Mother Teresa's sisters, but it wasn't the Mother House.

Finally, we arrived at the correct Mother House and I met Sisters Priscilla and Josma. I had brought my camera and diary with me and while I was registering, Sr. Priscilla told me that pictures weren't allowed within the Mother House without permission, but that she would try and arrange for me to meet and have some time with Mother Teresa. She warned, "Mother doesn't really do interviews." I told her that I understood and thanked her for her willingness to have the opportunity to see Mother Teresa.

Sr. Josma suggested I go back to the hotel and get some rest, but to return to the Mother House the next morning at 5:50 a.m. for Mass. Sr. Josma also told me I'd meet the other volunteers who were currently in Calcutta at Mass, and following Mass, the volunteers would travel to their assignments. My assignment, she told me, was Kalighat—a home for the sick, destitute and dying.

The next morning, I arose before 5 a.m. after getting very little sleep. I was concerned I would oversleep and miss the 5:50 a.m. Mass! I walked from the Lytton Hotel to the Mother House, having determined during my cab escapades that the hotel was actually quite close to the Mother House and I arrived quickly after a brisk walk.

The Mass was held in a large second-floor room in the Mother House and was conducted by a Canadian priest. There were many

THROUGH THE LENS OF HUMANITY

Missionaries of Charity Sisters present, all wearing the white sari with the light blue trim made so recognizable by Mother Teresa's presence on the world stage. I noticed a dozen or so volunteers sitting on the floor toward the back of the room, and I joined the group, trading introductions with several as the Mass got underway.

Just before the Mass started, Mother Teresa came into the room and sat on the floor in the midst of the Missionary of Charity sisters. She departed immediately after the Mass concluded. I was excited to see her and was told by the other volunteers that she was present at all the services when she was in town.

After the Mass, I went downstairs to a common room where all the volunteers had gathered and had tea and cookies before we headed out to our various volunteer locations that were scattered around Calcutta. Sr. Josma came up to me and introduced a young woman named Teresa, who was a volunteer from Spain. Teresa would help me my first day as a volunteer, Sr. Josma told me.

Teresa was an attractive young woman who was with a contingent of Spanish college students who were volunteering during their school break. Teresa spoke excellent English, and she explained to me that she and several of the Spanish group were also going to be volunteers at Kalighat this day. She indicated that she and her group were in their second week of volunteering and during that time, they had all rotated through most of the Mission Sites operated by the Missionaries of Charity order.

Teresa and I joined her Spanish colleagues and took a bus to a stop near Kalighat and then walked the remaining short distance to the building site.

Kalighat had been established as a Missionaries of Charity site by Mother Teresa in 1952, on her 42nd birthday. The building itself was a former Hindu temple to the goddess Kali. With permission of city officials, she had converted the former temple to a hospice center. It was now known as "Mother Teresa's Home for the Sick and Dying Destitutes." People who came to this free hospice center often had been picked up off the streets of Calcutta. Most had been abandoned and they possessed all manner of infirmities and chronic illnesses. Many had

"The Beauty of Holiness"

tuberculosis. Others had hideous open wounds and sores from injuries or illness. All shared a common bond of poverty.

People brought to the Kalighat hospice center received medical attention primarily from Missionaries of Charity sisters and "are given the opportunity to die with dignity with someone who cared," Mother Teresa has said. "A beautiful death is for these people, who lived like animals, to die like angels—loved and wanted."

As I stood on the outside of the building, I observed a multi-story structure that seemed to constitute the majority of the block. The walls were a faded yellowish and white color streaked with dirt, soot, and smoke from the teeming environments that surrounded the building. Atop the building was the notice:

> Missionaries of Charity
> Normal Hriday ESTD - 1952
> Mother Teresa's Home for the Sick and Dying Destitutes

I was appalled when I walked into the building. All my senses were assaulted. The interior was stiflingly hot and poorly lit. My vision was further impaired by a hazy smoke that hovered from ceiling to floor. The odors and stench were an overwhelming combination of unpleasantness that lingered stagnantly in the the stifling, barely circulating air.

When we entered the front lobby, we were met by one of the Missionaries of Charity sisters. I was assigned to work in the men's ward and the Spanish volunteer contingent was assigned to either the women's ward or to the kitchen area. My duties included working with the sisters and novices from the Missionaries of Charity and other volunteers in distributing food and water to the patients, helping move patients from their mattresses to examination areas, cleaning and rinsing mattresses and bedding, helping novices distribute medications, and assisting them in tending wound and sores. My duties also included changing dressings, washing and scrubbing dishes and clothes, and in several instances, helping remove patients who had expired in the men's ward out to ambulances in the rear of Kalighat for transmittal to a city health facility.

Through the Lens of Humanity

Many of the patients were emaciated and were clearly dying of starvation. Most were deformed, crippled, or blind. Some were likely suffering from HIV/AIDS. There were some, who after eating, insisted on leaving and left. The patients were all ages, from young children to the very old, although many were of an indeterminate age. I was told that the men's ward routinely handled about 100 patients a day. On this particular day, it appeared to me that all the mattresses were full and a number of patients were leaning against a wall or lying on the floor.

Basically, all the men patients were housed in one large room on one side of the building and the women's ward was essentially a duplicate unit on the opposite side of the building. In both areas, I noticed there didn't appear to be any segregation of patients in terms of severity of illness or medical need. It appeared that patients were placed in whatever area was available at the time. Emphasis was clearly placed on on reducing the present suffering as much as possible.

I did all that I was asked to do, although candidly, many times, I found myself physically repulsed by what I was seeing and doing in trying to help the patients. As an experienced hospital administrator, I was also bothered by the absence of skilled medical personnel to care for patients who clearly could have benefited from more organized medical services. It was concerning too only minimal efforts were made to clean and sterilize eating utensils and medical instruments; I saw no real efforts toward infection control. I worried about the risks the sisters, novices, and volunteers were taking through such intimate contact with so many patients who could be highly contagious. One of the novices, who noticed my discomfort, shared with me that many of the volunteers experienced similar levels of concern and discomfort. And yet, at that time and that place, we each tried to show compassion and grace to those who were suffering and alone.

I have the highest admiration and respect for the sisters, novices, and volunteers who committed themselves daily to Kalighat's ministry of caring and compassion under such difficult and challenging conditions. None of the systems at Kalighat were perfect, but it is an extraordinary place of loving kindness. In the Christian tradition, people take part in a practice known as "the passing of the peace." It is a bold

"THE BEAUTY OF HOLINESS"

act of declaring our reconciliation as children of God. Not only are we reconciled with God, we are reconciled with each other. I saw Kalighat as a demonstrable reflection of the practice of "the passing of the peace"—of individuals, through their acts of kindness and love, acknowledging the humanity of another, and in so doing, declaring that each of us, including the most vulnerable souls among us, are deserving of grace.

* * *

About mid-morning during my first day at Kalightat, I heard a great commotion and hubbub out in front of the building. After a moment or so, Mother Teresa walked through the front door and into the central lobby escorting a visiting cardinal from Rome. As she guided the cardinal through the building, she stopped in each section and talked with the sisters and volunteers working in those areas. When Mother Teresa came through the men's ward, she stopped and greeted me and another volunteer. We shook hands and she blessed me as we exchanged greetings. I was told it was the first time that Mother Teresa had visited Kalighat in several months and all the workers were excited to see her.

Mother Teresa and the cardinal stayed at Kalighat for about 30 minutes, but before she left, Mother Teresa stopped at one of the cots near the front door and spoke briefly to the man lying there. Later, one of the sisters told me and the other volunteers that this was what Mother Teresa always did when she visited Kalighat: she always stopped at the cot nearest the door, which usually was where the sickest lay. Mother Teresa said it was here at the front where she felt were those who were nearest to death—and nearest to heaven.

Shifts for volunteers at Kalighat were usually from 8 a.m. to 12 noon, and then from 3 p.m. to 5:30 p.m. Because of Mother Teresa's visit to Kalighat, the volunteers had extended our shift to 1 p.m. As our shift ended, I took the Metro back to the Mother House with the Spanish volunteers. When we arrived back at the Mother House, Sister Josma reminded us all to come back 5:30 p.m. for evening Mass, which was to be a service of Adoration. Bidding the other volunteers goodbye, I headed back to the Lytton Hotel for lunch and a much-needed nap.

Around 5 p.m. that evening, after resting, showering, and having a bite to eat, I started walking back to the Mother House. I'm guessing the distance was about a mile and the route was pretty direct from the hotel. My walk took me through a very impoverished area and I constantly encountered beggars asking for rupees or food. I had been told not to give anyone anything, otherwise the group of beggars would only get bigger and more insistent. Therefore, I basically kept my head down and just plodded forward toward the convent.

I arrived early for the service and made my way upstairs to the common room where the service was to be held. The room was spacious, one wall fronted the street and the sounds of traffic, car horns, and street life filtered through the windows into the room. A few wooden benches stood in the back of the room, but these were the only furniture in the room other than a solitary lectern in the front. The floor was grayish in color and concrete, and the walls I suspect had once been white, but were now faded and smudged with noticeable chipping and cracks throughout. A little light was visible through the windows, but the overhead lighting, while a bit dim, was certainly adequate to illuminate the room.

Being early, I was the first one in the room, and I sat down cross-legged on the concrete floor facing the lectern and the windows on the street side wall squarely in the middle of the room. Within a few moments, a few sisters came in, quietly sat down on the floor, and bowed their heads in meditation or prayer.

I, too, was quietly sitting and reflecting on my day at Kalighat when I heard someone sit down on my right just a foot or so behind me. I turned slightly to acknowledge the person and found myself face to face with Mother Teresa. She smiled and nodded at me and then bowed her head. It was electrifying and humbling to realize she was sitting right beside me. I sat up straighter!

Quickly, the room filled with sisters and volunteers and soon there were probably 100 or more people. The Canadian priest opened the service and began the Mass. During the course of the service, the congregation began reciting prayers of the rosary. Not being Catholic, I did not have a rosary and simply sat quietly while the prayers were being offered.

All of the sudden, I felt a nudging on my right side. I turned and Mother Teresa leaned forward and asked me in English if I had a rosary. A bit surprised and I'm sure red-faced, I whispered to her that I was not Catholic and I didn't have one. She smiled and nodded and turned and spoke to a young sister sitting near her. The sister stood up, left the room, and within moments returned with a pink plastic rosary, which she gave to me. I thanked the sister, then turned to Mother Teresa and thanked her. She nodded and smiled and continued praying.

There I was, holding a rosary in my hand, but feeling a bit self-conscious because I had no clue how to participate in the rosary prayers. As if she understood this, all of the sudden, Mother Teresa moved forward until she was sitting right beside me. Then she positioned her rosary so I could see it as the prayers were being said. When the prayers ended, she looked over at me, smiled, and patted my hand. I thanked her again. Quite honestly, I was speechless.

After the service, as we stood up, Mother Teresa put her hands together, bowed her head, and moved quickly out of the room. I lingered there and spoke with Sr. Josma, who asked how my day had gone. I shared some of my experiences and Sr. Josma told me she thought I'd be able to speak with Mother Teresa for a few minutes after Mass on Monday, August 26.

As we were speaking, Teresa, the young woman from Spain joined us and asked if it was okay if the volunteers prepared a cake for Mother Teresa to celebrate her birthday, Monday the 26th and her baptismal day on Tuesday the 27th. Sr. Josma indicated she would check with Mother Teresa and try to arrange a celebratory time with Mother Teresa and the volunteers on Tuesday, August 27th.

When I realized that I'd be speaking to Mother Teresa on her birthday, I was amazed at how the events of this trip were coming together. I walked back to the Lytton with my Spanish friends, many thoughts circulating through my head.

Through the Lens of Humanity

* * *

The following morning was Sunday and as I returned to the Mother House for morning Mass, I was assigned to work in a mission site in south Calcutta—an orphanage for street children, mainly young boys. The Spanish volunteers were also assigned to this site and once again, we took public transportation to the location.

Upon our arrival, every one of the volunteers was mobbed by young, filthy children eager to play. We were all quickly filthy ourselves after playing with the children. But then we got down to business; our tasks were to help wash, clean, and bathe the children, assist the children in washing their clothing, and then provided haircuts to many of the children. This was challenging since many of the children had lice-ridden, matted hair. All these activities—washing, cleaning, bathing, the cutting of hair—were all done outside. With the heat of the day and the scores of children to deal with, by noon, all the volunteers and the Missionaries of Charity Sisters were exhausted. But we had one task yet to go—feeding the children. We lined up the children in a couple of lines, and then passed out bread and a rice and stewy mix to the children. The children were clearly hungry, many had thin, gaunt faces, several had distended bellies. I'm quite sure this was the best meal they had had recently.

Almost as if on cue, just as we were finished feeding the children, Mother Teresa arrived to dedicate a new building for the orphanage. Teresa had alerted me that Mother Teresa might be coming, so I had brought my camera and was able to get several photos of Mother Teresa blessing the children and speaking to the sisters and volunteers.

After the dedication service, the volunteers and I left the orphanage and took the bus back across the famous Howrah Bridge to the Mother House. Then for me, a walk back to the Lytton Hotel for an afternoon respite.

"THE BEAUTY OF HOLINESS"

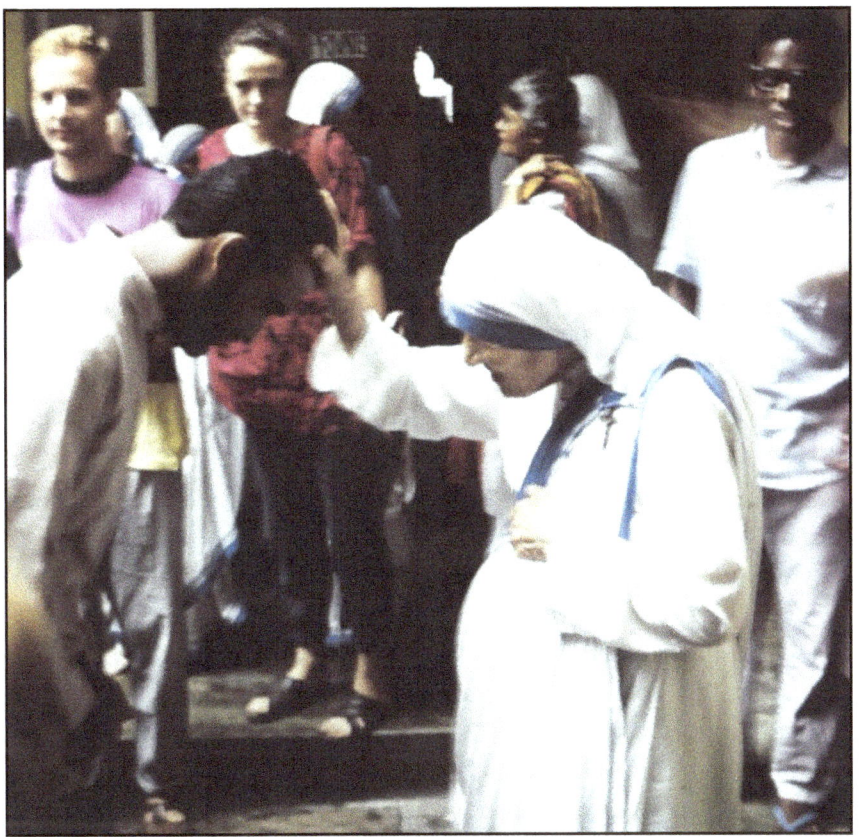

Mother Teresa "blessing" the volunteers and youth at an orphanage site

* * *

That evening, I walked back to the Mother House and ran into a contingent of volunteers staying at a nearby hotel and who were also walking to the Mother House. We arrived several minutes early, went directly up to the second-level common room, then seated ourselves in the back of the room on the wooden benches.

Entering quietly through one of the side doors near the front of the room, Mother Teresa appeared and on the table by the lectern, she set up an ornamental cross and flowers. She then moved to the back of the room and sat silently by herself with her head bowed for a few minutes.

Through the Lens of Humanity

Several moments before the service was to start, Mother Teresa got up and walked over and invited all the volunteers to move closer to the front. I was standing up at the time. She walked up to me, grabbed the front of my shirt, and gently started pulling me forward. She was smiling and said to me, "Come, get closer to Jesus."

We all moved to the front and seated ourselves on the floor in the front near the table and lectern. Mother Teresa conducted the service, which lasted about 20 minutes, and as she was leaving, clasped her hands together bowed her head in our direction and left.

After the service, volunteers milled around and Sr. Josma came up to me and again said I should be able to see Mother Teresa privately after Mass the next morning.

Monday morning, I met the Spanish volunteers outside their hotel and we walked together to the Mother House for the 5:50 a.m. Mass. Since Sister Josma had told me I'd have the chance to speak with Mother Teresa after Mass, I had brought with me the gifts I wanted to present her. That today also happened to be her birthday was quite an unexpected bonus—an act of grace one might say.

Because it was Mother Teresa's birthday, it seemed quite a few more people than usual were at the morning Mass. As the Mass ended, Sister Josma stepped up to me and told me to go on downstairs for tea with the other volunteers and she would come for me when Mother Teresa was able to see me. As morning tea was ending and the volunteers were about to depart for their assigned mission sites for the day, Sister Josma appeared and invited me to follow her upstairs, where Mother Teresa would meet me.

I followed Sister Josma upstairs, who she asked me to sit on a bench just outside the chapel and indicated Mother Teresa would be with me shortly. As I looked around, I noticed we were effectively in an open corridor area that had a roof but no walls, in a passageway that seemed to connect two different sections of the second level of the building. The bench I was sitting on, while near the chapel, was also close to what appeared to be an office area that had a hanging ceiling-to-floor curtain that seemed to function as the door into and out of the area.

"The Beauty of Holiness"

Mother Teresa emerged from behind the curtain, greeted me, grasped my hand, and sat down on the bench. As I held her hand, I could feel the tremendous energy this tiny woman exuded—an energy she seemed to pass on to all who meet her, an energy I seemed to absorb as I sat with her.

I had been apprehensive and nervous about meeting with her, but once we sat down, she made me feel completely at ease in her presence. We sat very close together on the bench, I leaned forward toward her to hear her better—she spoke very softly. Her face was very lined and she was a very small woman, stooped a bit at the shoulder. She was barefoot and wearing her white Missionaries of Charity sari with the blue trim. Her eyes were very lively, alert, and she turned her complete attention to me as we began speaking. Her intensity and presence were palpable.

I began by telling her who I was, what my vocation was, and that I had previously been to India as a volunteer at the Miraj Medical Center in 1987. She nodded and said she knew of Miraj. Then I mentioned that I had several gifts I wanted to present to her.

I told her that I was Presbyterian and that I attended Immanuel Presbyterian Church in Milwaukee, Wisconsin. I told her a little bit about Immanuel then presented her a blue sweatshirt that had the name of the church on the front along with an etching depicting the church's building. She told me that she had been to Milwaukee, that she had received an award from Marquette University and that she remembered the city. She unfolded the sweatshirt and looked at the front, and smiling, she said the blue of the sweatshirt matched the blue of her sari and that she'd wear it.

I then presented her with a paperweight medallion that had a raised rendering of the Children's Hospital of Wisconsin's building on it. She was fascinated by the way the medallion was constructed and she also asked a few questions about the children's hospital.

Finally, I gave her the bottle of oil and perfume that Greet Barthelemy had given me to present to her. I shared with her the story behind the gift and told her that I had just spent time with Greet and how Greet had used to work with Dr. Albert Schweitzer. Mother Teresa said she knew of Schweitzer and was thankful for the gift from Greet.

I then told her that I would soon be attending McCormick Theological Seminary, a Presbyterian seminary located in Chicago. I shared too, my interest in the concept of "call" and what caused people to follow what they perceived their call to be. I told her that I wanted to ask her about this if she was willing.

"I don't give interviews, " she said, "but I will talk with you."

I thanked her and then asked her how she thought people knew they were "called by God to do certain things and live a certain way."

Her reply was immediate.

"Before you can know your "call," you have to accept that life has meaning, that your life can have a purpose and that there is a Divine Presence. Then you have to empty yourself, give yourself to the Divine, and then follow what you think is right because it will be divinely inspired."

She then said that if you were in contact with God and at peace with God then the thoughts that come will give you the decision, show you the way. She said that when the call comes, you will be at perfect peace with the call. Then she said you should continue to pray for the decision and if you are completely at peace, then that is your way, that is your call.

She went on that God does not allow any disturbances. If you are not completely at peace with the decision, no matter what you might sacrifice, if you do not have the right intentions - then you do not have a valid call.

"Continue to pray," she said, "and once you are at complete peace, then you will know that it is God's way for you. To remain faithful, one must pray constantly for even stronger faith. Pray to Mary, Mother of Jesus; she is available 24 hours a day."

She said, "Pray. Mary, Mother of Jesus, be a mother to me now."

She repeated this several times very adamantly. She then said to me, "If you want to be a Presbyterian priest, then pray to God about it and see if you are at peace."

"THE BEAUTY OF HOLINESS"

She paused and then she said, "I will pray for you and you pray for me."

We had been speaking almost 30 minutes. Then she asked me if I had a charm of the Virgin Mary. When I said no, she got up and went behind the curtain and came back with several charms for a necklace or bracelet that were silver and had the image of the Virgin Mary on them. She kissed them, blessed them, and then handed them to me. Then she gave me a very beautiful rosary and kissed and blessed it for me. She saw that I had in my hand one of her prayer cards—a small card that had her picture on it with a prayer, and a smaller card that had a prayer and her name on it. I had picked the cards up off a table outside the chapel.

She took the prayer card with her picture on it and signed it, *"God Bless You—Mother Teresa."* Smiling, she said that the smaller card was her "business card" and she signed it: *"Be only all for Jesus through Mary."*

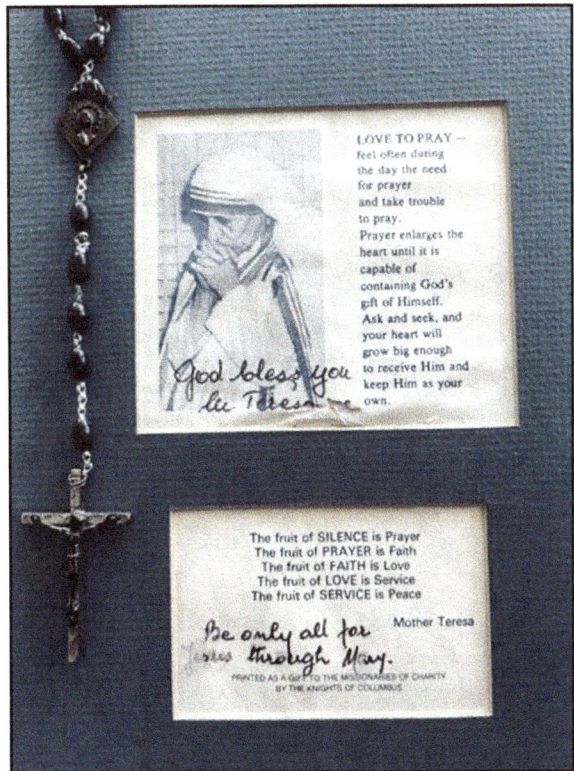

Mother Teresa's "Business Cards" and the rosary she gave me.

~ 115 ~

Through the Lens of Humanity

As we started to wrap up our conversation, she asked where I had volunteered, I told her that I had been to Kalighat and the orphanage and that I was going back to Kalighat that afternoon. She responded that she had remembered seeing me at Kalighat, and that it was "a very special place." I told her I was aware that Kalighat was the first mission she established in Calcutta. She nodded and repeated several more times, "Yes, it is a very special place."

The she squeezed my hand and said again, "I'll pray for you and you pray for me."

As we stood up, I thanked her for meeting and talking with me, and I wished her a "Happy Birthday." She smiled and nodded and then said again, "God Bless You" and then she went into the chapel.

After meeting with Mother Teresa, I went and found Sister Josma and thanked her for facilitating the meeting with Mother Teresa. Outside the Mother House was an ambulance that was headed to Kalighat and I was able to catch a ride.

I was thrilled to have spoken with Mother Teresa and felt very humbled by the experience. I also know that most volunteers don't get the chance to meet with Mother Teresa like I did and for this I also felt very, very grateful!

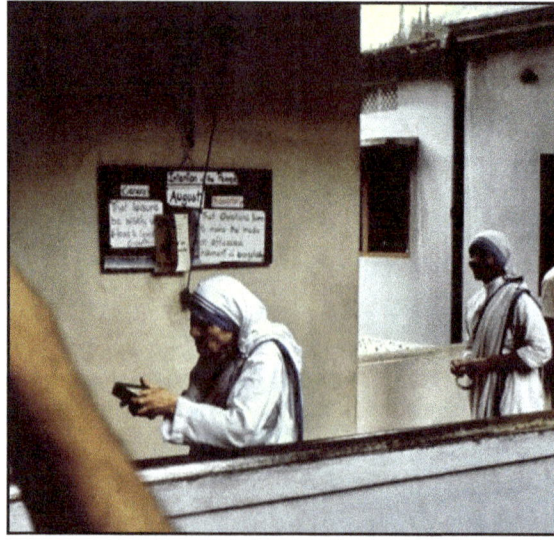

Mother Teresa on the balcony outside the 2nd floor chapel

"The Beauty of Holiness"

* * *

After I finished my shift at Kalighat, I returned directly to my hotel—the afternoon traffic was such that I wouldn't get back in time to make the evening service, hence my returning to the hotel. However, I did walk over to the Salvation Army Hotel, where the Spanish volunteers were staying. Teresa and her colleagues had been able to get a cake to celebrate Mother Teresa's baptismal day, which was the very next day the 27th. However, the air conditioning in their hotel had broken down so I went to the bakery to get the cake with them and then we took it to my room in the Lytton. My air conditioning was barely functioning itself, but at least we thought it might help prevent the cake from getting stale.

On the morning of the 27th, Teresa and the Spanish volunteers came by the Lytton and we took a cab to the Mother House since we were also taking the cake for the celebration of Mother Teresa's baptism day.

After Mass, the sisters sang celebratory songs to Mother Teresa, and she met with them while the volunteers went downstairs for tea and cookies.

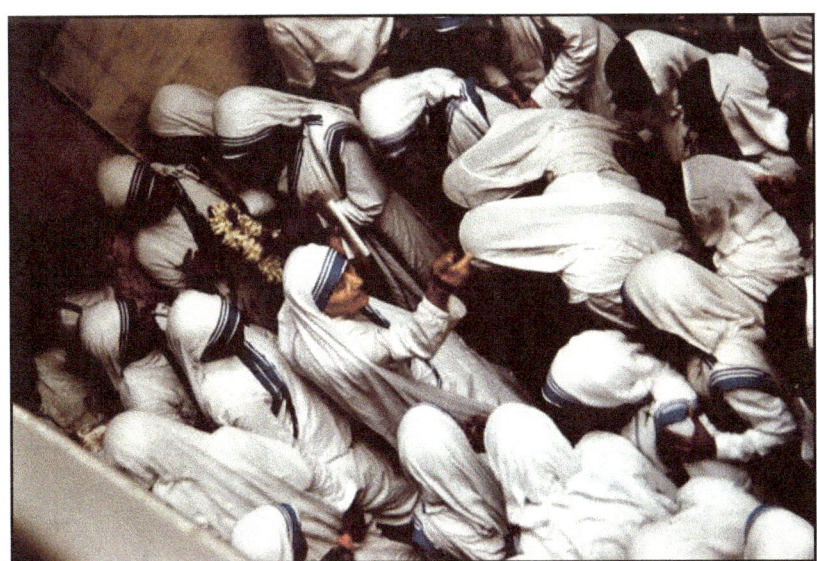

Mother Teresa celebrating her birthday with the Sisters of the Missionaries of Charity

THROUGH THE LENS OF HUMANITY

The volunteers then went to the chapel to meet and have cake with Mother Teresa. She sat on a stool in the chapel and spoke to us for approximately 20 minutes. She commented that our visiting and working with the poor was a gift to us from God, and how our lives would be blessed because of this. She spoke about doing small things with great love and hoped that when we returned to our homes we would continue to dedicate ourselves to helping others.

As she finished speaking, one of the sisters gave her a small box full of the "charms" of the Virgin Mary. She started passing them out to all the volunteers. When she got to me, she gave me another and laughed and said, "I think some of you might have two or three."

That Tuesday, many of the volunteers stayed at the Mother House due to torrential rains that flooded the streets and made travel virtually impossible to the mission sites. The rains and floods were so heavy that transportation was greatly impacted throughout the city. I walked back to my hotel in ankle-deep water. Fortunately, the power was still on in the hotel!.

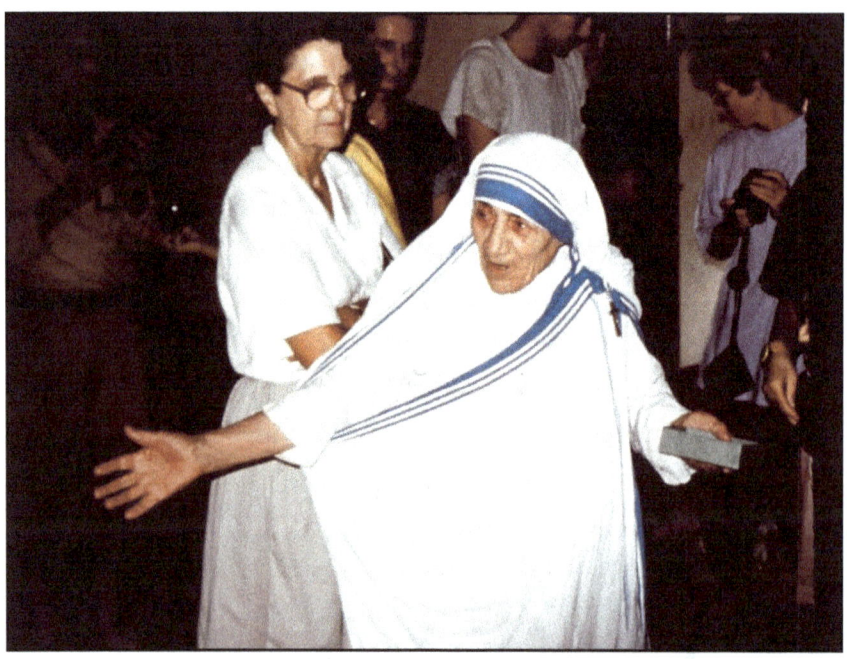

Mother Teresa handing out Virgin Mary "charms" to volunteers

"THE BEAUTY OF HOLINESS"

On Wednesday morning, I went to Mass as usual. On my way, I stopped by the Salvation Army Hotel because I was aware that the Spanish volunteers were all leaving early in the morning for home and I wanted to say goodbye and wish them all well.

After Mass, I stayed at the Mother House and spoke with the Canadian priest who conducted the morning Mass for an hour or so. Due to the rains, much of the public transportation system was still not functioning well, so many of the volunteer shifts were not possible to do due to the difficulty in getting to the mission sites.

Thursday was the regular day off for the volunteers so I spent most of the day touring the city of Calcutta and doing some souvenir shopping.

Friday morning, I attended Mass and afterwards I approached Mother Teresa. As I walked up to her, she laughed and said , "Oh, the Presbyterian priest. You're still here, I haven't seen you and I thought you had left."

I told her I was actually leaving Calcutta the following day, and I thanked her again for speaking with me. She reiterated some of what she had said before: "Humble yourself and you will become a holy person—this will be my prayer for you." We talked some about the possibility of my sending her some medical supplies for use in her projects, and she told me how to do that. Then we clasped hands in a very friendly goodbye, and as she left she said, "God bless you. I'll pray for you and you pray for me."

I repeated the same words to her.

A number of years ago, an article entitled "I Believe in Mother Teresa" appeared in the *Saturday Evening Post*. It was excerpted from Robert Fulghum's book *All I Really Need to Know I Learned in Kindergarten*. In the article, Fulghum admiringly writes of Mother Teresa:

> "To cut through the smog of helpless cynicism; to take only the tool of uncompromising love; to make manifest the capacity for healing humanity's wounds; to make the story of the Good Samaritan a living reality; and to live so true a life as to shine out from the back streets of

Calcutta takes courage and faith we cannot admit in ourselves and cannot be without."

Fulghum concludes his article with these words:

"If ever there is truly peace on earth, goodwill to men, it will be because of women like Mother Teresa. Peace is not something you wish for; it's something you make, something you do, something you are, and something you give away!"

On September 5, 1997, at the age of 87, Mother Teresa passed away after suffering a heart attack. Nineteen years later, on September 4, 2016, Mother Teresa was canonized as Saint Teresa of Calcutta by Pope Francis in Saint Peter's Square, Vatican City.

As the years have passed and I have reflected on my time in Calcutta with Mother Teresa, now Saint Teresa, I find myself asking, as we do with other great personalities of history, how can I/we benefit? What can we learn today in our time and place from this unique individual?

Christian Feldman, an international best-selling biographer, answers this question about what Mother Teresa's example can mean to us in this manner:

.... to deal mercifully with oneself and attentively, respectfully, and lovingly with others, especially with the weaker ones - who not infrequently reveal themselves to be the really strong ones, and richly benefit those who have decided to cast their lot with them. Perhaps we can learn a whole new equilibrium between giving and taking, and acquire the courage to open up our anxiously broken hearts. And we might remember heaven too, which often enough, busy as we are with all those other things, we forget."

—Christian Feldman, *Love Stays*

CHAPTER 5
"BLESSED ARE THE PEACEMAKERS"

When Archbishop Desmond Tutu won the Nobel Peace Prize in 1984, he joined Dr. Albert Schweitzer, Mahatma Gandhi, Dr. Martin Luther King, Jr., and Mother Teresa as one of the great inspirational leaders of the 20th century. His eloquence, humor, and passion during the midst of a decades long struggle against apartheid in South Africa established him as an international presence and one of the great moral leaders of our time. Despite his fame, Tutu never aspired to the public acclaim he received for the pivotal roles that he played as a leader, liberator, and healer as South Africa freed itself from the shackles of apartheid. Indeed, Doug Abrams, who coauthored a number of books with Tutu, insists that Tutu, rather than accepting elevation to some exalted status, was instead "the most human human I have ever met: the extraordinary example of what is possible for each of us if we are willing to answer the call of our times and turn to one another with the laughter-filled, tear-stained eyes of the heart."

On the occasion of Tutu's 80th birthday, the book, *Tutu: The Authorized Portrait*, was published. In an introductory Editor's Note, Abrams shares a touching and poignant moment in Tutu's life that speaks directly to Tutu's character as one of the great moral leaders of our time:

> Desmond Tutu looked out from the raised pulpit at St. Mary's Cathedral in Johannesburg unable to speak. The standing-room-only crowd of more than a thousand had gathered to hear him preach on the occasion of his seventy-fifth birthday. He gazed out at the congregation that he had led during the struggle to end apartheid, and the rest of us who had gathered from around the world. Three-quarters of a century of his impossibly rich life was flashing before him and it

rendered him speechless. From the self-described "township urchin" to the Nobel Peace laureate, archbishop, and healer of a nation, his life had been as unimaginable as the transformation of his beloved country. And yet, he had imagined it, believed in it and orchestrated it with a fist-pounding confidence that this is a moral universe.

The man who is known around the world for his laugh—that warm chuckle that deepens into a belly roar and concludes with a mischievous giggle—began to sob deep body-shaking sobs. The congregation spontaneously broke out into song, singing their love for him. His wife Leah, without pause, left her pew and despite her aching, aged knees, hobbled up the stairs and into the pulpit. Tutu turned around to face her and buried his head in her chest as she wrapped her arms around him. He continued to sob, the congregation raising them both up with their song. After several minutes, he was finished. Leah stepped down out of the pulpit and Tutu turned back to the congregation, completely renewed, and proceeded to deliver a passionate and brilliant sermon on the struggle to end apartheid, and this particular congregation's role in ending that oppressive system. During those moments, we witnessed a kind of leadership for which our world is desperate: a leadership based on recognizing our shared humanity and our shared vulnerability, and on recognizing that our need for one another is not weakness but strength.

I first met Archbishop Desmond Tutu in August 1992. He was delivering the confirmation address at St. Paul's Church in Rondebosch, a suburb of Cape Town, South Africa. I was visiting Cape Town for the first time after a mission trip to help deliver a donated ambulance to Embangweni Hospital, a small, remote Presbyterian Church U.S.A.-sponsored bush hospital in the central African country of Malawi.

My trip to Africa had been set up in Spring of 1992. Similar to my trip in 1991 to France where I met with Dr. Margrietha van der Kreek, a colleague of famed theologian and Nobel Peace laureate Dr. Albert

"Blessed are the Peacemakers"

Schweitzer, and to India where I had the opportunity to meet Mother Teresa, I had arranged to meet with Archbishop Tutu in Cape Town following completion of the ambulance delivery to Malawi.

I had sent a letter to Bishop's Court, the Archbishop's residence in Cape Town in early June 1992, indicating my plans to travel to Africa in August, first to deliver the ambulance in Malawi, and inquiring about the possibility of meeting Archbishop Tutu in Cape Town afterwards. I was initially advised that the Archbishop would be in Swaziland attending to synod business over the dates I suggested for my visit and consequently he would be unable to meet with me. However, as planning for my trip to Africa continued to unfold, I realized I could be in Cape Town earlier than I originally thought, so I called Bishop's Court with the hope that my earlier arrival in the city might enable me to visit with the Archbishop.

I was able to speak with Lavinia Browne, the Archbishop's personal assistant, who indicated that the Archbishop's schedule was still full, however, Lavinia did mention that he was preaching at Rondebosch on Sunday, August 9th. Lavinia suggested my best bet to meet the Archbishop was to attend the service and speak with him afterwards. I thanked Lavinia profusely for her help and we agreed that once I arrived in Cape Town, I'd call her again to confirm that the Archbishop was still preaching at Rondebosch and if she still felt it possible the Archbishop would have a few moments after the service to speak with me.

Following an incredible two-week adventure through southern Africa to deliver the ambulance to Embangweni, Malawi, I arrived in Cape Town late on the evening of Thursday, August 6th. Early the next morning, I called and spoke with Lavinia and she assured me that the Archbishop would be in Rondebosch on Sunday and that he was willing to meet with me after the service!

After two relaxing days of sightseeing in Cape Town, I arose on Sunday morning, had breakfast, and then took a 20-minute taxi ride form my hotel to St. Paul's Church in Rondebosch. The church sits in the heart of the community and is a beautiful stone building built in the mid-1800s with a single belfry erected in 1875. It is partially hidden by a row of trees, and behind the church is a beautiful, picturesque mountainside view.

The service Archbishop Tutu was to preach was scheduled to start at 9:30 a.m. I arrived at the church about 8:45. As I walked into the church, I met the parish priest and one of the lay ministers. I explained who I was and why I was there and asked if they would mind if I audio and video taped the service with my palm-sized video and audio recorder. They suggested that I sit in the balcony in the back of the church with the choir where I would have a bird's eye view of the service.

This was beyond my expectations and I was delighted when they introduced me to the choir director, who readily agreed with the plan and placed me alongside the choir in the balcony with a clear view of the pulpit and front of the church.

As the 9:30 hour approached, the church began to fill up and was completely full just prior to the appointed time. The organist seated at the magnificent, old organ in the choir loft began playing a hymn, and as the congregation rose and sang, Archbishop Tutu, in colorful, clerical garb befitting an archbishop, and the other service participants processed in and took their seats.

The service commenced in a traditional service format with the singing of hymns, welcoming statements and announcements, but as the time of the sermon approached and Tutu stepped into the pulpit, it seemed to me that the whole congregation leaned forward in eager anticipation of his words. He began:

> It is a very great joy to be here with you this morning on this precious occasion when these young people are to be confirmed.
>
> I hope you don't get to feel too much like that little boy who went to church with his mommy. In the sanctuary there was a red lamp and when the service went on and on, he turned to his mom and said, "Mommy, when it turns green can we go home?"

"Blessed are the Peacemakers"

As the congregation chuckled, Tutu proceeded to deliver a brilliant sermon on our shared humanity, our shared vulnerabilities, on our preciousness in God's sight, and on what it meant to be made in God's image.

In words that ring true at any time and in any place Tutu said:

> What does it mean to be made in the image of God? Dear friends, it means that you are God's representative, you are God's Viceroy. You are God's stand-in. Strictly, if I wanted to know what God is like I ought to look at you and say that you are a revelation of God for me. You see, it means now you, dear children, to the extent that you are able to do this, represent God. Represent God at home. Represent God at school. Represent God at play. You represent God so that the others may see God's desire for justice, for peace, for reconciliation. You represent God so that those who are hurting may receive the healing of God. The goodness of God must shine forth through you. The generosity of God must be experienced through your generosity and so others will be touched by you and if they are touched by you - they are touched by God.
>
> Students wrote an exam and as often they will do there are those who don't quite know the answers, but they have a go. And the question they were asked was, "What did John the Baptist say to Jesus Christ when Jesus came to him to be baptized?" This particular student didn't know the answer, but he would have his shot so he said, "John the Baptist said to Jesus 'Remember you are the Son of God and behave like one' "
>
> Remember, you have been created in the image of God. Remember, you have been redeemed by the precious blood of Jesus Christ. Remember, you are indwelled by the Spirit of God. Remember that you are God's Viceroy - and behave like one!

Through the Lens of Humanity

In his sermon and in his greeting of parishioners after the service, Archbishop Tutu exhibited grace, humor, and most of all, love and compassion for all. As I greeted him at the church doorway following the service, I introduced myself. He immediately said, "Yes, yes, welcome! I look forward to speaking with you." Lavinia had clearly let him know that I was going to be present and hoped to speak with him.

After most of the congregants had departed, Tutu changed out of his clerical garb and he and I sat together on a bench in a semi-secluded portion of the church's grounds. The archbishop had an inviting, enchanting, and charismatic personality, and an unflinching buoyancy that seemed to ooze from him in a way that makes one feel they are truly in the presence of grace.

It has been said that if you wish to glimpse inside a human soul and get to know a person, watch them laugh. Tutu's laugh is famous the world over. We laughed often as we sat on the grounds of St. Paul's Church. I shared with him stories of the adventures my colleagues and I experienced as we traveled through south Africa delivering the ambulance to Malawi. I shared with him too, the fact that I was undertaking theological studies at McCormick Theological Seminary. He indicated one of his daughter's was involved in theological studies as well.

As I had done the previous year with Mother Teresa, I presented the archbishop with a blue sweatshirt from Immanuel Presbyterian Church. With a squeal and giggle of delight, he jumped out of his seat and put on the sweatshirt. "How do I look?" he asked, laughing, "I like it!"

As our time together started to dwindle, we walked back to the front of the church and he introduced me to his wife Leah. Leah, the archbishop, the parish priest, and I spoke together for a few moments and then the Tutus excused themselves to return to Bishop's Court to prepare for the upcoming synod meetings in which the archbishop would participate the following week. The parish priest called me a taxi from his office and I returned to my hotel, realizing how fortunate I was to have just spent the morning in the presence of one of the world's most remarkable persons.

"Blessed are the Peacemakers"

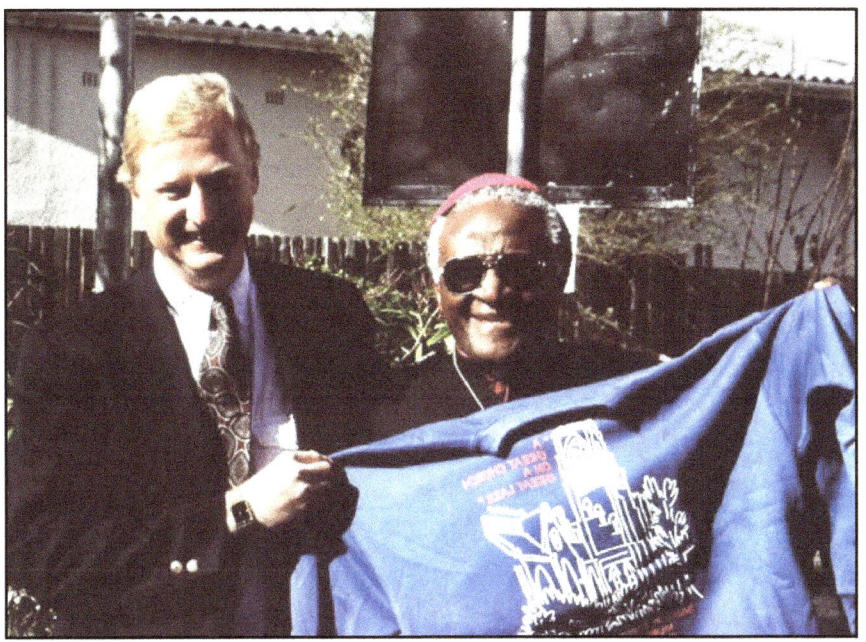

Meeting with Archbishop Tutu after church service in Rondebosch (1992)

Shortly after I returned to my home in Milwaukee, I wrote a letter to the archbishop, thanking him for taking the time to meet with me in Cape Town. I've included a portion of the letter below:

> ... My entire trip to Africa was very meaningful to me—not only the opportunity to help deliver an ambulance to Embangweni Hospital in Embangweni, Malawi but certainly the opportunity to hear your sermon on August 9th and to speak with you afterwards as well.
>
> My volunteer trip to India last year to work in Mother Teresa's missions and the opportunity to speak with her about her life's work, coupled with this year's trip to Africa and the opportunity to meet with you are experiences I will always cherish. As I mentioned to you, I have begun seminary training, and it is my intent as part of this training to write of

> the Christian ethics you and Mother Teresa bring to your life's calling and to the people you serve.
>
> I certainly hope I may keep in contact with you, and look forward to a chance to meet with you again.

Archbishop Tutu's response, which I received within days of my letter, is framed and hangs in my study and includes the following personal note:

> ... I wish you well in your studies. May you continue to be an instrument of God's healing of body, mind and spirit and may He bless you now and in the future.

Little did I realize that after this initial exchange with the Archbishop that I would be seeing him again quite soon in Milwaukee. What an extraordinary impact he was going to have on my life and the City of Milwaukee as well.

Indeed, the next time I saw Archbishop Tutu was the result of a remarkable series of events initiated in the summer of 1993. The Right Reverend Doctor Patrick Matolengwe was a former Bishop Suffragan of the diocese of Cape Town. His tenure in this role coincided with the many crises caused by the South African apartheid government as it sought to enforce numerous oppressive political and social policies directed at black South Africans. His service as Bishop Suffragan also coincided with Desmond Tutu's tenure as Archbishop of Cape Town. However, in 1988, Bishop Patrick moved to Milwaukee, Wisconsin, where he had accepted an appointment as Dean of All Saints Cathedral and also as an Assisting Bishop in the Episcopal diocese of Milwaukee.

In the summer of 1993, Bishop Patrick received a phone call from Reverend Paul Bodine, Interim Executive Presbyter of the Presbytery of Milwaukee inquiring if Archbishop Tutu could be persuaded to visit Milwaukee. The desire was to invite the Archbishop to Milwaukee in the spring of 1995 for a series of inspirational and cultural exchange activities within the City of Milwaukee, which would culminate with the Archbishop featured as the keynote speaker for the 25th Anniversary of the Interfaith Conference of Greater Milwaukee.

The phone call from Paul Bodine spawned a series of meetings between Bishop Patrick, Paul Bodine, Jack Murtaugh, Executive Secretary of the Interfaith Conference of Greater Milwaukee, and myself. Our initial goal was to determine if we could raise sufficient funds to pay the expenses for the Archbishop to travel from South Africa to Milwaukee and be in residence for four to five days. The upshot of these discussions was an agreement that the Interfaith Conference and Children's Hospital of Wisconsin (where I was serving as Executive Vice President) would provide the majority of funding for the visit, along with additional fund-raising efforts as required.

With the knowledge that funding was available, Bishop Patrick, on a visit to South Africa in 1994 to visit his ailing mother, met with his old friend and colleague and extended an invitation to the Archbishop to come to Milwaukee in 1995. The Archbishop agreed to come in May, and after some shuffling of dates to accommodate the Archbishop's schedule, the dates of May 12th to May 16th, 1995, were agreed upon for the Archbishop's visit, with the evening of May 15th being designated as the date for the 25th Anniversary of the Interfaith Conference.

Following the Archbishop's agreement that he was willing to come to Milwaukee, many planning meetings occurred relative to the precise activities that the Archbishop would attend and participate in during his visit. As 1995 dawned and the 25th Anniversary drew closer, we (Paul Bodine, Bishop Patrick, Jack Murtaugh and I) decided that the best course of action to complete the plans for the Archbishop's five-day visit was to meet directly with him and his staff to finalize all preparations. I volunteered to undertake this task and in early April 1995, I flew to Cape Town to meet with the Archbishop and members of his staff.

It was a whirlwind trip. Prior to undertaking the trip, I had advised Lavinia Browne, the Archbishop's personal assistant of the purpose of my trip and as before, she was extraordinarily helpful in setting up the meetings I required. I arrived on a Sunday evening and on the following Monday morning, took a taxi to Bishop's Court and spent the morning with Lavinia and John Allen, press secretary to the Archbishop who would also be accompanying the Archbishop and his wife Leah to the States.

When I arrived at Bishop's Court, the Archbishop came out of his office and greeted me warmly in the same jovial mood I had seen almost two years earlier in Rondebosch. He asked how Bishop Patrick was doing and shared a bit of how the two of them knew each other and some of their experiences together opposing apartheid. I told him how thrilled we were that he was coming. I also mentioned to him that one function we hoped he'd participate in was a commissioning service for a youth group from the Presbytery of Milwaukee that was going on a two-week mission trip to Mwandi, Zambia. He said he was looking forward to the trip to the States, and shared that prior to arriving in Milwaukee, he was going to visit one of his daughters who was studying in the the northeast part of the United States.

Intermittently during the morning, the Archbishop would pop in for a few moments and we'd brief him on the trip's plans, but he seemed perfectly content with Lavinia and John handling all the details. Late in the morning, he announced he was driving into Cape Town to run errands. Lavinia asked if he wanted a driver, but with his trademark laugh/giggle and looking at me he said, "They don't like me to drive, but I like to." He bid me farewell and said he looked forward to seeing me in Milwaukee.

In the midst of the flurry of this trip, I had the opportunity to spend some time with Lavinia Browne and her husband, Terry Crawford-Browne. Lavinia had worked for the Archbishop since 1985 as his personal assistant (and continued to do so throughout the entirety of his tenure as Archbishop and beyond including his appointment by President Mandela as Chair of the Truth and Reconciliation Commission. She has also served in varieties of roles within the Desmond Tutu HIV Foundation).

Terry had had a banking career in South Africa, but from 1985 to 1993, he had advised Dr. Allan Boesak and Archbishop Tutu on the

"BLESSED ARE THE PEACEMAKERS"

banking sanctions campaign against apartheid. Terry also was an activist seeking to expose corruption in the South African government relative to bribes alleged to be billions of dollars paid by foreign governments to secure arms procurement deals.

Lavinia and Terry were kind enough to take me on a full day's driving tour of Cape Town and the surrounding areas, and then over dinner in the evening, they shared with me what it was like for them as white South Africans to live and work in Cape Town during the apartheid era. With both of them being associated with Archbishop Tutu and his outspokenness and involvement in the anti-apartheid movement, they indicated they had both received death threats and were subjected to ridicule, criticism, and abuse by white South Africans and certainly by members of the South African government.

However, they were completely committed to the fight against apartheid and understood the personal risks and sacrifices they faced each day. With the release of Nelson Mandela and the subsequent peaceful transition to democracy, attitudes started to change for the better throughout South Africa, particularly after Nelson Mandela's election as president. As I got to know Lavinia and Terry, I understood how fortunate the Archbishop was to have these two as colleagues and friends. [Over the years I have returned several times to Cape Town, and each visit has included a dinner with Lavinia and Terry.]

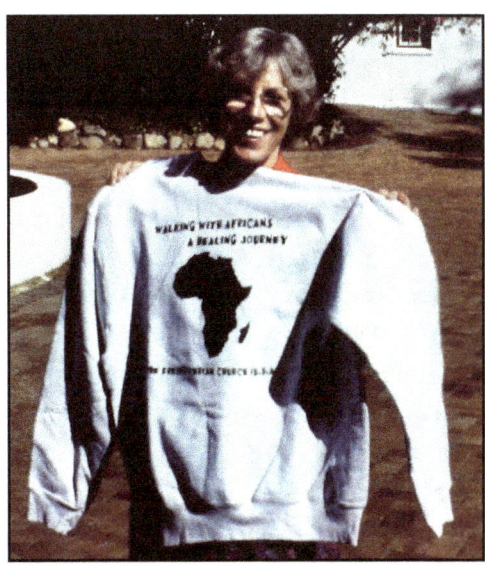

Lavinia Crawford-Browne,
Executive Assistant to the Archbishop
Photo taken at Bishop's Court in
Cape Town, South Africa

Through the Lens of Humanity

* * *

I returned to Milwaukee with an agreed-upon agenda—a packed, five-day itinerary comprising eight presentations by the Archbishop in a variety of community venues, each geared towards the theme of his visit: "Celebrating the dignity of every person and the solidarity of the human community."

Approximately a month later, on Friday morning May 12th, Bishop Patrick, Leigh Morris, Director of Public Relations at Children's Hospital, two hospital security officers, and I drove to Chicago's O'Hare Airport in a Children's Hospital multi-seat van to meet the Archbishop, his wife Leah, and the Archbishop's press secretary, John Allen.

The Tutus and John Allen arrived on time on an American Airlines flight from the East Coast, where the Tutu's had been visiting their daughter for a few days. As we greeted the Archbishop, he hugged Bishop Patrick and me; we could feel the tremendous energy this man exuded, an energy that he would pass on to all who met him during the following four days in Milwaukee.

We secured a wheelchair for Leah; she had recently twisted her ankle, and while she was able to walk with a cane, it was easier for her mobility to be in a wheelchair. Barry Sanders and Stan Romanowski, Children's Hospital security officers, assisted in gathering bags and getting us all loaded in the van for the 90-minute journey to Milwaukee.

Barry and Stan provided security and transport for the Archbishop throughout his stay in Milwaukee and grew quite close to the Archbishop during that time. The Archbishop constantly joked and talked with them as they ferried him from location to location.

From O'Hare Airport, we drove directly to Children's Hospital of Wisconsin for the first of the Archbishop's appearances.

Welcomed by hospital president Jon Vice and a large contingent of employees, patients, patient families, and of course, the news media, the Nobel Prize laureate quickly captured the hearts of all who saw and heard him.

"Blessed are the Peacemakers"

The entire hospital was embraced by this man. He talked with nurses and doctors about the complexities of their work. He talked with parents and relatives about the stresses of dealing with a sick child.

Tutu thoroughly enchanted the children. He gave a "high five" to a seven-year-old in for a bone marrow transplant. He charmed a three-year-old on a respirator. An 11-year-old girl had made the Archbishop a medallion; the youngster beamed with pride as Tutu placed it around his neck. In return, Archbishop Tutu gave her an autograph and a kiss. And every child received a silent prayer from this remarkable man of God.

Later, at a hospital sponsored luncheon, there were stern words, words filled with wisdom and warning: "It is ghastly to hear that every two hours, one child is killed with a gun in this country," he told his audience. "It is adults who teach them to hate, who teach them to hurt.

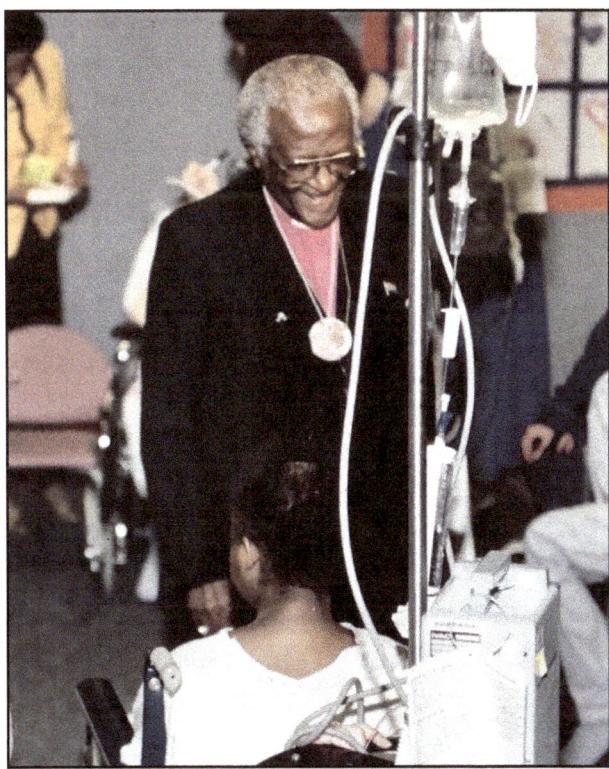

Archbishop Tutu touring Children's Hospital of Wisconsin

We have to change the hearts of adults so the world can become hospitable to children." He charged the audience with this message, "If you are quite serious about the survival of human society, then you're going to care about the children."

One could tell Tutu was deeply moved by his visit to Children's Hospital. He was deeply impressed by the physicians and other caregivers "who do incredible things every day." In a moment of reflection, Tutu continued, "God looks at this and rubs his hands and says, 'Hey, aren't they neat? They really justify the risk I took in creating the world.'"

"Yes," Tutu said, "they (Children's Hospital caregivers) do make up for the awfulness. When you see these people, you know there is a great deal of beauty in this world. You know that we are made for something better."

And so it went with Tutu's visit to Milwaukee. Whether he was addressing an audience at an inner city church, commissioning youth for a mission project to Africa, meeting with school children in a central city school, meeting with city and business dignitaries and clergy from all denominations, celebrating a mass at the Sunday service of All Saints Episcopal church, attending receptions or sharing the speakers podium with the Catholic Archbishop at the Interfaith Conference's 25th Anniversary dinner—here was a man who appealed to people from all walks of life. In all of his presentations, he connected with people by expressing his gratitude for their support to end apartheid in South Africa. Through his humor, he put people at ease.

Jack Murtaugh, executive director of the Interfaith Conference, reflected on Tutu's visit in this manner:

> Each of his presentations was tailored to a specific audience, yet still had a common theme. He challenged us to be caring, compassionate people. He spoke of the refugees of the world and raised up the needs of children, saying that they are our future. We were called upon to make his dream of a humane and just society a reality. He spoke of the beauty that exists in our multi-racial, multi-cultural society.

"Blessed are the Peacemakers"

> There was no doubt that in meeting Archbishop Tutu, one was in the presence of a person of faith who has a passion for justice. He did not hide his religious motivation nor his Christian roots. From his confidence in his own religious identity, he acknowledged the value and the need for inter-religious collaboration. He extolled the contributions of other faiths to end political and economic apartheid, not only in South Africa, but throughout the world and including our own country as well.
>
> We were moved by how he reached out beyond dignitaries in the audience he was addressing to the people who stood off to the side and in the rear. People who serve and are generally unrecognized - maintenance workers, clerks, nurses, security guards, drivers, waiters and waitresses. Through words and actions, he extended the circle to include everyone there. ... His presence and words nourished our spirit to go forward and to "uphold the dignity of every person and the solidarity of the human community."

During his visit, there were also whimsical and poignant moments. The Tutus and John Allen stayed in a suite at the elegant Pfister Hotel, the oldest hotel in the state of Wisconsin. They were on the 22nd floor in room 22 ("Tu-Tu"). When I was in Cape Town, I had asked Lavinia if there was anything special that the Archbishop liked that we could provide for him. She thought for a moment and said that he really liked rum raisin ice cream. I conveyed that information to the hotel and each evening, they delivered several dishes of rum raisin ice cream to the suite. The Archbishop, teasing me one morning, asked if I'd please arrange to have ice cream delivered to him nightly in Cape Town.

One evening, I was accompanying him up to his room and expressed how pleased we all were that he had come to Milwaukee and thanked him for his time with us. He had been walking just a step or so in front of me and he immediately stopped, turned to me, grabbed one of my arms, and spoke very passionately, "How could I not come? Your country and people the world over supported us in the dark days of apartheid, you were with us, I come to be with you, we should always be for each other."

On Saturday afternoon the 13th, the Archbishop presided at the commissioning of 20-plus youth destined for a summer mission trip to the village of Mwandi, Zambia.

After the service the Archbishop, the clergy from Immanuel Presbyterian Church (where the commissioning took place), and I, adjourned to the English Room a restaurant located in the lower level of the Pfister Hotel. Reverend Johnstone, one of the clergy from Immanuel Presbyterian Church, asked the Archbishop about some of the most meaningful moments for him over the last several years.

"I experienced the most astonishing sense of freedom last April, in 1994," Tutu said. "At age 62, I was able to vote for the very first time in my life. It is hard to explain that sense of freedom after so, so many years of oppression, turmoil, and violence." His eyes grew misty as he continued. "The moment that I and so many others had waited so long

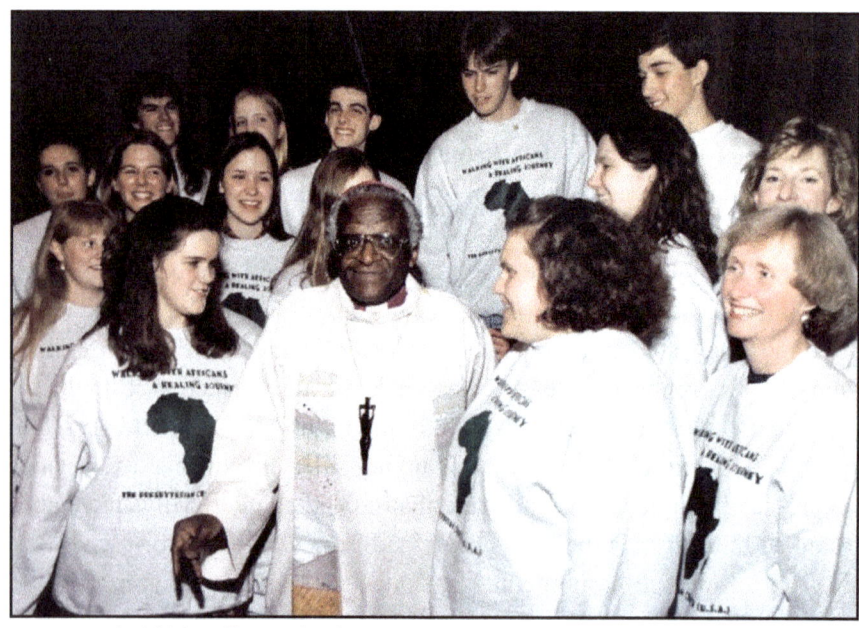

Archbishop Tutu at the Commissioning Service for Youth and Adults at Immanuel Presbyterian Church

"Blessed are the Peacemakers"

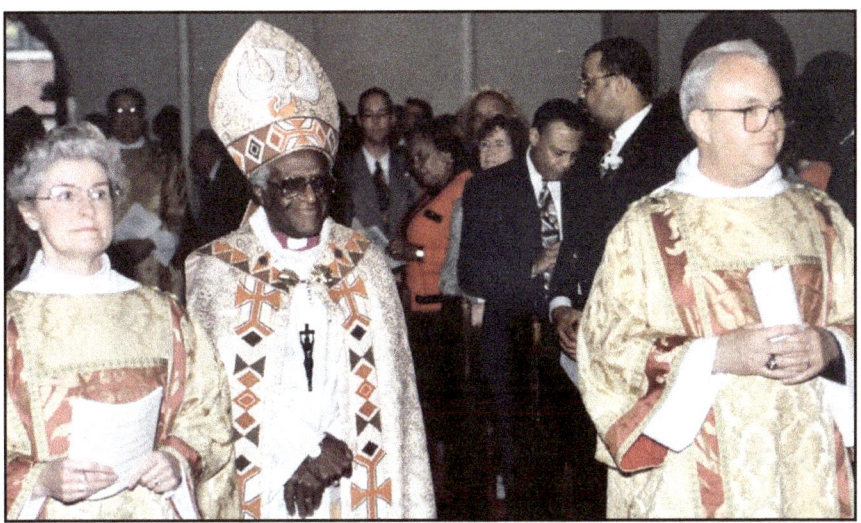

Archbishop Tutu processing into Milwaukee's All Saints Cathedral for Sunday Services on May 14th, 1995

for had finally arrived. I remember taking my paper ballot and placing it in the box. I remember shouting and singing and doing a little jig."

As he spoke, it wasn't just the Archbishop's whose eyes were misty. This was a very remarkable and revealing moment.

"And that day in April, April 27th, we elected Nelson Mandela President of South Africa. It was dreamlike how so many changes are beginning to occur after so much oppression and violence."

Looking around the table, he said, "We really do have a God of surprises, don't you agree?"

Monday, May 15th, the date of the 25th Anniversary Celebration for the Interfaith Conference arrived. I was amazed at how well all the events over the preceding days had gone—all the ceremonies and activities had been extraordinarily well received and everything seemingly had gone off without a hitch. That was about to change.

Early on Monday afternoon, the Archbishop's press secretary, John Allen, notified me that they had word from South Africa that President Mandela was asking the Archbishop to return to South Africa immediately.

Through the Lens of Humanity

On May 10th, a mining accident in the town of Vaal Reefs, South Africa, had resulted in the death of 104 miners when an elevator carrying the gold miners plunged approximately 1,500 feet to the bottom of the shaft. The Vaal Reefs tragedy was history's worst ever elevator disaster. President Mandela was declaring Wednesday, May 17th a national day of mourning and prayer and he wanted the Archbishop to be present for these events.

Given the duration of travel between Milwaukee and South Africa, our challenge was to figure the best way to have the Archbishop participate in the 25th Anniversary Celebration and still get back to South Africa for the services for the miners. After spending several hours on the phone, Leigh Morris, Director of Communications for Children's Hospital, and I were able to arrive at a solution.

After the 25th Anniversary Celebration ended, we would transport the Archbishop to a private airport where a local corporation, Harnischfeger Industries, had a private jet that would fly the Archbishop to New York, where he would catch a direct flight from JFK airport to Cape Town. Harnischfeger was donating all costs associated with the flight to New York. John Allen and Leah Tutu would remain in Milwaukee and return to South Africa according to their original travel plans.

When I shared this news with the Archbishop, he was deeply moved that we were able to accommodate President Mandela's and his desire to be present in South Africa for the national day of mourning and prayer for the deceased miners and the families.

Riding with the Archbishop to the airport after the 25th Anniversary Celebration, we talked and joked about the various events of the last few days. When we got to the airport, he apologized for the hectic way he was leaving without a "really proper goodbye" for everyone. We embraced right before he boarded the flight, and I knew this man of God, of peace and love who had blessed us with his presence for four days, was off to where he was currently needed the most.

* * *

"Blessed are the Peacemakers"

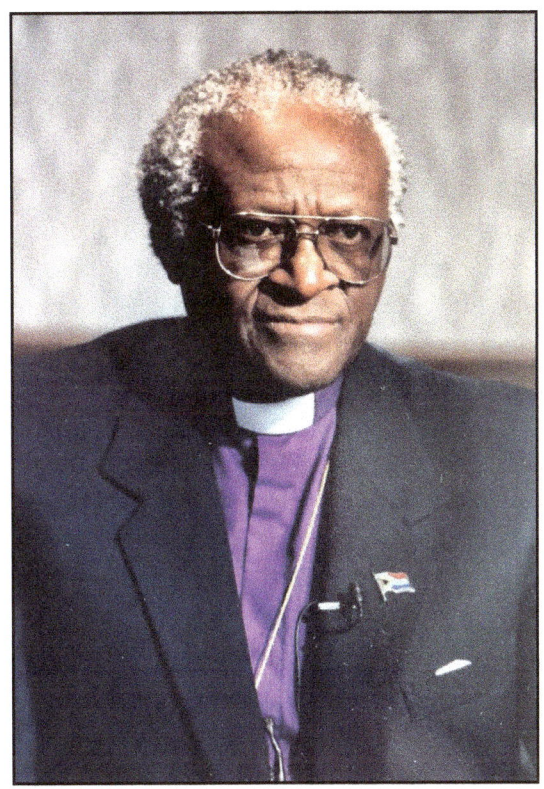

The Archbishop preparing to address Milwaukee's Interfaith Conference's 25th Anniversary Celebration.

In September 1995, four months after his visit to Milwaukee, Archbishop Desmond Tutu and sixteen others were appointed by President Nelson Mandela to the Truth and Reconciliation Commission. Tutu has stated, "… that it was the commission's goal to reach out to as many South Africans as possible, offering amnesty to all, both those who had been victims and those who had been perpetrators during apartheid's long reign. Our slogan was: The truth hurts, but silence kills. Our aim was to engage all South Africans in the work of the commission, ensuring that all would have the chance to be part of any serious and viable proposal for healing and reconciliation."

In 1996, Tutu's term as archbishop ended, but he continued to assume other roles, pre-eminent among those being the Chairmanship of the Truth and Reconciliation Commission (TRC), which had begun public hearings early that year.

Through the Lens of Humanity

In 1997, I was in Cape Town in late June with colleagues following a visit to Zambia, and I contacted Lavinia Browne (Lavinia was still functioning as Tutu's personal assistant; she was now working with him as part of the TRC) about the possibility of seeing the Archbishop during my time in Cape Town. She suggested that I attend a Mass at St. George's Cathedral in downtown Cape Town on Thursday the 27th at 7:30 a.m. The Archbishop, she said, was planning on being there and she was sure I could greet and chat with him after the service. She also mentioned that former staff members of Tutu's during his tenure as Archbishop would be at the service, and "Arch" as she called him, would be taping interviews with them as a series of remembrances of their years together. She also mentioned he would be meeting with an organization that was working on human rights issues in Tibet on Thursday morning as well. So while I hoped to meet briefly with the Archbishop, it certainly sounded as if he had a very busy schedule that morning.

St. George's Cathedral is a magnificent Gothic edifice in downtown Cape Town. It is the oldest cathedral in southern Africa and is the Mother Church of the Anglican Diocese of Cape Town. It is known as the "People's Cathedral" for its role in the resistance against apartheid. The Mass that Thursday morning was held in a small alcove next to the main sanctuary. About 20 people were present, including the Archbishop, Lavinia, John Allen, several clergy (some of whom I assumed were formal staff members of Tutu's), a dozen or so parishioners, and myself. The service lasted about 30 minutes and afterwards, when I walked up to the Archbishop, he gave me a hug and said a little prayer. We talked for a few minutes about his Milwaukee visit, he expressed how much he enjoyed it, despite, he chuckled, his rapid departure at the end.

We went downstairs for coffee and cookies and people milled around for 15 or 20 minutes. Then Lavinia walked up to the Archbishop to say it was time for him to go for his interviews. Taking that as my cue that it was time to leave, I started walking over to the Archbishop to say goodbye. To my surprise, Lavinia stopped me and said I too was invited to attend the session with the Archbishop and his former staff!

"BLESSED ARE THE PEACEMAKERS"

We walked about one and a half blocks to the Regis Hotel, where, on the 4th floor in a small conference room, a conference table had been set up in a horseshoe fashion with several microphones scattered around the table. Tutu sat at the head of the horseshoe with his former staffers (mostly clergy) on either side of him. Lavinia and John Allen sat on one side of the table and I sat in the back of the room.

One of the clergy introduced the session. My impression was that this was one of a series of discussions/interviews that the Archbishop was conducting with former staff to memorialize many of the activities and events during his tenure as Archbishop to discern his thinking relative to decisions he made and to explore the impact of these events on his life and ministry. Part of the discussion also seemed to be an attempt to capture Tutu's theological perspective on a number of topics, specifically the Truth and Reconciliation Commission, and what the consequences of the TRC would be for South Africa. But clearly part of

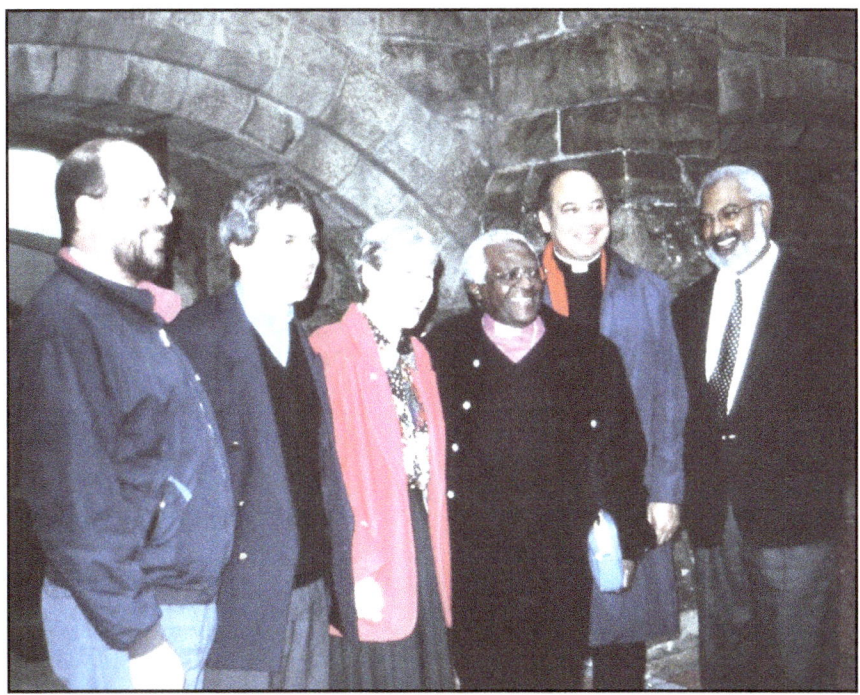

Retired Archbishop Tutu and former members of his staff

the session was simply colleagues and good friends reliving shared memories and experiences with an abundance of laughter and tears.

The session went about an hour and a half, primarily with Tutu responding to staffers' questions. The Truth and Reconciliation Commission had already held public forums for over a year and one of the first questions posed to Tutu was whether reconciliation and forgiveness in South Africa was really possible. And what was Tutu's theology concerning this issue?

Tutu's responses were fascinating. "Why," he said, "should humans be surprised at the dastardly things, the heinous acts that people do to each other? Our theology acknowledges the concept of original sin, humans are sinful and will do brutal things, things some would even call demonic. However, our theology also acknowledges that people can change, people are created in the image of God." He continued. "We can't consign anyone to hell—it is possible for people to change."

As to whether there can be forgiveness and reconciliation, Tutu expressed frustration over people "splitting hairs in the face of the government's generosity in offering amnesty. Why do people have to become so legalistic. Why must we look for retributive justice?"

"Forgiveness," he said, "is not, cannot be cheap or easy, but South Africa has the opportunity for something truly great to happen. So we mustn't get so legalistic. This is a universe of a righteous God where lies cannot prevail forever. We can't just let our sense of purpose be to put people on the carpet."

"That is why people, white and black, should be together. People don't understand how liberated they will be through forgiveness and reconciliation. If our country is to be healed, everyone must say be willing to say 'we're sorry,' and we're with you in times of trouble." This is why, he said, he went to Botha's funeral—for reconciliation. Whites and blacks both hunger for forgiveness and reconciliation. "Remember," he said, "the foolishness of God is the foolishness of love."

One of the former staffers asked Tutu to explain his concept of the image of God, which drew a very emotional response.

"Blessed are the Peacemakers"

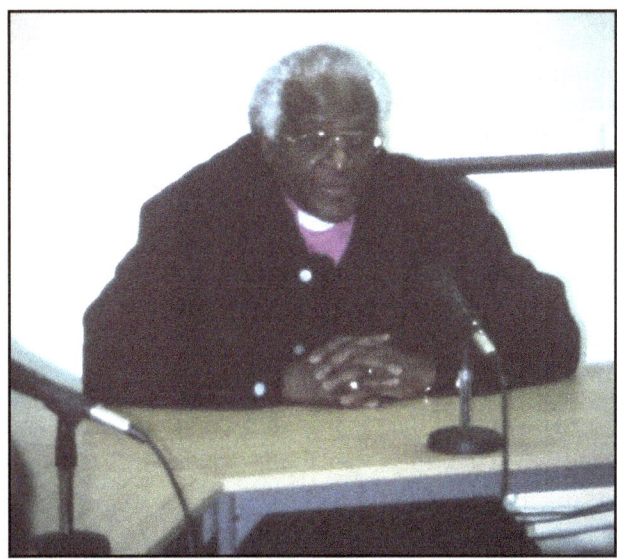

Retired Archbishop Tutu reminiscing moments from his decade as Archbishop of Cape Town.

Tutu spoke about the Apostle Paul's phraseology about the nursing and nurturing aspect of God. But then he painted a fascinating illustration of his concept of God. He asked those in the room to visualize sitting next to a fireplace and then he said, "As you sit next to the fireplace, you begin to assume its attributes. You become warm, you begin to glow in its warmth … Spiritually, if you allow yourself to become accessible to God, then you can assume attributes similar to God, as one assumes the fireplace's attributes by becoming close to it.

Tutu was emotional as he spoke of what he feels it is like for one having the experience of God. He described it as a mother folding her arms around an infant. Her love is always present, even in the infant's most troublesome behavior. In this way, God is saying, 'I love you'— all we have to do is accept this love."

[**Author's Note**: P.W. Botha served as South Africa's Prime Minister from 1978 to 1984, and as South Africa' ceremonial executive State President from 1984 to 1989. Botha was a fierce opponent of Black majority rule and the apartheid years under his leadership were among the most brutal.]

THROUGH THE LENS OF HUMANITY

Tutu said several times that his imagery of God includes a sense of returning home, always returning to love. "But unfortunately," he said, "our whole business is always trying to impress God, and this is not necessary."

At the time of this session, Tutu had just recently been diagnosed with prostate cancer [he was actually leaving for treatment in the United States later in the week], and he said at this point in his life, he was trying to "be there with God." "Perhaps," he continued, "for him this aspect of his life-threatening disease had been a good thing."

When asked about what was on his mind when he was told of his prostate cancer diagnosis, Tutu grew reflective and talked about times past when he knew he might face death. He spoke of the numerous death threats he had received during the apartheid era and the real possibility of his assassination. He talked about being told to leave the country or else he would be killed. He said he knew that if he did this just once [left the country], his effectiveness in calling for reform and change would be over. His credibility would be lost, he said.

He spoke movingly and with obvious emotion of a special service his staff held for him in the event of his assassination: "Sort of a handing him over to God." He spoke with some humor about receiving a death threat one day and a policeman saying to him, "Can't you just stay in bed for a few days?"

And, with a great deal of emotion, he spoke of how he had told his family how he wanted his funeral. I noticed many in the room had tears in their eyes as he spoke of these things. I sat there thinking what incredible courage he had, as well as his family and his staff.

Tutu chuckled when one of the staff mentioned how "God-driven" he was and responded by saying that was because he desired God's presence and knew that he and his staff must have the highest standards. But he also spoke of how angry he could get with God and his own questions of "how could God allow some things to happen." These were the times he mentioned when he most sought "the qualities of the fireplace," i.e., when he sought to assume the attributes of God's spirituality.

"Blessed are the Peacemakers"

Tutu also expressed his belief that people were "God-carriers." "Others must see God in us," he said. And, he said if we are God-carriers, then we must represent God in a certain way. When we see things that are wrong—oppression, for example—we must say that is not who God is and we must not permit oppression to occur.

As the session was drawing to a close, one of the clergy said to him, "We felt that you were the 'future in our presence. "What future are you looking for?" he asked Tutu.

Tutu acknowledged he had been reading a book by noted theologian Walter Brueggemann entitled *Hopeful Imagination.* Tutu said he believes that God is seeking restoration of the beginning of creation, a more caring and just society where "lions do lie down with lambs." Tutu said he is a dreamer. "We must dream of a society where there is no poverty, there are no wars, why not "beat swords into plough shares?"

"If God's dream is to be actualized, it will be because we agree to be God's co-workers. Can you imagine what an incredible privilege it is to be God's co-worker?" he asked.

As the session was winding up, I thought of a statement a South African newspaper reporter had made regarding what it felt like to meet Tutu. "It was like having a direct line to God," he said.

I think all those present in the room with the Archbishop this morning would certainly have agreed with that statement.

As he was leaving, the Archbishop stopped and as we exchanged goodbyes, I thanked him for allowing me to sit in on such an intense and intimate conversation. He said he was glad I was there, and apologized we didn't have more time to talk. He also asked me to give his greetings to his friends in Milwaukee. I left thinking what an incredible privilege it was to have been included in this remarkable conversation.

It was a number of years later when I next saw the Archbishop. It was 2006, and I was in South Africa on behalf of a Milwaukee-based non-for-profit organization, the Center for International Health (CIH), which I had joined as president in 2003.

Through the Lens of Humanity

One of our projects was a collaboration with the Philani Maternal, Child Health and Nutrition Project. Philani had been established in 1979 and delivered community-based services that addressed maternal, child health, and nutrition problems in the informal settlements on the outskirts of Cape Town. Archbishop Tutu was a patron and long-time supporter of Philani.

Lavinia Browne had alerted me to the work of Philani, and by working with Lavinia and with a letter of support from the Archbishop, CIH had applied and received a United States Agency for International Development (USAID) International Food Relief Program (IFRP) grant to distribute ready-to-use supplementary food and dried soup mix for the clinics, schools and community centers affiliated with Philani. Two million individual meals were provided via the award and the primary beneficiaries would be mothers and their young children.

When I arrived at the offices being used by the Archbishop and Lavinia in his post-Archbishop days, I was greeted by Lavinia. She informed me that "Arch" was in and would be with me shortly. It gave me an opportunity to catch up Lavinia about her and Terry's current endeavors.

Within a few moments, "Arch" came out and invited me into his office. As I walked through the door, he grabbed my hand and said, "Let's say a little prayer." Afterwards, for the next several moments, I shared with him what I had been doing since I last saw him. The Truth and Reconciliation Commission had produced its final report and I mentioned what an incredible effort that had been for not only South Africa but for the world as well. He nodded and thanked me for that acknowledgment.

I had brought with me a copy of his book, *No Future Without Forgiveness*, and asked if he'd sign it for me. He took the book and joked he was glad someone bought it and wrote a nice message in the inside cover of the book. As I was about to depart, I asked him if he'd mind if Lavinia took our picture. He agreed, and this photo remains one of my prized possessions.

"Blessed be the peacemakers, for they shall be called the children of God," says Jesus as recorded in the Gospel of Matthew. Throughout his life, Desmond Tutu sat at the very center of bitter moral and

"Blessed are the Peacemakers"

political conflicts, yet he followed his convictions and his faith with tireless dedication. If there is ever to be truly peace on earth, it will be because of people like Archbishop Tutu. Throughout history, it seems someone comes along who shows us who as humans we really want to be. Desmond Tutu was one of these people.

And as the Archbishop would say, "Let us turn into the stillness and listen to God speak with the voice of the heart:

> And God says, I have a dream. I have a dream that all of my children will discover that they belong in one family—my family, the human family in which there are no outsiders. All, all belong, all are held in the embrace of this one whose love will never let us go, this one who says that each one of us is of incredible worth, that each one of us is precious to God because each one of us has their name written on the palms of God's hands. And God says, there are no outsiders - black, white, red, yellow, short, tall, young, old, rich, poor, gay, lesbian, straight - everyone. ALL belong. And God says, I have only you to help me realize my dream.
>
> Help me.
>
> —Archbishop Desmond Tutu

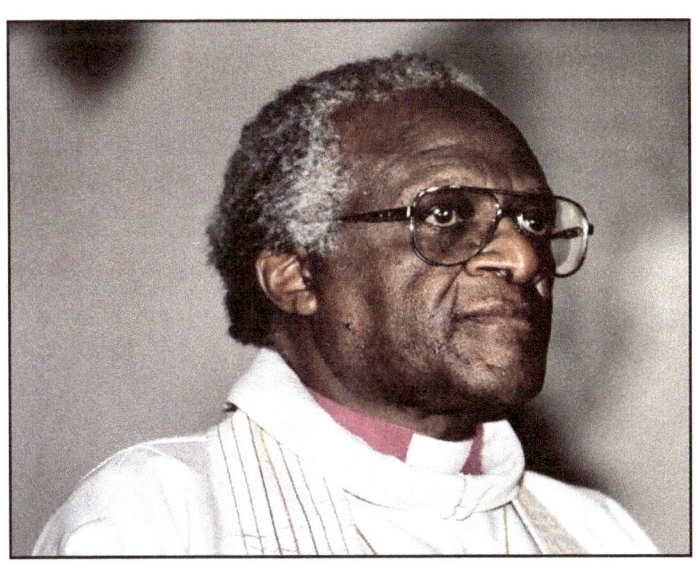

Archbishop Desmond Tutu
(October 7, 1931— December 26, 2021)

[**Author's Note**: After Archbishop Tutu's death in December 2021, I reached out to Lavinia Crawford-Brown to ask if she had any special remembrances of the Archbishop she'd like to share. Below are her comments.]

Dear Mark

Thank you for this memoir of Desmond Mpilo Tutu, the Arch, or Father – as he liked staff to address him. I had the immense privilege of serving him for twenty-two years. I had worked for his predecessor Archbishop Philip Russell and, typically, the Arch said, "I would like you to stay on, and if we don't get along, one of us will have to go."

You refer to the vulnerability of Father Desmond. I was at a small lunch party in his home, celebrating his 90th birthday. I said, "Father, I am sure you never believed you would live to be 90!" He took my hand and we laughed and laughed together. As with many public figures, elaborate funeral arrangements were in place for the eventuality. But when the time came, 26th December 2021, the Covid pandemic was upon us. Travel restrictions prevented overseas friends from attending the State Funeral in St George's Cathedral, Cape Town and the Tutu family were allowed only 100 personal guests. To me, it was a relief not to have the crowds – the simple pine coffin on which Leah had strewn a few white carnations – and close family and friends.

Shortly after he had been diagnosed with prostate cancer in 1996, the Arch was invited to preach in St George's Cathedral, his closing words were how he wished to be remembered, "I laughed, I hoped, and I loved".

Part Three

Uncommon Journeys

CHAPTER 6

SAFARI!

A CHRONICLE OF ADVENTURE FROM SOUTH AFRICA TO MALAWI

After my travels in 1991 to France and India to visit and work with Dr. Margrietha van der Kreek and Mother Teresa, my travel wanderlust was reinvigorated and I was eager to explore additional options for overseas travel coupled with medical mission opportunities.

In late 1988, I was delighted and excited when Dr. Paul Jewett, who along with his wife Judy, were the Presbyterian Medical Missionaries I had worked with in 1987 in Miraj, India recommended me for an appointment to the Board of Trustees of the Medical Benevolence Foundation (MBF). MBF is a designated medical missions organization of the Presbyterian Church USA, whose mission essentially was to support Presbyterian medical missionaries and medical mission sites abroad.

This was a perfect vehicle for me to participate in my dual passions of travel and medical mission work. Being on the Board of MBF afforded me the opportunity to know and work alongside dedicated medical missionaries whose lives were devoted to the health and welfare needs of literally millions of impoverished, destitute and neglected peoples around the globe. Church-sponsored and -supported medical missionaries have brought physical, emotional, and spiritual health to countries for centuries, but alas, these days, full-time medical missionaries are a fading breed, though the care they provide even with their dwindling numbers is still substantial in many remote areas of the world.

Through the years, I have been fortunate to know many Presbyterian medical missionaries whom I believe have been the "best of the best".

During my tenure on the MBF Board, I was honored and privileged to work with medical missionaries Dr. Archie and Huldah Fletcher who served for decades in India, Dr. Paul and Judy Jewett who served in Haiti, India, Malawi and Central America, Drs. Cherian and Kalindi Thomas who served as missionaries for both the Presbyterian and Methodist Churches in India, and Dr. Salvador and Irma de la Torre who served in Haiti, Zambia, Kenya, and Malawi.

The following is both an adventure story and a medical missions story - a story of three colleagues who purchased an "ambulance" for a remote bush hospital and drove it several thousand miles across multiple African countries to deliver it!

* * *

It was a bright, sunny morning in late July, 1992. I sat in a departure terminal at Milwaukee's General Billy Mitchell Field airport, waiting to board a flight to Chicago, where I would connect to a flight to Paris and ultimately fly on to South Africa. I reflected on events that had occurred over the previous three months that had brought about this new journey abroad. Here's what had happened.

In May 1992, I was having dinner in Evanston, Illinois with Medical Benevolence Foundation (MBF) board members Dr. Paul Jewett and Tom Logan. The spring meeting of the Board of Trustees of MBF, a medical missions organization supported by the Presbyterian Church USA, had just concluded and the three of us were preparing to return to our respective homes. Paul and his wife Judy were Presbyterian medical missionaries whom I had first met in 1987 in Miraj, India, and they had attended the spring board meeting to provide the trustees with an update on their activities in Embangweni, Malawi, where they were currently serving. Tom and I had traveled together to Malawi in 1990 to visit Presbyterian mission hospitals and clinics in the rural Malawian communities of Nkhoma, Ekwendeni, and Embangweni, and knowing of each others ongoing interests in mission projects in Africa, we had stayed in touch. Paul knew of Tom's and my specific interests in Africa, and he had invited us to dinner to share his concerns about several major issues confronting Embangweni Hospital and how they might be addressed.

As we dined, Tom looked over at me and asked, "What do you think of the idea of buying an ambulance, shipping it to Africa and then driving it to Embangweni and donating it to the mission hospital?"

Before I could respond, Paul chimed in and said, "Tom and I spoke earlier today about this. You've been to Embangweni. Given its remoteness, there is no reliable transport for medical emergencies, or a rapid and safe means of getting medical personnel and emergency supplies and equipment from one location to another out in the bush. Having an emergency vehicle like an ambulance would significantly assist us in providing care to all our patients and not just those in emergent situations. It'd give us a medical transport and capability that would enable us to open and operate clinics and preventive education programs out in small villages and bush locations."

Paul and Tom had my attention after their buying, shipping, and driving an ambulance through Africa comments, and as our dinner progressed, it was obvious we were all enthusiastic about trying to acquire an ambulance for Embangweni. Slowly we began to hatch a plan. Due to Tom's prior work with building wells in Malawi, he had expertise in shipping equipment to Africa and in dealing with African import taxes and registration information.

We agreed that Tom and I would look into the costs associated with purchasing and shipping a vehicle to Africa. We were aware we wouldn't be shipping an "ambulance" *per se*—we knew we needed to purchase a vehicle that was sturdy and capable of surviving the wear and tear of Malawi's virtually nonexistent rural and bush roads. We also felt buying a vehicle in the United States afforded us with more options to find a vehicle that was not only economical, but more likely to meet the quality, safety, and durability standards that ensured the vehicle could withstand the rigors of Malawi's topography and terrain.

Finally, we all tasked ourselves with raising funds to purchase and ship the vehicle to Africa.

I was surprised at how quickly all our plans came together. Tom and I explored what type of vehicle to purchase and with input from Paul, we agreed upon a Toyota Land Cruiser. We felt we could strip out the back seats to accommodate stretchers and medical equipment and modify the Land Cruiser enough to make it a very viable emergency medical vehicle. While Tom and I went about acquiring the vehicle, Paul successfully petitioned MBF for partial funding for the ambulance. With this funding in hand, Tom and I secured contributions from churches and other donors and within weeks, we had fully raised the amount required to not only purchase the vehicle, but to pay for the shipping and African import costs as well!

From the very outset of our conversations, Tom and I had planned to travel to Africa, clear the vehicle through customs, and then drive it ourselves to Embangweni. As our plans progressed, given that Malawi is a landlocked country, we had to decide exactly where we wanted to ship the vehicle. South Africa had always been top of mind due to its major ports and more reasonable import and duty taxes. Paul, upon returning to Malawi, had mentioned to Dr. Nico van Velden in Nkhoma our plans about buying an "ambulance" for Embangweni. Nico, whom I'd met a couple years earlier when I visited Nkhoma, suggested that we import the vehicle into South Africa and then have it transported to Johannesburg, where he had family. He would meet us in Johannesburg and the three of us would drive the vehicle to Malawi. The real advantage of this was that Nico was logistically familiar with the best routes from South Africa to Malawi. And the clincher was he suggested that as we traveled, we take the time to visit renowned national game parks and safari camps along the way!

As I sat in Milwaukee awaiting my Chicago flight, I mentally reviewed my itinerary—a flight from Chicago to Paris, then onward to Johannesburg to retrieve the vehicle, then a drive through the Kalahari Desert that would include the countries of South Africa, Botswana,

SAFARI!

Zambia, Zimbabwe, and finally Malawi. And it didn't end there. Once the ambulance was safely delivered to Embangweni, I would return to South Africa—Cape Town specifically—where I was scheduled to meet with Archbishop Desmond Tutu. And finally, I would ride the renowned Blue Train from Cape Town to Johannesburg before returning home. Not a bad summer's vacation, eh?

First up was Paris. As Tom and I had prepared our travel itineraries, we selected Paris as the European connection point to South Africa. We did so because stopping in Paris afforded the possibility of a very pleasant reunion. A year earlier, in 1991, I had visited Dr. Margrietha ("Greet") van der Kreek, a physician who in had worked with Dr. Albert Schweitzer in the 1960s in Africa. I had visited Greet the previous year at her home in southern France and when I shared with her that I would be traveling to Africa to help deliver an ambulance to Malawi, she insisted that we stop and see her and her husband Guy in Paris. They kept a small apartment in central Paris, she said, and they'd enjoy meeting us in Paris if we were able to layover for a while.

I had shared stories with Tom about my visit with Greet the previous year, and he was not only agreeable to Greet's request, but eager to meet her. So we scheduled a 36-hour layover in Paris before continuing our journey to Johannesburg, South Africa.

After the short flight from Milwaukee, Tom and I met in Chicago's O'Hare Airport before our respective flights to Paris. Tom was booked on an Air France flight, I was on a United Airlines flight. Both of our flights arrived in Paris about 10 a.m.. Once we re-connected, we took a taxi to the Ceramic Hotel in Paris, which was just a stone's throw from the Arc de Triomphe. Greet and Guy arrived at the hotel around noon. I had brought Greet a copy of the transcripts of all our conversations I had recorded during my visit the previous year, and I brought Guy a Bill Moyer's book he had requested, *A World of Ideas*. Greet was very excited to get the transcripts of our conversations and Greet, Guy, and I enjoyed a few moments of reminiscing about last year's time together.

After a few moments at the hotel, we walked to the Metro station and rode the subway to Greet and Guy's small, but cheerfully and tastefully decorated apartment. Scattered around the apartment were family photographs and mementos and photographs of their time in Africa with Albert Schweitzer. We only stayed a few moments at their apartment and then walked a short distance to a favorite Vietnamese restaurant of theirs for lunch.

Our lunch conversation was filled with talk of Africa and Schweitzer. Tom shared with Greet and Guy that he had also met and had direct experiences with Dr. Schweitzer. Tom also spoke about how he had hitchhiked through Africa after college graduation and had stopped and volunteered for several weeks at Schweitzer's Lamborene Hospital.

Greet and Guy then recounted how they had worked with Schweitzer at Lamborene for a number of years, Greet as the hospital's chief surgeon and Guy managing construction projects for the hospital and helping procure medical supplies. As they conversed and exchanged stories, Greet, Guy, and Tom concluded that they had not been in Lamborene at the same time. It was delightful, though, to see Guy and especially Greet come alive as they spoke with someone who had also experienced Schweitzer's Lamborene as they had.

As we enjoyed our meal, there was much laughter and even some tears as we all traded travel stories and experiences. Some were humorous anecdotes, or touching and moving experiences with patients and families, and even dangerous situations we each had been in where literally life and limb were at risk.

The next morning, Greet showed me the Bible Schweitzer had given her when he had baptized her in Lamborene. As she had the previous year, she became teary-eyed as she shared what that experience had meant to her, and how precious the Bible that Schweitzer had given her was to her. We all were moved and teary-eyed as she recounted the story.

Early in the afternoon, Tom and I went with Guy and Greet to the main train station to see them off on their journey home—first to Marseille and then Tourve. With hugs and kisses all around, we bid them farewell with wishes for their safe travels home and for their upcoming trip to India. As she left, Greet said what has become such a meaningful phrase for me—"*In thoughts with you*"—a wonderful thought of presence with another, no matter how far apart the distance.

SAFARI!

From the train station Tom and I made our way back to the Ceramic Hotel, picked up our bags and went to the airport for our evening flight to Johannesburg. Our airline was Union de Transports Aeriens (UTA), which at that time was being merged into Air France. Our flight route that evening was from Paris to Brazzerville, Zaire for a short one-hour layover and then on to Johannesburg. In Brazzerville, Zairian military personnel armed with machine guns and rifles encircled our plane and I saw one or two armed military personnel in the front cabin of the aircraft. When I asked the flight attendant after we were again *en route* if the military presence was common, she responded yes, there were domestic protests occurring within the government and the government was unstable and all international flights were boarded during a layover to deter incidents involving planes or passengers.

[Author's Note: Zaire was the name of the country from 1971 to 1997; the country is now known as the Democratic Republic of the Congo, (DRC)]

Approximately seven hours after departing Brazzerville, we landed in Johannesburg. It was a 11:30 a.m. on a sunny, clear Sunday morning. We cleared customs without incident and were met in the arrivals lounge by Dr. Nico van Velden. As we piled our belongings into his car, Nico assured us that the Toyota Land Cruiser had arrived and he felt certain that we could begin our "trek" to Embangweni on Tuesday morning.

Pulling out of the airport, Nico began to share with us the current political environment in South Africa. Things in the country were still very tense despite the release of Nelson Mandela from prison almost two years earlier. The country, he said, was still openly and unashamedly operating under the policy of apartheid. South Africa was divided into four racial groups: whites, coloreds, Asians, and Africans. Under the policy of apartheid, he continued, there is a denial of civil and human rights to all peoples in South Africa who were not accepted as white. In essence, there were dual patterns of white and non-white life in South Africa.

Through the Lens of Humanity

We headed north towards Pretoria as we left the airport's parking lot. Nico indicated we were going first to drop off some packages he had brought from Malawi for his brother and sister, who both lived in Pretoria. As we turned north, Nico pointed toward a sign giving directions to Soweto. Nico stated that Soweto was likely the largest black township in South Africa. It was home to several hundred thousand black men, women, and children. Townships were a way of segregating the blacks from white urban centers, and Soweto had been the focal point of many riots and protests against apartheid, most notably in 1976 when several hundred protestors, many of them school children were killed by heavily armed police. Over the years, periodic clashes between blacks and police have continued in Soweto primarily over economic and social issues. Ironically, Nico said, the blacks in Soweto probably have better living conditions in strict material terms than most blacks in African countries outside of South Africa. Apartheid supporters have tried to use this fact to justify the continuing oppression that black South Africans endure.

In Pretoria, we had tea with Nico's brother, sister, and brother-in-law, and then continued traveling north to Rustenburg to Nico's parent's house where we were going to be housed until we departed for Malawi on Tuesday morning. Nico had been staying with his parents for a few days awaiting our arrival from the states.

Nico's parents' home was a beautiful ranch-style house in a nice area of the city. As I looked around the neighborhood, though, the common denominator of all the houses was their extensive security—all the windows and doors had fitted metal bars and the walls surrounding each house had ground-up glass and metal imbedded on the top of the walls to prohibit climbing over the top. Nico's parents stated that house robberies were unfortunately common and virtually everyone had taken similar precautions to try and discourage home invasions.

During our first night at the van Velden home, Nico laid out his proposal for our drive to Embangweni. We would leave early Tuesday and cross the border into Botswana. Once in Botswana, we'd take several days and visit several game parks before crossing into Zambia. Zambia is also known for its wildlife and Nico suggested spending a

SAFARI!

few days around the Zambia-Zimbabwe border—the location of Victoria Falls. During part of our trip, we discussed renting a plane for a fly-over of the areas we'd be in—Victoria Falls was one of the areas where this would be particularly appealing. From the Falls, we'd drive into Nkhoma and drop off Nico and spend a day at Nkhoma Hospital. Then Tom and I would drive from Nkhoma to Embangweni and present the Toyota "ambulance" to Paul and Judy Jewett and all the staff at Embangweni Hospital.

As we talked about this itinerary, Nico declared he felt we would have excellent game viewing throughout the trip. Primarily this was because the entire area was in the midst of a drought, which meant that the animals would be out looking for water. Unfortunately, the drought was also having a devastating effect on the people, particularly in Malawi, where the population was suffering severely and food and water supplies were becoming more and more scarce as the drought persisted.

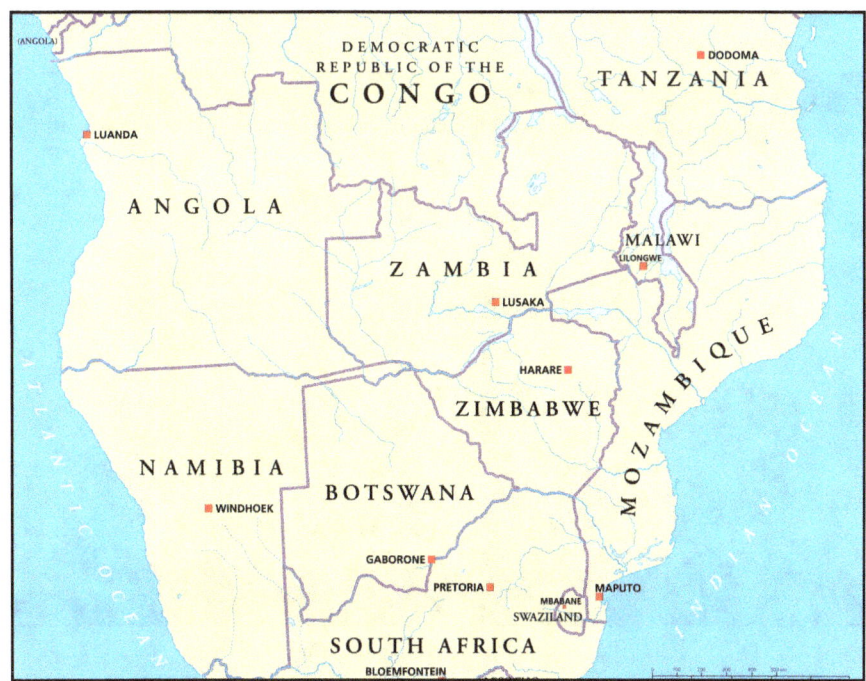

Trip Itinerary: South Africa, Botswana, Zimbabwe, Zambia, Malawi

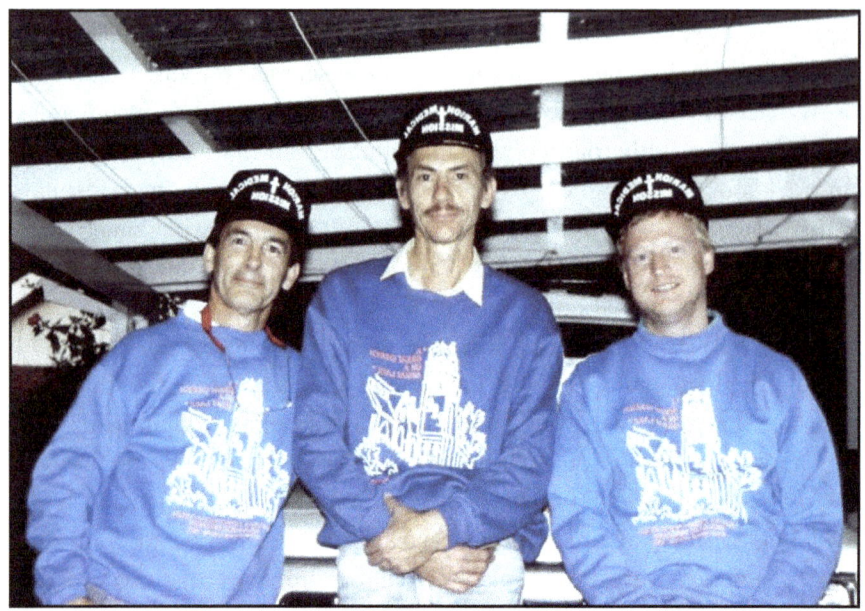

The three intrepid travelers the night before our journey began.
Left to Right: Tom Logan, Nico van Velden, Mark Anderson

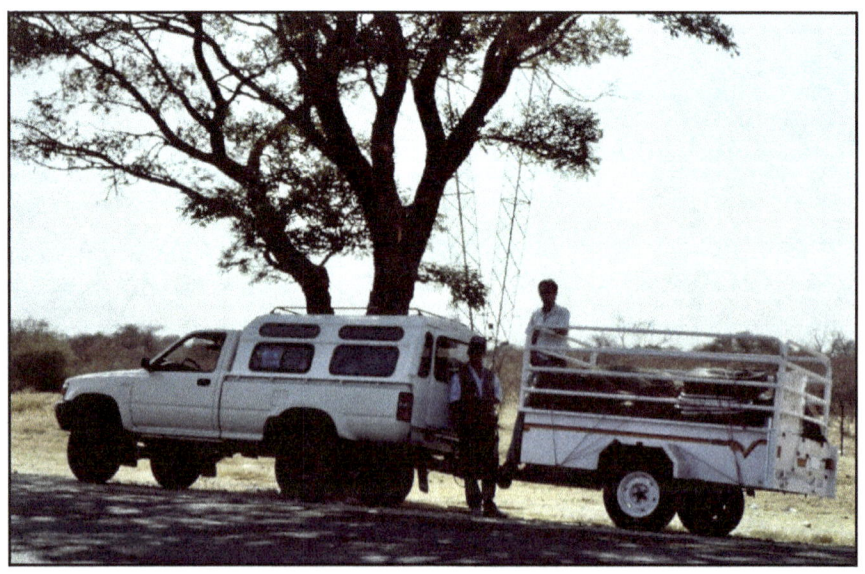

The "ambulance" loaded and ready to go!

SAFARI!

Monday, the next day, we spent the day running errands—to the bank, to the grocery store, but most importantly, to pick up the Toyota at the dealership where we'd asked it to be delivered. In addition to the Land Cruiser, we had also bought a trailer, which we had attached to the Toyota. That evening we loaded our bags, supplies, a tent, and a few spare parts for the Toyota into the trailer and targeted a 5:00 a.m. departure time for the next morning.

The next morning, we noted that the Toyota's odometer read 1027 kilometers. We were all eager to see what the reading would be in Embangweni and what adventures would befall us on the way.

Two hours after leaving the van Velden home, we reached our first destination, a South African police control point where we registered the Toyota and declared our intent to cross over into Botswana. After registering the vehicle in South Africa, we drove into Botswana and spent about an hour registering the vehicle there and clearing all our possessions through Botswanan custom processes.

A common practice at border crossings was for the border officials to have the travelers take all their possessions out their vehicles and open every bag for their inspection. This often meant the clearance process could take hours, and many times if the officials saw items they might want, they would simply confiscate those. If anyone protested, the clearance process was extended and even more items were put at risk for confiscation. Fortunately for Tom, Nico, and I, the border crossing wasn't busy when we arrived, and though the officials examined some of our bags, by and large they paid little attention to us and we cleared the crossing with relatively minimal scrutiny.

The three of us alternated driving. Once we were in Botswana during my turn at the wheel, I noted that we were running low on gas. We drove miles and miles without coming to a town and we were all getting concerned because we weren't carrying any spare gas. Finally, when it seemed we were running practically on fumes, we came to a small town with a gas station and filled up. The experience encouraged us to purchase several spare containers of gas!

Breathing a sign of relief, we continued our journey. The kilometers seemed to zip by as we headed for the small town on Nico's itinerary called Nata. Nata's claim to fame was that it was a small town midway between larger Botswanan towns. As such, it had gained notoriety as an important refueling and stop-over location before travelers headed on to more significant Botswanan cities, like Kasane or Maun, or prestigious tourist destinations such as the Chobe Game Reserve and the Okavango Basin. That was exactly our purpose in stopping as we arrived in Nata in the late afternoon. It was to be our campsite prior to entering several of Botswana's game reserves. We found a campsite/lodge, rented a four-man tent, and grilled our dinner over a campfire. No surprise—we turned in early after a long day of driving.

We were now in the Kalahari Desert and the distinctive features of the area surrounding Nata were white sands, dozens of towering termite mounds, and Mokolwane palm trees.

Literally dozens of termite mounds dotted the sandy landscape, some with massive diameters and heights approaching that of two-story buildings. Nico was our "resident" Africa expert and he told us the mounds themselves are elaborately built structures of sand, clay, wood chips, and the saliva secretions from thousands, perhaps in some cases, even millions of termites. The really large mounds might have taken as long as a hundred years to build. The mounds are like icebergs, Nico said. "You see the mound above the ground but the structure itself also can extend deep into the underground." Basically the mounds' purpose is to protect the termites from predators, provide shelter from the elements, and offer a breeding location. Along our journey, we were to come to realize that the mounds had many other useful purposes in the Kalahari Desert savannah.

Nico also explained the importance of the Mokolwene palm trees. The trees grow naturally in the savannah and they are a source not only of shade, they also produce an edible fruit. Many people eat the stems of young Mokolwene palm trees like a vegetable. The tree branches are also the key ingredients in the weaving of baskets, hats, and ornamental items we saw displayed in the tourist shop at the campsite.

We had decided to make Nata our "base camp" while we toured the Moremi and Chobe game reserves. Nico had advised that we'd

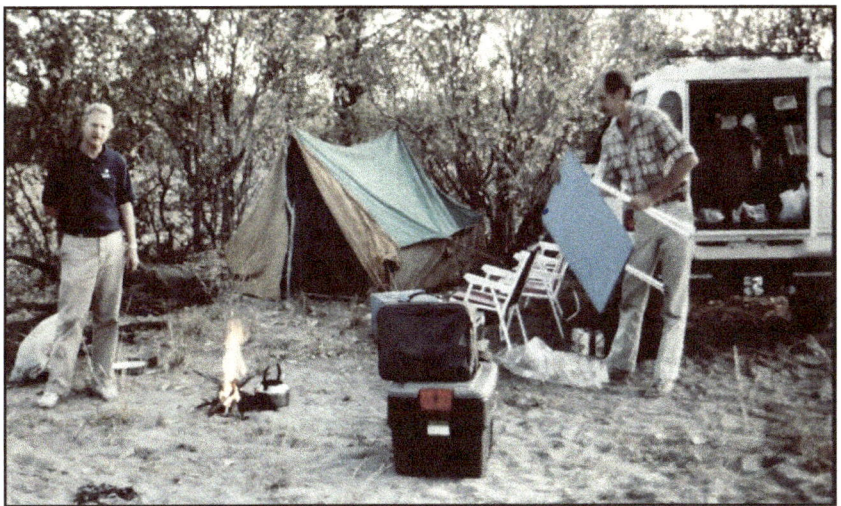
One of our several Kalahari Desert campsites

never be able to navigate the dirt and sandy roads in the game reserves towing a trailer, which would only increase our chances of getting stuck. Before turning in for the evening, we chained the trailer to a tree and completely locked everything up—and hoped and prayed it'd still be there in several days' time!

Early the next morning, we departed the Nata campsite with Nico at the wheel and drove the approximately 300 kilometers from Nata to Maun, arriving there around lunchtime. The signpost for Maun said the population was a little over 45,000. We could see that it was a town whose economy was based primarily on tourism given its proximity to several major game reserves.

Maun had a small airport and our intent had been to charter a small aircraft for an hour or so, but unfortunately, no charter flights were open until late in the afternoon. Since we hoped to drive to our next planned campsite before dark, we decided to forego the flight.

Pulling out of Maun, I was at the wheel on our way to Moremi Game Reserve, a distance of approximately 150 kilometers. While not the largest game reserve in Botswana, Moremi does possess a diversity of habitats, and consequently is inhabited by a vast array of animals including elephants, hippos, giraffes, zebras, lion, rhino, Cape buffalo, and hyenas.

About 50 kilometers from the Moremi entrance, we had a flat tire.

Quickly it became clear that there was good news and bad news. The spare tire provided with the vehicle was locked in the well beneath the Toyota's under carriage. The bad news was that the key to the lock provided by the dealer didn't unlock the lock. The good news was that we had purchased an additional spare before the trip and had it packed in the Land Cruiser, so we were able to change the tire.

After we changed the tire we continued our journey, but we realized we wouldn't reach the reserve entrance before dark, so we pitched a camp about a kilometer off the road and settled in for the night. As we ate dinner and shared stories around our campfire, we talked of the animals we had already seen—elephants, giraffe, impala, zebra, and kudo. We turned in early. Tom and Nico shared the tent, while I slept in the back of the Land Cruiser. My allergies were in full bloom and I got very little sleep.

After awakening a bit after dawn, I put on a jacket to combat the chill of the early morning and crawled out of the back of the Land Cruiser. I took in the campsite and the soft winds that were blowing and listened to the noise of the bush. I was reminded of Isak Dinesen's words from her book *Out of Africa*, "Here I am, where I ought to be."

After a few cups of coffee, it took us no time to load up our gear and began our exploration of Moremi. We entered through the south gate and paid the park fees, self-drive safari fees, and camping fees for the several nights we'd spend in the reserve.

Leaving the entrance area, we were rewarded almost immediately with views of grazing zebra and herds of impala. As we passed the Khwai River, we saw dozens of bathing hippos and numerous crocodiles sunning on the riverbank.

Late in the morning, as I was driving along one of the dusty, sandy trails, we came upon a bend in the road. As we pulled closer, the view was obscured by acacia trees and bush undergrowth. As I rounded the bend, roughly 20 yards in front of us was a herd of about ten elephants—big elephants, with a few "baby" elephants tagging alongside

SAFARI!

the larger elephants. They were just taking a leisurely morning stroll down the sandy road. The three largest elephants, which happened to be the three closest to us, all turned to face our vehicle. Each possessed an impressive pairs of tusks, snorted, and then emitted a loud trumpeting sound as they tossed their long trunks into the air and flapped their ears. Again, quite impressive!

They then stamped their massive front legs and lurched forward several yards toward us, kicking up sand and dust which swirled in the air. Then they stopped. Then they repeated it all again. And now they were only about ten yards away.

My mind flashed two brilliant thoughts: One— "This is not good." Two—"Oh, shit."

"Back up, back up, back up!" Tom and Nico were screaming.

Easier said than done. The vehicle we had bought had the steering column on the right side instead of the left which I was used to. The vehicle was stick-shift and I was attempting to quickly manipulate the gears with my left hand instead of right. I ground the gears a bit, and though the vehicle was four-wheel drive, it took a few moments for the tires to find good purchase.

Trumpeting. Ears flapping. Leg stamping. Charging. The elephants repeated their routine. Now the largest of the three was only about five yards away.

Time seemed to move in slow motion as I worked the stick shift and pushed and depressed the clutch, but finally, the gears and tires caught and in a cloud of dust of our own, we were moving backwards— slowly, but then more rapidly. The largest of the elephants continued to trumpet, dip its head and tusks up and down, and flap its ears, but it didn't charge again.

When we were about 25 yards away from the beasts, I stopped and Tom, Nico, and I watched the elephant just stare at us. Then it turned, strolled back to its two comrades and the rest of the herd, and they all leisurely resumed their morning promenade down the dusty trail.

Tom, Nico, and I looked at each other, shook our heads, and let out nervous laughs. We got out of the vehicle and watched as the elephants turned off the trail into the underbrush and after a moment or two, passed out of sight. We got back into the vehicle and continued down the trail. I let Nico take over the driving.

Over lunch and with the help of a few beers we began to laugh about the morning's experience and plotted our afternoon's excursion. We were in for another magnificent experience.

Nico was somewhat familiar with the reserve's trails due to previous visits to Moremi with his family. He suggested taking a trail that would take us out into the savannah where he thought we might have a better opportunity to see either lions or cheetahs. With Nico at the wheel, we turned onto a trail where after a short drive, we looked out over a huge, flat expanse of the savannah. We parked the Land Cruiser and peered at sand dunes, rough, yellowy shrubs, and wiry, waist-high grasses. Scattered throughout the savannah were the ubiquitous termite mounds. Way off in the distance, we saw the craggy edge of the river bank.

Nico spotted them first. About a quarter mile away on a series of rounded termite mounds that looked more like small hills were several lions. Nico started up the Toyota and we slowly edged toward the lions. As we drew closer, we saw six lionesses sitting and sunning themselves on the termite mounds. Tom and I were amazed that Nico kept driving closer and closer to them.

"They can't smell us if we're in the car," Nico explained. "And they're not scared of the vehicle as long as we don't drive directly at them or honk the horn or draw undue attention to ourselves," he added.

Nico slowly nudged the Land Cruiser up to about 20 feet from the lions. "They're all very young," Nico stated. "They're still staying together as part of a pride."

Nico turned the engine off and for the next 30 or 45 minutes, we took photos and videos of the lionesses. Their selection of the termite mounds to sit and recline on became clear. The height of the mounds provided them a better view of the savannah in all directions. They were able to see the comings and goings of other animals from their vantage point.

One of the lions was sitting erect on the mound and seemed to be observing the savannah more purposefully than the others. As I

SAFARI!

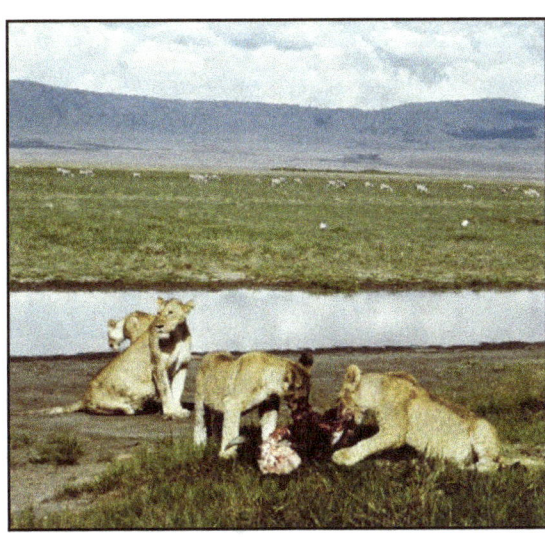

Hungry young lions "dining" on a zebra

watched, almost imperceptibly at first, the lion seemed to sit even more erect, her attention focused on a specific area. I pointed this out to Nico, and he grabbed the binoculars and followed the gaze of the lion.

"Ah," was all he said for a moment. "She's spotted something."

It took a few moments, but far off in the distance, we slowly saw movement and spotted a solitary animal moving in our direction perhaps a quarter of a mile or more away.

The lioness roused herself and moved into a crouched position, and with her movement, the other lions intuitively followed her gaze.

"I believe it is a blue sable antelope," Nico said as he peered through the binoculars.

Ever so slowly, the sable moved closer and closer. It was being cautious. It would take a few steps, stop, pause, and after a few seconds, move forward again. Nico passed the binoculars around and I could distinguish the characteristic long curved horns atop its head.

Without making a sound, the lioness on the mound slipped off the mound and crouching low in the grass around the mound, began moving slowly toward the sable. At almost the same time, the two other lionesses moved off the mound. The first lioness was moving slowly directly toward the sable, while the other two lionesses separated in

THROUGH THE LENS OF HUMANITY

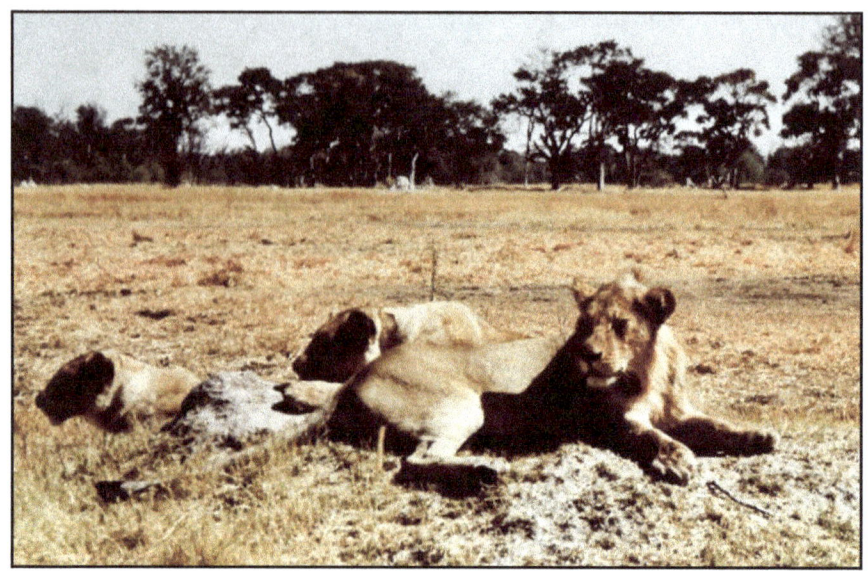

Three lionesses sunning themselves on a termite mound
when they spot movement in the distance.

soundless synchronistic harmony, one moving to the lead lion's left, the other to the right.

Seemingly oblivious to the danger ahead, the sable moved forward in its own dance-like cadence. One step, two steps, three steps, pause. One step, two steps, three steps, pause.

In the meantime, the two lions on the left and right were expanding the "trap," moving outward so that as the sable continued to move forward, it would be confronted on three sides, head on and from the left and the right.

We watched fascinated as the hunt unfolded. I was filming with my hand-held video and Tom and Nico were using the long-range lens on their cameras to record the scene.

By now, the distance between the animals had closed considerably. While cautious, the sable gave no sign of awareness of the lions' presence.

I was focused on the lead lion. She was crouched so low her movements more accurately might be described as crawling toward her prey. I could see the tension in her muscles. Our excitement and tension in the cab of the Land Cruiser was palpable.

It seemed the "hunters" were almost in position. The three lionesses that had remained near the mound were motionless and almost entirely invisible as they had quietly moved off the mound and into the wiry grass.

The sable's cadence suddenly changed. One step, two steps, pause. Head bops up and down. One step, two steps, pause. Head bobs up and down. One step, sees the lion on the left and bolts to its right and begins to bound away. The lion on the right races forward, forcing the sable to turn, only to be confronted by the lead lioness.

As we watched, it appeared the trap had been expertly sprung on the sable. Suddenly, as one of the lionesses charged forward, the sable literally bounded high in the air and over the lioness. The lioness spun herself in the air and slapped the side of the sable, almost knocking it down, but the lioness was off balance and miraculously, the sable now had an open path to run. And run it did—with three lions in pursuit. As this was happening, the three lions by the mound all charged forward but they were too far away from the action to make a difference.

With a burst of speed, the antelope was able to outrun the lionesses. After a short chase, the lions realized their continued pursuit was fruitless.

The lions moved back toward the mound. The lead lion was flicking its tail as if disgusted or angry. Then the lions returned to their vigil on the mound.

In the cab of the Toyota, we slumped back in our seats. It was clear that the three of us were disappointed that the lionesses had been unsuccessful in their hunt. Nico summed it up beautifully, though, when he simply said, "It's life and death in the Kalahari. Today for the sable, life won."

After the excitement, we continued our "self-drive" safari and drove from Moremi Game Reserve to Chobe National Park, about 30 kilometers, or roughly an hour's drive given the sandy and dusty roads. We were being vigilant as well, and sticking to the speed limit. We didn't want to be surprised again by elephants or other animals

THROUGH THE LENS OF HUMANITY

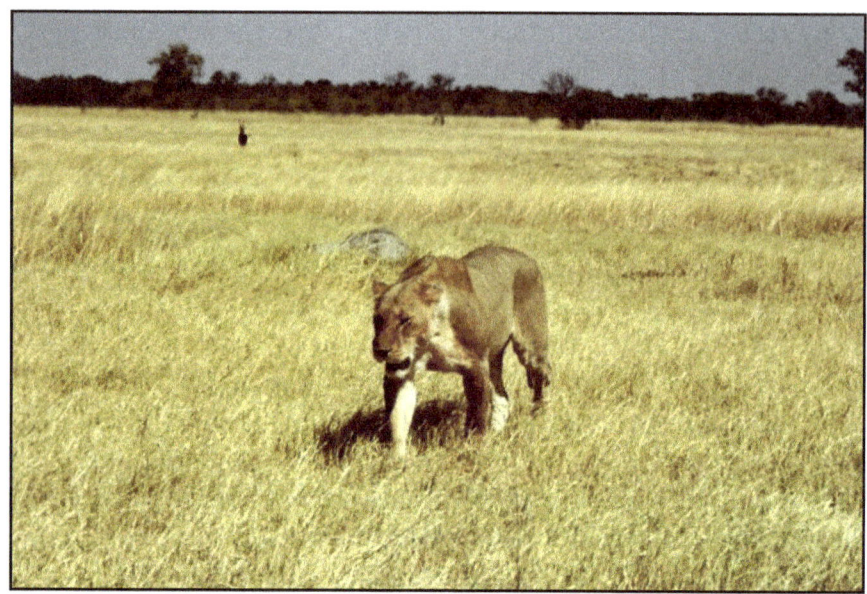

A disappointed lioness returning to the termite mound after an unsuccessful hunt. The "lucky sable" is visible in the upper left portion of the photo.

appearing suddenly out of thick bush alongside the roads. Our route was very picturesque through woodlands and past several lagoons known as the "hippo pools," named of course after the numerous hippopotami that called the ponds home.

At the Chobe entrance gate, we again paid all the necessary fees for camping and for our "self-driving" safari tour. As darkness was approaching, we decided to find a campsite and settle in for the evening. We found an area that had fire pits and what we hoped were working showers and toilets. Alas, the showers and bathroom stalls had been pushed over by elephants in their search for water.

Tom and I began putting the tent up while Nico started a campfire. All of us were aware of two very large and curious spotted hyenas lurking about 25 yards away. As we were setting up our camp, they became emboldened and trotted a little closer. Clearly they had become accustomed to seeing tourists in the campsites and their curiosity was not easily dissuaded by our efforts to shoo them away. With their distinctive barking noise that sounds like cackling laughter, they withdrew to the bush after a few moments.

Dinner that night was stew and a few South African beers that we liberated from our stash of adult beverages. Sitting around the campfire, Nico told stories of growing up in South Africa and how he ended up after medical school in Nkhoma with his wife and family. We also marveled at our experiences of the day, first with the elephants and the lions and the spectacular scenery we saw throughout the day.

Darkness was falling as we were talking and we watched as the sky turned a deep blue with violet hues as the sun set. With the darkness came a light cool breeze, and once in the darkness, we observed stars that seemed closer, brighter and more glorious than I had ever experienced them.

The darkness also brought the evening music of the Kalahari—the cackling laughter of hyenas, the long, deep reverberating roars of lions, the yelp of jackals, the deep *woohoo* of the spotted owl, and the repertoire of various calls, noises and alarms of other animals and birds.

As I lay in the back of the ambulance listening to the cacophony of animal sounds, I was aware in many ways of the hypnotic effect that not only the sounds, but the experiences of Africa, can have on people, and were certainly having on me. I thought again of Dinesen's phrase: "Here I am, where I'm ought to be." With these thoughts swirling in my brain, I drifted off to sleep.

Just before dawn we were all awakened by the shrill shrieking laughter of hyenas. They were in the midst of our camp nosing around, apparently looking for scraps of food. I heard Tom and Nico from the tent shouting to try and get them to move on, but to no avail. So I crawled into the cab of the vehicle and started honking long blasts on the horn, which did the trick. We heard the hyenas scamper off, the shrieking laugh echoing in the distance.

Since we were up, we decided to tour the Savute section of Chobe at dawn's early light and then return to camp for breakfast afterwards. Savute was in a rather remote area of Chobe and when we arrived, we were rewarded with a visual of huge herds of zebra and impala. Sprinkled in the background were a few giraffe standing on termite mounds, their necks stretched to the tops of palm trees feasting on the fruit hanging there.

We drove around Savute and noticed three giraffes in the distance strolling along the treeline. We pulled close to them, and I'm sure against every park rule, we got out of the vehicle and approached them. Surprisingly, we were ignored. The giraffes paid us almost no attention until we were within about twenty yards or so from them. And then, they simply turned and loped away, with us in hot pursuit.

I don't know what possessed us to get out and "run with the giraffes," but it was a very liberating and enjoyable feeling of freedom and connectivity with nature. Perhaps it was part of the hypnotic and mysterious feeling I had experienced the evening before—that we, along with all creatures, are part of a deeper, larger, more mysterious and vital creation than we can ever fully know or truly comprehend. For my part, there is something about Africa that had touched my soul's essence. It seems it is the nature of Africa to draw humans back to the past, to their roots, to *"Here I am, I am where I ought to be."* Perhaps here in Africa, we are all seeking to remember what remembers us.

Our afternoon was spent near the Linyanti River and Linyanti Reserve in the northern part of Chobe National Park. Game viewing was excellent here too. Near the river, we observed numerous hippos and water birds. A memorable sight was watching a crocodile snagging the hoof of a careless impala crossing the river. As the impala struggled to free itself, the crocodile propelled itself out of the water and twisted its scaly body in midair. In doing so, the crocodile landed atop the impala pushing it underwater. A few moments later, the crocodile came to the surface and slowly dragged the dead impala ashore. To paraphrase Nico's phrase of the day before: "It is life and death in the Kalahari. Today, for the impala, death won."

The roads around the river were exceptionally sandy and deep rutted, and during my time behind the wheel, we got mired in the sand. While Tom and Nico pushed, I was able to maneuver the vehicle out of the rut, but from that moment on the teasing was incessant about how my turns driving yielded trouble: charging elephants, flat tires, getting stuck in the sand. I simply responded that my driving enhanced our travel experiences.

That evening, on the way back to our camp in Chobe, we stopped at a market and bought some bread and other items for our dinner. While Nico was laying out the food items in front of the campfire and tent, he walked back towards the vehicle to get a few things. Quick as a flash, two rather large baboons who had been observing us from the trees dropped to the ground, raced over, grabbed the bread, and skipped and hopped their way back into the trees, leaving Nico helplessly yelling at them and chasing after them. But, there was really nothing we could do but laugh and be a little more vigilant.

That evening, the "music" of the Kalahari played again, this evening though, the grunting of hippos was added to the ensemble, and it was delightful to just sit and listen.

The morning before we had been awakened by hyenas. This evening, the shuddering roars of lions kept us awake and alert and seemed much closer to our camp. However, none of us felt compelled to go look to see if the lion happened to be visible.

Early the next morning, we were awakened by a pair of elephants strolling near our camp. Peeking out of the back of the ambulance where I was sleeping, I saw both elephants pausing to tear bark and leaves off trees for their breakfast. As we arose and were fixing our breakfast, we saw that the elephants hadn't been our only night visitors. One of the bags of trash we had tied up and set aside had been ripped open and its contents strewn around camp. The prime suspects were hyenas and baboons.

We had another "perfect" morning of game viewing in Chobe. This morning, we chose to stay near the river and saw many Cape buffalo and hippos. Cape buffalo are the target of many professional hunters, but these are shrewd, tough, and mean beasts.

"Cape buffalo might be the most dangerous of all animals when wounded," Nico said. "If they are not killed initially and only wounded, they will fight to the death. There are many stories of hunters wounding buffalo and then following the animal in the bush to finish the kill, only to be ambushed by a charging buffalo who lay in hiding, waiting for the hunter to appear. They are ferocious beasts."

In the river itself were dozens of hippos. Their coarse grunting sounds filled the air. We watched many animals carefully and cautiously move toward the river for a drink. A small herd of elephants appeared for a drink but then began filling their long trunks with water and spraying themselves and others with water to cool themselves. The most interesting sight were the giraffes bending their long necks and carefully splay out their front legs to get down closer to the water.

We parked the vehicle under a tree on the riverbank and ate sandwiches for lunch, all the while enjoying the sights and sounds of the Linyanti River. After lunch, we loitered for a while, just watching the animals. It seemed we were viewing a self-contained slice of creation that was oblivious to our human presence, or actually that we were unnecessary interlopers in the Kalahari dramas of life unfolding before us.

As I reflect on these scenes now, I recall the words Laurens van der Post attributed to a wise old African hunter: "Should the last man vanish from the earth tomorrow, there is not a plant, or bird, or animal who would not breathe a sigh of relief."

> [**Author's Note**: Laurens van der Post was a South African humanitarian and philosopher who was advisor and friend to British Heads of State, who wrote numerous works on Africa and the world of nature.]

After sitting a while, with a bit of sadness, we piled into the vehicle for the drive back to Nata to pick up the trailer and then resume our journey onward to Embangweni. We returned to Nata right around dusk, and to our relief, found the trailer chained to the tree as we had left it. For us, Nata was a bit of a return to civilization and we enjoyed refreshing showers and then sat down at the Nata Lodge for a delicious steak dinner. Our agenda for tomorrow was to arise early, depart Botswana, and cross the border into Zambia.

Four a.m. in the morning came early, but it was our agreed-upon departure time.

SAFARI!

Tom drove the entire distance of approximately 300 kilometers from Nata to the Botswana/Zambia border. It was a relief to get back on tar-paved but pot-hole-riddled highways. Clearing customs into Zambia posed a problem A Botswana clerk stated we didn't have the appropriate documents for the trailer and directed us to another crossing several kilometers away to fill out the required documentation. Fortunately, we were able to do so and were cleared out of Botswana without further ado. The Zambian side presented no delays, and once cleared, we traveled the 90 kilometers to Victoria Falls in short order. While Nico serviced the vehicle, cashed checks, and purchased a few items for the trip to Nkhoma, Tom and I toured the falls.

We were greatly disappointed. Two years earlier when I had visited the falls, they had been overpoweringly spectacular. At that time, the whole area around the falls seemed to thunder and roar with the rush of water cascading over the cliffs of the mile-long mountainside. A spewing, watery mist caused by the surging water literally climbed hundreds of feet into the air and hung there like a ghostly vapor as if seeking to cling to the sunlight. Sadly, that was not the case this day, as the year-long drought afflicting multiple countries within central Africa had depleted the waters of the mighty Zambezi, reducing the water flowing over the falls to a mere trickle, exposing the rocky face of the cliffs in a manner not commonly seen.

Tom and I were both happy that we had visited the falls previously and had seen it in all its majesty. But this day due to the drought, we walked briefly to the fall's main observation points and then met Nico at noon at the Musi-O-Tunga Hotel restaurant for lunch. (This was the hotel where I had stayed two years earlier).

Lusaka is the capital city of Zambia and it was our next destination. This leg of the trip was almost 400 kilometers and our hope was to arrive in Lusaka in the early evening. We were making good time until we came to a roadblock. Officials were stopping traffic and requiring all passengers to walk through a sanitation zone to ostensibly kill some sort of virus the officials were afraid was spreading. It seemed ridiculous but we complied in order to continue our journey.

Through the Lens of Humanity

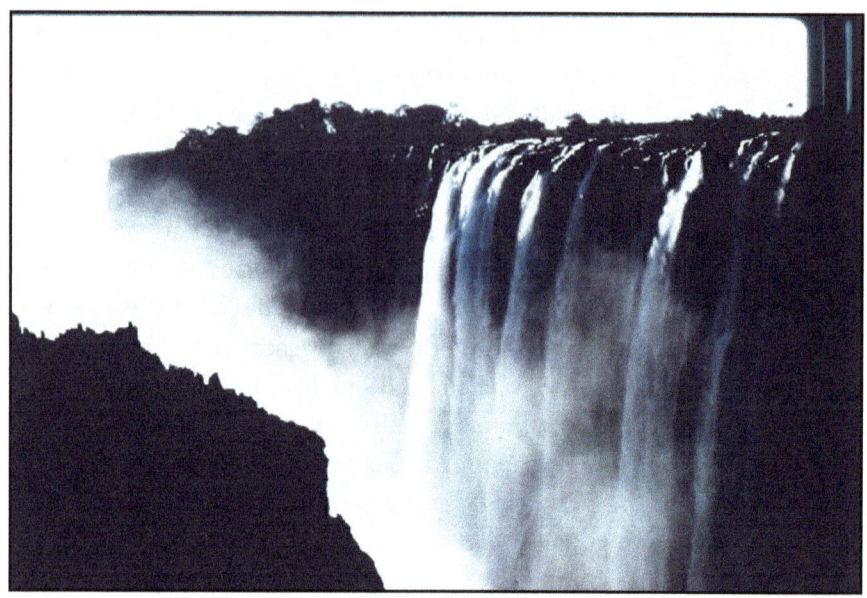

Even with reduced water flow due to drought,
Victoria Falls is still a magnificent and imposing sight.

The last 100 or so kilometers into Lusaka were on potholed roads, which slowed our progress considerably. We didn't pull into Lusaka until well after dark, about 9 p.m. Nico knew of a bible college in Lusaka that had a guest house where we intended to stay the night. Fortunately, when we got there, they not only had rooms available but were still serving dinner!

After we had settled in our rooms, the three of us joined a couple Nico knew, a pastor and his wife from the bible college, and a gentleman visiting from Zimbabwe, for dinner.

The major topic of conversation as the six of us dined on a late evening meal was the devastating drought that had plunged many countries into chaos.

"Millions of people need relief,", said the pastor. "Millions in Zambia, millions in Zimbabwe, millions in Malawi. And at the same time, the AIDS epidemic is impacting thousands of people. The police, army and governmental officials—so many of them are sick with AIDS that the whole structure of governments in these countries are at risk.

Safari!

The countries' leadership is so crippled by the AIDS epidemic, they certainly aren't able to do much to help with drought relief."

The wife of the pastor told the horrifying story of a family whose parents went to search for food at the market and food relief stations. While they were gone, their three children were so hungry they ate swill and dirt from the street and then drank water. The mud and the swill solidified within them and they suffocated from the internal pressure within their bodies and they died. When the parents came home and found their children dead, they were so distraught, they committed suicide. After her story, we silently finished our meal and somberly went to bed.

At 4:30 the next morning, we left Lusaka. Our day's objective was to drive to get across the Zambia/Malawi border and get to Nkhoma before dark, a distance of about 625 kilometers. The border crossing took less than a hour—we were pleasantly surprised at the ease of entering Malawi, and it greatly improved our timetable of making Nkhoma before dark. The rest of the drive to Nkhoma was uneventful, though every few hundred kilometers or so, we had to stop at Malawi police control-point roadblocks, but at each we were permitted to proceed without delay.

Late in the afternoon, we pulled into Nkhoma. Nico was ecstatic to be home and be reunited with his wife Muriel and their three young children. We helped Nico unload the trailer of his possessions and the medical equipment which he had picked up during his visit in South Africa.

The evening was relaxing with a lot of joy and jokes as we shared tales of our travel experiences. We tried to keep the embellishments to a minimum. During the evening, Nico placed a call to Embangweni, and while the connection was poor, he as able to discern that the Jewetts were not in Embangweni at the present time but would be returning in several days. Tom and I decided to proceed with our original intent to leave the next day for Embangweni. We hoped the Jewetts would arrive while we were there, but we had our own schedules we needed to be attentive to, so we departed the next day for Embangweni about noon.

THROUGH THE LENS OF HUMANITY

In the morning, Tom and I toured the Nkhoma Hospital with Nico and spent the morning there taking photos and talking with the medical staff. After bidding Nico farewell at the hospital, Tom and I walked through the town a little and then returned to the van Velden home and had tea and lunch with Muriel and the children. At noon, we began the 250 kilometer trip to Embangweni.

We alternated driving and Tom was behind the wheel when we reached the turnoff for Embangweni. About 5 kilometers from Embangweni we came upon about a dozen Malawians who were walking to Embangweni. We offered them a ride, which they quickly accepted; they all stood in the open-air trailer as we drove slowly toward Embangweni. Within minutes, the Malawians in the trailer began singing, shouting, and clapping. We must have been a sight as we entered Embangweni, almost like a traveling choir of sorts!

We drove to the residents' quarters, which were behind the hospital and learned that Paul and Judy Jewett would be gone for several more days. They had the unexpected opportunity to meet with some of their children in Zimbabwe, so we certainly understood their absence. It did mean, however, that neither Tom or I would actually see them this trip. While we were disappointed, we were delighted to meet some of the new medical missionaries who had arrived in Embangweni.

Foremost among these was Dr. Rebecca (Becky) Loomis. Becky was quite used to and committed to a medical missionary life—her parents had been medical missionaries to both South America and Ethiopia. Sarah McCullough was a nurse at Embangweni Hospital and she and Becky were sharing the residence that Paul and Judy lived in when I visited previously. Paul and Judy had relocated to a recently remodeled residence. Tom and I were assigned a residence that was vacant at the time and was primarily used for visitors.

We had a wonderful dinner that evening with Sarah and Becky at their home and thoroughly enjoyed the evening. Becky was a little fidgety during dinner; she had told us she was going back to the hospital for a while after dinner to continue to treat a young Malawian child who had been severely burned in a cooking fire accident. Becky indicated she loved her work but it was very stressful at times when she

SAFARI!

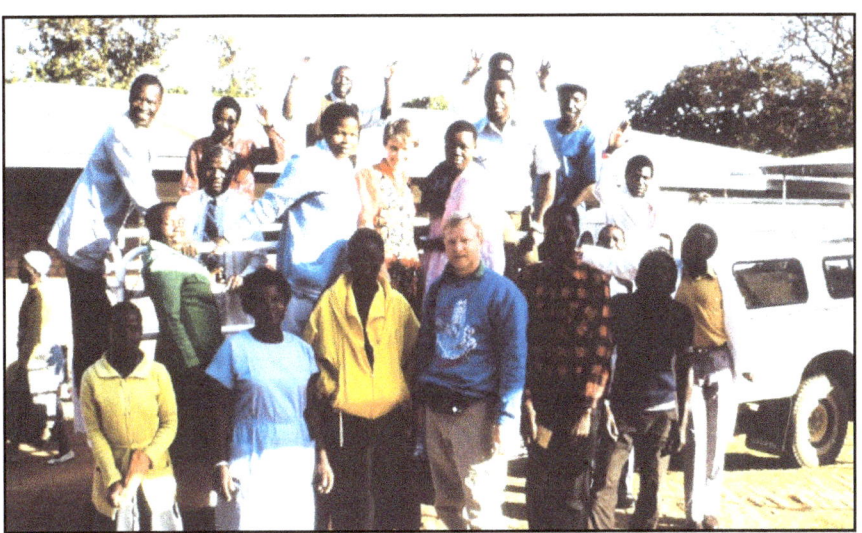

Embangweni villagers welcoming the ambulance. Dr. Rebecca (Becky) Loomis was the on-site Presbyterian Church U.S.A. medical missionary

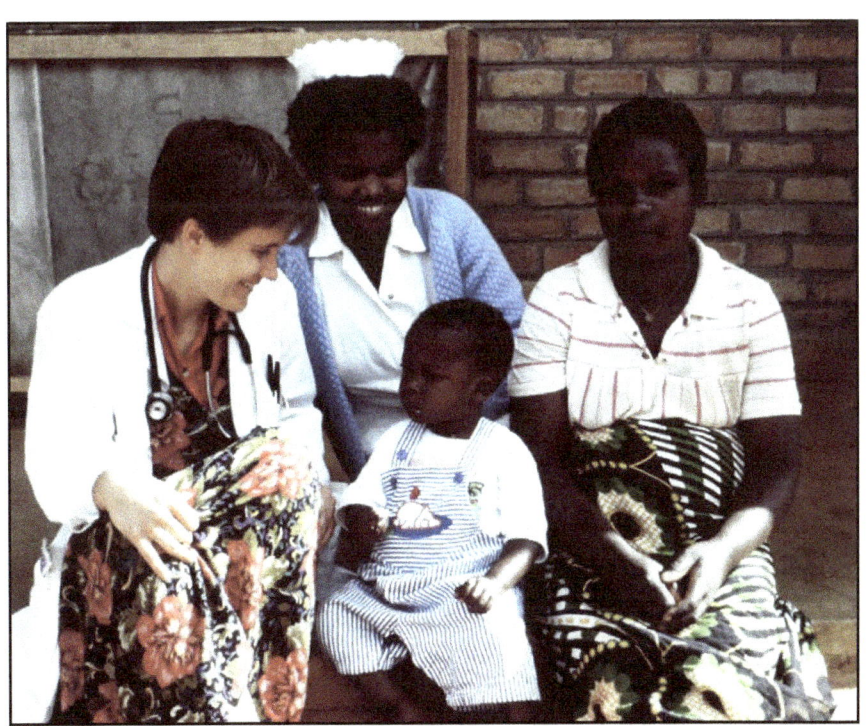

Presbyterian Medical Missionary Dr. Becky Loomis, a hospital nurse, and mom and toddler

knew she was the only physician at the hospital. And with Paul having been gone for several days, she admitted she was a little harried.

She was delighted to have American visitors and Paul had certainly briefed her regarding the ambulance!

Paul had prepared a letter for us to show governmental officials when we registered the vehicle, and part of our conversation with Becky and Sarah at dinner was all the logistics of getting the vehicle registered and doing other tasks while we were there that might be of assistance to Becky, Sarah, and the hospital staff.

The next morning we attended the 7 a.m. chapel service with Becky and Sarah. The service occurs daily and is attended by hospital staff and patients and family members if they desire. It is usually led by a hospital staff member and generally lasts about 15 minutes. This morning, though, Becky introduced Tom and me; we talked about the ambulance and how we hoped it would be utilized and useful for the hospital. Most of those in attendance had seen us arrive in the ambulance and they were all eager for us to bring it to the hospital for a dedication ceremony.

After the service, Tom and I drove the ambulance to the hospital and quickly a crowd of both staff and patients gathered. Soon the songs started, and it was quite lovely as the rich, clear voices singing *a cappella* filled the air. Tom and I both said a few words and then Becky thanked us on behalf of the hospital and the people of Embangweni. It was a wonderful feeling, realizing that just a few short months earlier, an idea had taken shape and culminated this day with the hope and promise that the lives of Malawians in Embangweni might be improved through this gift.

After a number of photos, we unloaded the footlockers of supplies and equipment we had brought with the ambulance and after we had unloaded everything Becky asked that we take another photo with the staff all standing around the ambulance or in the trailer That was the best part: the handoff to those that would use the ambulance in service of others.

In the late afternoon, we adjourned for tea and dinner, again with Becky and Sarah in their home. I was getting a little melancholy, knowing I was leaving the next day to return to South Africa and realizing how much that this journey's experience had meant to me. Bidding Becky and Sarah good bye, Tom and I left to prepare for our 5 a.m. departure the next morning.

Our early-morning departure enabled us to reach Lilongwe mid-morning. I was departing for Cape Town, South Africa, while Tom was going to remain in Malawi another couple of days to officially register the vehicle; he was scheduled to depart two days hence.

We laughed and talked about our experiences as Tom drove me to the airport. Though Tom, Nico, and I had not known each other well prior to this trip, we agreed that we had become "brothers-in-arms" along the long and dusty roads. We had shared a journey and experiences each would remember all our remaining days. He wished me well on the remainder of my journey; he knew I was heading to Cape Town for a scheduled meeting with Archbishop Desmond Tutu. We got to the airport early and had lunch, toasted our success with the ambulance delivery, and agreed to speak again when we were both again in the States.

I boarded a flight to Johannesburg at noon, and from Johannesburg, took a connecting flight to Cape Town and then a taxi to my downtown Cape Town Hotel.

I was ready and eager for the next part of this incredible journey - meeting Archbishop Tutu.

> [**Author's Note:** I arrived in Cape Town Thursday evening, August 6, 1992. I had petitioned Archbishop Tutu's office to see if I could visit with the Archbishop during my stay in Cape Town. Lavinia Browne, the Archbishop's special assistant indicated the opportunity to meet with the Archbishop could occur on Sunday, August 9th. Indeed I was able to meet the Archbishop at this time and my account of my visit on August 9th, and subsequent meetings with the Archbishop is detailed in described in the chapter entitled "Blessed are the Peacemakers."]

CHAPTER 7
THE MWANDI ROAD

In the mid-1990s, I was the Chair of the Presbytery of Milwaukee's Mission and Stewardship Committee. In the Presbyterian Church USA, a "presbytery" is an administrative body that represents all the congregations of a defined district. The Presbytery of Milwaukee in the mid-90s consisted of 50+ churches in and around the greater Milwaukee metropolitan area and several nearby communities.

At the time, one of the goals of the Mission and Stewardship Committee was to organize and coordinate an every other year overseas mission trip through which adults and youth from the various churches within the presbytery could have an opportunity to participate. Three of these presbytery-wide overseas mission trips occurred during the years I served on the committee. In 1993 a contingent of 16 individuals spent two weeks in Hungary and the Netherlands, in 1995, 24 individuals spent two weeks in the African country of Zambia, and in 1997, a group of 25 traveled to Chile for a two-week mission experience.

While each of these experiences were incredible and meaningful to the travelers involved, the 1995 journey to Mwandi, Zambia was unique in that the mission trip was to a long-established Presbyterian supported site and its participants worked alongside dedicated medical missionaries who were giving their lives in service to others.

In this chapter, I describe the origins of the 1995 Zambia trip, how it came about, the special commissioning service that was held for the group and led by Nobel Peace Prize Laureate Archbishop Desmond Tutu, the enduring effect this trip has had years later, and the long-lasting relationships between faith communities that were created.

Through the Lens of Humanity

Mwandi, Zambia is a small town located approximately 90 miles west of Livingstone in the western province of Zambia and in the mid-1990s, was home to about 8,000 members of the Lozi tribe. The village sits on a tributary of the Zambezi River, and its Lozi name means "place of fish" or "plenty of fish."

Mwandi and its surrounding area are part of the region known as Barotseland. Renowned missionary physician and explorer Dr. David Livingstone is credited with first bringing Christianity to this region, and French missionary Francois Coillard was responsible for establishing a Christian mission station, including a hospital in the village of Mwandi, in 1884.

I first heard of Mwandi, Zambia in early 1994. At the time, I was Moderator of the Presbytery of Milwaukee's Mission and Stewardship Committee. One of the presbytery's goals for mission was to actively engage in mission trips and exchanges, with an emphasis on involving the presbytery's youth. The committee had initiated an informal process of an every-other-year mission trip abroad, with the intervening year offering a domestic mission experience. In 1993, I had helped chaperone a 16-person trip to the Netherlands and Hungary, and in 1994, the committee was deliberating locations for the presbytery's 1995 mission trip.

While attending a Medical Benevolence Foundation (MBF) conference in Pittsburgh in April, 1994, I was encouraged by MBF's Executive Director to speak to Dr. Salvador de la Torre, who, with his wife Irma, were the medical missionaries in residence in Mwandi, Zambia. Riding on a shuttle bus in Pittsburgh to MBF's dinner venue, I met Dr. de la Torre and broached the subject of a mission group from Milwaukee traveling to Mwandi in the summer of 1995.

Speaking with a rich and thick Mexican accent, Salvador was immediately receptive to the idea and in short order, we had agreed upon the basic parameters for a youth-oriented mission trip. He felt they could accommodate up to 20 individuals for roughly two weeks. Both he and Irma supported and encouraged mission groups to come to

Mwandi and he mentioned it was not uncommon for groups this size to visit Mwandi one or two times a year.

Salvador suggested we use an organization called Medical Missions, which was based in Columbia, South Carolina, to assist in the preparation and planning of our mission trip. Francis Burriss, a former Presbyterian minister and founder of Medical Missions, had previously arranged travel for mission groups to Mwandi and could assist in determining travel costs for our proposed journey.

With an "invitation" from Salvador in hand, and an agreement with Francis Burriss of Medical Missions to assist with trip preparations and logistics, I was able to secure approval from the Presbytery of Milwaukee to proceed with planning for a Mwandi mission trip.

The Mission and Stewardship Committee notified churches that a mission trip to Mwandi, Zambia was being planned for summer 1995. Presbytery-wide informational sessions were held and stressed that interested individuals would be required to fill out an application and participate in an in-person interview. Estimated costs of the trip were projected to be $9,000 per participant, inclusive of all expenses except personal souvenirs. The per-person costs of the trip would be shared so that one third of the cost would be paid by the Presbytery, one third paid by the participant's home church, and one third by the participant. Applicants were asked to attach letters of recommendation from their clergy as part of the application process.

Applications were due in early fall 1994. The application itself was pretty basic; it asked for general demographic information about the individual, any potentially disqualifying health issues, which church they attended, previous participation in mission trips or church projects, and so on. The most important component of the application was a short essay by applicants describing why they wanted to go on the trip, what skills and attributes they felt they would bring to the group, and how they felt the trip would contribute to their own faith development.

Including my own, we received 24 applications. As the Mission and Stewardship Committee reviewed the applications, it was obvious the committee felt all 24 applications were worthy of selection and we felt in a bind. We didn't want to exclude anyone, but Salvador had indicated that 20 participants would stretch their accommodation space and resources. I contacted Salvador and Irma and after some negotiations, we agreed that our mission group's upper limit would be 24.

So our mission group comprised six adults and eighteen youth, eight males and sixteen females. The youngest amongst us was a 13-year-old female, the oldest a 51-year-old male. We represented 13 different congregations. Seventeen of the youth were high school students; one was a college freshman. Many of the youth had previously been active in youth-oriented presbytery projects and most knew each other prior to being selected for this mission trip. The six adults were clergy, nurses, health and business executives. Of our group of 24, only two, Bovhi Musengwa, a pastor originally from South Africa, and I, had ever been to Africa.

In January 1995, we began to meet monthly on Saturday mornings to get acquainted with one another. We began planning and coordinating fundraising activities to help generate funds to offset traveler costs and to purchase medical supplies or clothing we'd take to share with Mwandi villagers.

One Saturday, we viewed a 30-minute video of Mwandi that had been created by Medical Missions, the organization that was assisting us in our preparations for our visit. The video revealed an African village situated in a region that is relatively flat, and distinguished by lush coverings of greenery along the river near where the village is located. Sandy and dusty dirt paths lead into and through the village, which is comprised of several hundred thatched huts. Blackened and aged cooking pots and utensils and cooking fire pits decorate the sparse area between huts.

The village itself has no electricity, which is available in the adjacent medical facilities that are uniformly constructed of cement to discourage termites. Through the hard work of a decade of Presbyterian church groups primarily from the Carolinas, a series of guest houses had been erected and surround the mission hospital and clinic buildings, and which, as do the hospital and clinic, have electricity and indoor plumbing.

The Mwandi Road

The video illustrated the poverty of the villagers. The villagers are of Lozi ethnicity and are primarily semi-nomadic cattle herders and fishermen. Malaria, HIV, cholera, and other disease are widespread in the village and surrounding region.

After viewing the video, one adult traveler commented, "There is much we and others can do in Mwandi. Our work will help nudge the village another increment toward the modern world we take for granted in the United States."

Coinciding with the planning for our mission trip to Mwandi was making arrangements for Archbishop Desmond Tutu to travel to Milwaukee to participate in a series of interfaith and community events. (Please see the chapter entitled "Blessed are the Peacemakers.") The timing of both these events was propitious.

I volunteered to travel to Cape Town, South Africa, to meet with the Archbishop and his staff to help coordinate and finalize his Milwaukee agenda. In addition, going to Cape Town gave me the opportunity to add Mwandi, Zambia, to my travel itinerary. I would go and see firsthand where our mission group would be living and working and determine with Salvador and Irma de la Torre what projects would be best for our group to undertake while in Mwandi. It would also give me a chance on my return to allay any concerns the travelers or their families might have about living conditions, creature comforts, and safety issues while in Mwandi.

In early April, I flew to Cape Town and met with Archbishop Tutu and Lavinia Browne and John Allen of his staff, and we outlined and tentatively agreed on a five-day Milwaukee schedule beginning on the 12th of May. The Archbishop and his wife Leah were adding Milwaukee to the tailend of a previously planned visit to the United States. The Archbishop told me he was looking forward to visiting Milwaukee, as his colleague Bishop Patrick Matolengwe was currently serving in Milwaukee at All Saint's Cathedral, and Marcus White, son of Milwaukee's Episcopal Bishop Roger White, had spent time working in Cape Town with Tutu's staff. The Archbishop also was delighted to be involved in commissioning our mission group. "It is how we build peace and understanding among peoples," he said.

Through the Lens of Humanity

After my short but productive trip to Cape Town, I boarded a flight that took me first to Harare, Zimbabwe, and from there, on to Victoria Falls. We deplaned on the tarmac, and I and the other passengers walked through the doorway that was both the entry door into the airport, and the exit door to board aircraft. Our bags were delivered to a small dusty room and placed on a long table for passenger retrieval. It was here that I was met by Salvador and Don Holmes. Salvador introduced Don as a mission associate who helped with the daily operations of the mission site.

We tossed my bags in the back of a white Land Rover and pulled out of the airport.

"Get your passport ready," Salvador said. "We're going to have to cross the border into Zambia just down the road."

Victoria Falls is part of the boundary line between Zimbabwe and Zambia with a section of the falls in each country. The city Victoria Falls is in Zimbabwe, and shortly after departing the airport, we reached the border crossing building. We went in the door on the Zimbabwe side and Salvador and I filled out the requisite forms while Don did what was necessary for the vehicle. Then we walked a short distance to the Zambezi side and repeated the process. All in all, processing took about 20 minutes. Salvador said we got through in record time. "It can take up to an hour or more sometimes," he said.

Once we cleared the border crossing, we drove for several miles on a nice paved road toward Livingstone, Zambia, and Don, who was driving, said, "Keep your eyes open for there are often elephants and zebra in the brush alongside the road."

We didn't bother to stop in Livingstone but rather took a left at a sign that proclaimed it was the road to Sesheke. Salvador turned in his seat and said, "Now the fun begins. Mwandi is only about 90 miles from here but it'll take us about four hours to get there."

And so it is with the road to Mwandi. You head west out of Livingstone on the Sesheke Road. The road is reasonably paved for probably 40 miles or so, but the road is fatigued by age and the lack of adequate maintenance and is replete with potholes, many the size of small craters and appear unexpectedly. The road winds through a rural

THE MWANDI ROAD

area and is dotted with small clusters and enclaves of thatched huts that form small villages.

Roughly 40 miles out of Livingstone, there is a turnoff to the south to Kazungula, which is a small border town in the southern province of Zambia. Its claim to fame is that the territories of four African nations—Namibia, Zambia, Botswana, and Zimbabwe—come together at a point in the Zambezi River just outside of Kazungula.

The road changes dramatically after passing the Kazungula turnoff, becoming even more treacherous. As a matter of fact, the designation "road" becomes an exaggeration. The "road" can more accurately be described as dirt tracks created as the pavement has become so frayed and crumbly that it is easier to drive in the dirt ruts alongside the road

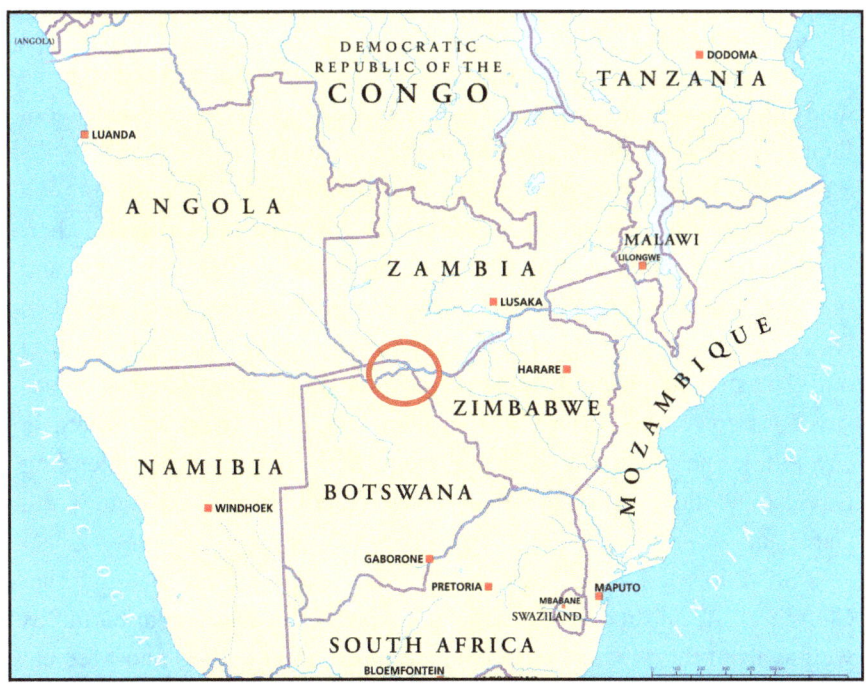

Map of Central Africa: The red circle designates the border town of Kazungula, Zambia, and the area of the Zambezi River where four countries —Namibia, Zambia, Botswana, and Zimbabwe—come together. Kazungula is approximately 40 miles from Mwandi, Zambia, and is halfway between Livingstone, Zimbabwe and Mwandi, Zambia.

and attempt to avoid the potholes and battered pavement fragments altogether.

With the exception of passing the occasional big-rig, multi-ton freight trucks—these huge, heavy rigs by the way, were clearly responsible for the destruction of the road—there was very little vehicular traffic on the road. The majority of the traffic we encountered was foot traffic.

Many of the pedestrians we saw were tribal children walking and skipping down the road, and I swear they seemed to giggle with delight each time they saw our Land Rover bounce into and out of the road's crevices. We passed adults and children driving their scrawny cattle toward their villages. We passed people riding bikes; they too were precariously navigating the dirt ruts along the road. We passed villagers clutching fishing poles and proudly displaying strings of fish. Two young children struggled to carry a huge catfish down the road and through the bush.

As Don zig-zagged the Land Rover down the road, avoiding as many potholes as he possibly could, Salvador and Don told me about themselves and what had brought them to Mwandi.

Salvador and Irma were originally from Mexico. He was a surgeon by training, Irma a surgical nurse. It was Irma who had sparked their interest in international medical missions work. After they met and married, they left Salvador's lucrative surgical practice and moved to Haiti, where they worked in a mission hospital for several years. During our visit, they had been in Mwandi for almost ten years. Their daughter AnaRosa and son Rodrico, both in their late teens, lived with them in Mwandi. AnaRosa and Rodrico were both planning on attending Davidson College, a Presbyterian-sponsored college in Davidson, North Carolina.

Salvador and Irma were mission associates of the Presbyterian Church USA, and received financial support from the denomination as well as from the Medical Benevolence Foundation (MBF) and Medical Missions.

Don and Marlene Holmes were from South Carolina and had been in Mwandi for a couple of years. They worked for Francis Burriss and Medical Missions, Inc. One of their primary center of attention was to help host the various mission groups sponsored by Medical Missions who came to Mwandi.

Don coordinated the maintenance tasks for Mwandi Hospital, including the hospital and clinic buildings, the staff residences, and the various vehicles owned by the mission hospital. Marlene assisted Irma with many of the administrative tasks of the hospital, and helped coordinate many of the humanitarian efforts, such as food relief services that the hospital received from international donors, including the Presbyterian Church, USA.

"Mwandi is a very special place," Salvador said in his heavy Mexican accent. "It has become Irma's and my home away from home. There was so much to do and build here when we first came. We've made a lot of progress. We've built a new hospital, a clinic building and even small houses for the hospital staff. But there is so much more to do. And you'll see how poor the villagers are and how devastating the disease. Malaria, dysentery, and now AIDS have taken so many. Too many of the villagers we've known over the years have died from AIDS."

"Marlene and I love it here too," piped in Don. "When the opportunity to come to Mwandi came up, we were at a time in our lives when we wanted to do something different and unique and we jumped at the chance and haven't regretted it at all!"

Salvador and Don told me that our group would be the largest they'd hosted, but they were comfortable that all would work out. After having spent a brief time with them, I was confident our group would have a magnificent and memorable experience as well.

Approximately 3½ hours from Livingstone, Don announced that the turn-off to Mwandi was just up ahead. Minutes later, we came to an intersection of sorts. To the left was the final leg of the road to Mwandi. Salvador motioned Don to pull over on the right side of the road, where a small electrical substation was located.

"Several years ago," Salvador began, "we had a team of physicians and volunteers visit from several churches in the Columbia, South Carolina area. They were appalled by the conditions in the hospital, especially the lack of electricity, and they went back to their home churches and raised over $300,000 US to pay the Zambian government to build this substation and string electrical power lines from Livingstone, and through this substation into Mwandi. Therefore, the hospital, clinic building, and the guest houses all have electricity. But not the village itself."

"Except for the chief's palace," added Don.

"Yes, the chief has lights and cable TV," Salvador said as he and Don laughed. *It is good to be the chief*, I thought.

"We pay for the electricity primarily through donations to the hospital. The villagers can't afford to pay for electricity, which is why with the exception of the chief, the village isn't on the electrical grid," said Salvador.

We made the left turn toward Mwandi and our pace slowed even further because there was no pavement on this road, just deep, sandy dirt that rose skyward in clouds as we passed.

"Mwandi is about two miles down this road," Salvador said. "This is the main (and only) entry road into the town."

After we had traveled about a mile, the pedestrian traffic of villagers really increased, and as I looked out my window, I saw a scene that instantly became an endearing and enduring memory for me of Mwandi.

A woman of indeterminate age, dressed in bright colors—a red scarf tied around her head and she wore a multi-colored *chitenge*—was singing as the walked along the roadside. [A *chitenge* is a piece of cloth that measures several yards in length that Zambian women, particularly in rural areas, wear as a garment that wraps around their body. The width of the cloth essentially covers the body from the waist to the ankles).] A white maize-filled bag was balanced perfectly on her head. She was carrying one small child on her back and holding hands with two other small children.

She was framed by a deep blue sky, the thick green foliage abutting the roadside, a touch of blue on the horizon where the Zambezi River met land, and the earth tones of the pock-marked, dusty Mwandi road.

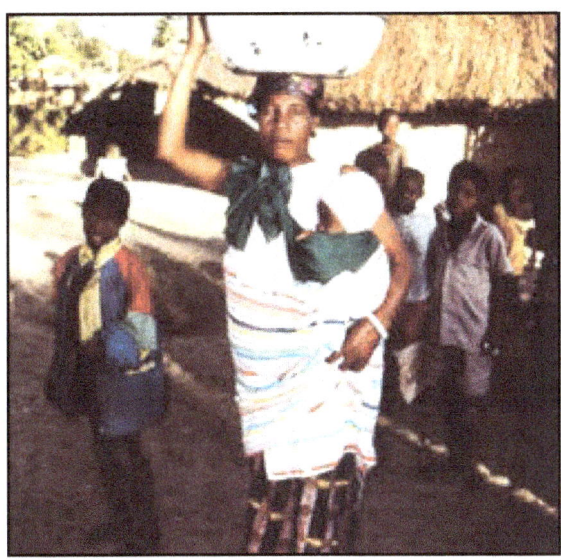

Mwandi village woman with children and maize in the basket on her head

This image immediately became my quintessential "African postcard" and I became enchanted with Mwandi before I ever set eyes on the village or the mission hospital.

As we approached the village, the first thing I saw in the distance was a tower. It was supported by four wooden posts and rose approximately 40 to 50 feet in the air. At the top was an enclosed platform with about a four-foot-high guard rail. Don called it the village lookout and I could tell immediately that it provided a bird's eye view of the village and the surrounding landscape.

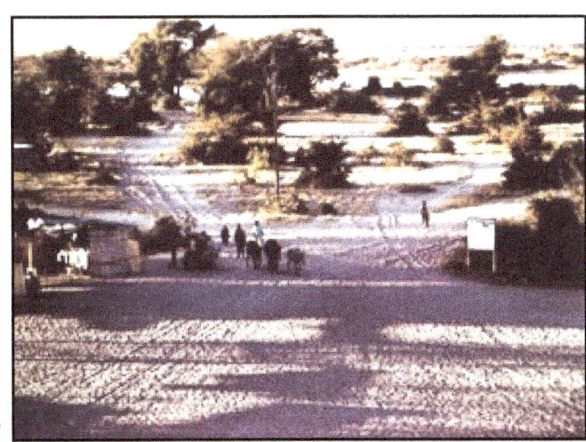

Mwandi Village viewed from atop the "Tower"

THROUGH THE LENS OF HUMANITY

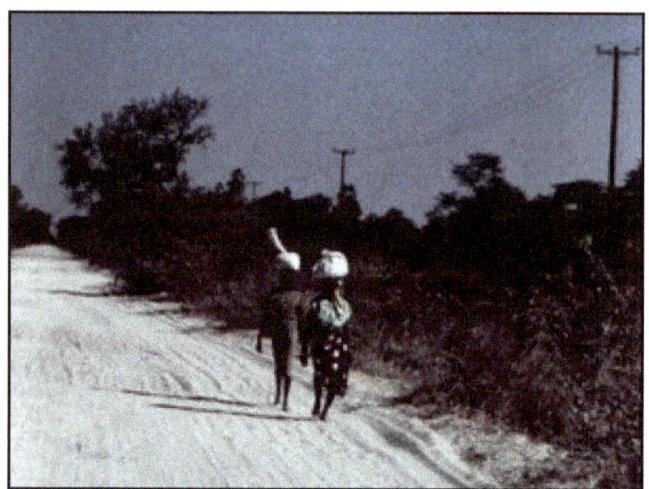

Mwandi villagers heading to Mwandi's open-air market

As we approached the "Tower," we drove through Mwandi's business district—a post office, the police station, a small trading post that served cold drinks and local food, and an open-air market. I could see villagers haggling over fish, chickens, *chitenges,* and other items. Adjacent to this area was a large field with worn and torn soccer goals at each end; children were playing in groups.

Salvador stated that we were passing by an important part of the village. He pointed out the palace of the chief, a fairly nondescript building other than its large size and yes, the electrical wiring leading into the facility.

Beside the palace was a long, narrow structure with a thatched roof but without walls. The roof was supported by a series of six or eight wooden posts above a floor that appeared to be cement.

"That is the where the *kuta* meets," explained Salvador. "The *kuta* is the tribal court and the members are the village elders and chief's councilors. They are the Lozi aristocracy; they hear and make recommendations to the chief about issues facing the tribe. This is one of the oldest types of governing structures among African tribes, going back hundreds of years."

Salvador continued. "The chief in the village is Chief InYambo Yeta. He is young and has been educated abroad as a lawyer. He has also been active in the Zambian governmental affairs in Lusaka and it is rumored he desires to have a political career within the Zambian government. He is the eldest son of the *Litunga*, the monarch of Barotseland, which is the Lozi tribe's homeland. The *Litunga* lives in the village of Lealui, which is in the lowlands and about 240 miles from Mwandi. Lealui is the traditional home for the Litunga."

I learned later that the term *Litunga* means "keeper of the earth," and that the Barostse state was founded by Queen Mbuywamwambwa over 500 years ago.

"You and your group will learn a lot about the Lozis while you're here," Salvador said. "You'll be doing projects and working with them so you'll get to know their culture and traditions very well."

Don drove slowly past the mission hospital and clinic buildings to give me a look at them, and then pulled up to the guest house where I would be staying for the next several days. I dropped off my bags then Salvador and I walked from my guest house to the mission house, where Salvador, Irma, and their children lived.

Over supper at the de la Torres, Salvador and Irma shared stories of their experiences at Mwandi. The building of the new hospital and clinic building. The multi-year project of getting electricity into the mission facilities. The building of guest houses to accommodate medical, healthcare, and church volunteers in mission to raise the health, educational, and social status of Mwandi's villagers. All this happened, they said, because they encouraged and sought the help and support of volunteers and donors to come to Mwandi and participate in its development.

We began to plan how our mission group would contribute to the continuation of Mwandi's evolution!

Thanks to Don and Salvador, the next day I toured Mwandi: the mission grounds, including the hospital and clinic; the mission learning/educational center; the primary school; *Kandiana,* a homeless center in the village for elderly "orphans," *Kalane,* an area in the village where the mentally disturbed lived; and the village itself.

The tour was extremely enlightening and gave me a perspective of what the living conditions would be like and what work assignments would be available for a group our size over the approximately 15 days we'd be in Mwandi.

That evening, Salvador, Irma, and I plotted next steps. Having seen the guest house lodgings, using age and sex determinants, we agreed on basic room accommodations. Given we had 24 people, we knew we'd have to stretch the accommodation space, but we all felt confidant we could house everyone. Irma introduced me to Lontia, a Lozi woman whom Irma over the years had taught to cook for large international groups like ours. Based on the meals I had had in Mwandi, I knew we were in good hands with "Chef" Lontia. I made arrangements with Irma to get some of our trip funding to her prior to our arrival so they could stock the cupboards with some of the food products we'd require.

It seems that one of the project staples for fundamentally unskilled mission groups is painting. And it was to this old standby that Salvador and I leaned heavily upon as we planned our projects. We decided our group would take charge of painting the exterior surfaces of all staff houses, paint the exterior of the hospital and clinic building, and selectively a few of the interior rooms of the hospital. In the village, we'd clean up the grounds and paint Kandiana, the homeless center, and Kalane, the center for the disabled and mentally challenged. Additionally, we'd have members of our group work in the mission's learning/education center and the sewing center.

My time in Mwandi was short, but it was a reassuring visit in allaying concerns about our mission trip expectations, in terms not only of creature-comfort issues for a group of 24, but also with respect to who we would be working with, how we could most meaningfully contribute to the mission in Mwandi, and how this experience would contribute to the growth and development of our participants.

I departed Mwandi convinced of the life-changing possibilities for Mwandian and Milwaukeean alike our upcoming mission trip.

As told in more detail in "Blessed are the Peacekeepers," four weeks after I returned home from Mwandi, Archbishop Tutu and his wife Leah arrived in Milwaukee and took the city by storm. For four days, his visit was a *tour de force* of appearances that challenged his audiences to be more caring, compassionate people, and to work toward a more humane and just society.

One of these appearances was on Saturday, May 13th at Immanuel Presbyterian Church, where he preached the commissioning service for the Presbytery of Milwaukee's 24 mission travelers. After the service, the Archbishop met privately with our group and encouraged each of us to participate fully in this multi-racial, multi-cultural experience.

Six weeks later, on Friday, June 23rd, our group met at Milwaukee's General Billy Mitchell Field for our departure. All 24 travelers, with families in tow, arrived early for our 4 p.m. departure. We checked in 51 pieces of luggage (24 pieces of personal luggage and 27 "action packers." The "action packers" were sturdy plastic storage bins about two feet wide, four feet wide, and ten inches deep. We packed gifts, toys, and clothing for the villagers, plus small tools like paintbrushes, toolkits for our projects. We were three bags over the limit. The airline graciously waived overage charges for weight and baggage limits when we told them our destination and trip's purpose. With hugs, kisses, and waves goodbye from family and friends, we boarded the first of several flights for the 8,000-mile-plus journey to Mwandi.

Our outbound itinerary included a planned eight-hour layover in London with two reserved dayrooms in the Gatwick Airport complex. Two of our group had made arrangements to meet with friends they knew in London, the remaining 22 of us took the Gatwick Express into Victoria Station and then the "Tube" into London's Piccadilly Circus. We landed right in the middle of a gay pride parade with huge crowds, which made moving around the area pretty difficult.

The entire group reconvened at Victoria Station at the designated time to take the Express train back to Gatwick. Except one. Jennifer, one of the youngest of the youth, had told another youth she was going to quickly go to the restroom and then rejoin the group.

We waited and waited and a couple of the adults went out looking for her, to no avail. We had her paged—no response. We called the hotel in Gatwick—no one had seen her. After searching for an hour, two of the adult travelers and I stayed at the Station, while the remaining members of the group returned to Gatwick. I kept paging her at the train station and at the hotel.

Finally and thankfully, she answered a page—at the hotel. The three of us still at the train station quickly boarded a train to Gatwick. Jennifer was apologetic, saying that she got turned around in the Station due to the crowds and then got scared. She didn't hear the pages but said she did see the signs for the return to Gatwick and thought that was her best option. I was thankful we hadn't lost someone before we even got to Africa! It had been a long day in London, so with a deep sigh of relief, my 23 traveling companions and I boarded our evening flight to Harare, Zimbabwe.

From my trip to Mwandi in April, I knew that we had a tight connection in Harare to catch our flight to Victoria Falls. The challenge we faced was landing in Harare's international terminal and having to transfer to the domestic terminal, which was a separate building several hundred yards from the international terminal. The problem was going to be retrieving our 51 bags and action packers, clearing customs in the international terminal, then transporting by hand all the bags and action packers to the domestic terminal and getting issued our tickets for the Victoria Falls flight. This is a fairly easy process in the US and Europe, but not nearly as simple in Africa, where luggage transporters are virtually nonexistent and the pace of life is slower, particularly it seems you're the ones in a hurry. We weren't aided by fact we were a little late arriving in Harare and our 2½-hour threshold was down to about an hour and 20 minutes.

Prior to this leg of the journey, I had warned the group that this transfer was going to be a challenge. We had tried to delegate tasks so that we'd navigate the transfer process quickly as possible. All was going well until one of our adult travelers got into an argument with a Zimbabwean customs official. It is never a good thing to get into an argument with a customs official whose country you're trying to enter! Fortunately, when I explained to the official why we were in Africa and what our time dilemma was, he began assisting us, not only in clearing customs, but he went with us to the domestic terminal and helped expedite our check-in process for Victoria Falls as well. As we were

The Mwandi Road

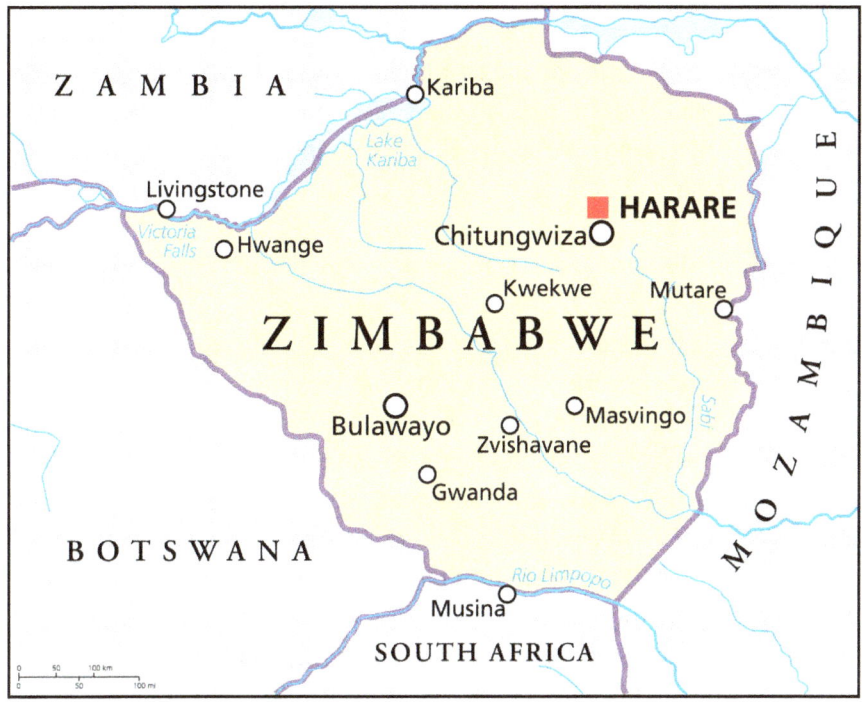

Our group landed in Harare, Zimbabwe, then flew from Harare to Victoria Falls, then on to Mwandi by land transport!

called to board our flight, I expressed my sincere thanks to him and left him with a generous tip!

An hour after departing Harare, we landed in Victoria Falls. As we deplaned, I immediately saw Don and Marlene Holmes—our welcoming committee. They were prepared and had come with a flatbed truck for all our luggage, and an air-conditioned bus they had rented to transport our group. We loaded up everything and everyone and headed for the Zambian border just outside of Livingstone. We cleared customs into Zambia without incident and were on our way to Mwandi! After 24 hours of air travel, that meant only four more hours to go—four long, dusty hours on the road to Mwandi.

We drove straight into Mwandi and to the Simba House, Mwandi mission's principal guest house. Salvador and Irma met us there and we all enjoyed a late lunch buffet prepared by Lontia. Then Salvador, Don, and I directed everyone to their rooms in the guest houses, which were all named for African animals: Simba House, Kudu House, Hippo House, Elephant House, etc. All the guest houses had electricity; most had indoor plumbing. We assigned the teenaged boys to those houses where the bath and bathrooms were adjacent to the house; they didn't seem to mind at all.

Late in the afternoon, I stopped by all the rooms to make sure everyone was okay and settling in. All were happy. Simba House was the largest of the guest houses. It had a large living room and a patio and backyard that overlooked the Zambezi River. It was our designated group gathering place. Tables were set up in the back for our meals and it was a central location among the mission facilities.

That evening, a few folks straggled back for dinner but most had already "crashed" after nearly 30 hours of travel. We agreed the next day, Monday the 26th, would be a day of acclimation and touring of the mission sites and the village.

It was a tired and rough-looking group of people that gathered for the tour Monday morning. The pleasant surprise was the breakfast of eggs, bacon, biscuits, and pancakes that Lontia had whipped up for the group. Lontia was an immediate hit; no one had expected this quality of cooking in the middle of a rustic African village!

Don and Marlene were our tour guides. They took us through the hospital, the clinic, the learning center, the primary school, and the staff houses compound. All along the way, Don and I pointed out the areas where we'll be doing painting and projects. Then we walked through the village and saw the living conditions of the Lozi. We went by Kandiana and Kalane, the centers for the abandoned elderly and mentally disturbed. I could tell our tour was an eye-opening experience for the group, particularly for the teenagers. I'm certain most had never seen the level of poverty that existed in the village. In the hospital, we saw many individuals who were afflicted with AIDS, and as I watched their faces, I could tell by their expressions that many were stunned by the sights.

Once we were in the village, I felt like our group was seen as Pied Pipers; many village children were laughing and waving and following along with us on our tour. They'd shout, "*Mukuwa, mukuwa,*" as we passed and then they'd erupt with giggles and laughter.

The Mwandi Road

Mukuwa, I had learned from my earlier visit to Mwandi, was the Lozi word/phrase for white person. The children shouting it at us as a means of greeting and friendship, and then waved and giggled. We smiled and laughed and waved back. Marlene advised us to be careful if we shared sweets with them, for they would encircle us asking for candy whenever they saw us.

We finished the tour in late morning and returned to Simba House for lunch. Afterwards, we divided ourselves into three work groups, sorted out the painting supplies that Don had prepared for us, and returned to the staff house area and began painting the houses.

We quickly slipped into a work pattern. Breakfast in the morning, paint till noon, stop for lunch, paint till about 3 or 4 p.m. in the afternoon. Some people took breaks from painting so they could visit the primary school or the learning center or observe the activities in the hospital and clinic.

Stopping work around 3 or 4 p.m. gave the youth a chance to spend time with young people from the village and explore each other's cultures. A favorite activity was for our youth to play soccer with village youth in the big field next to the market and the chief's palace.

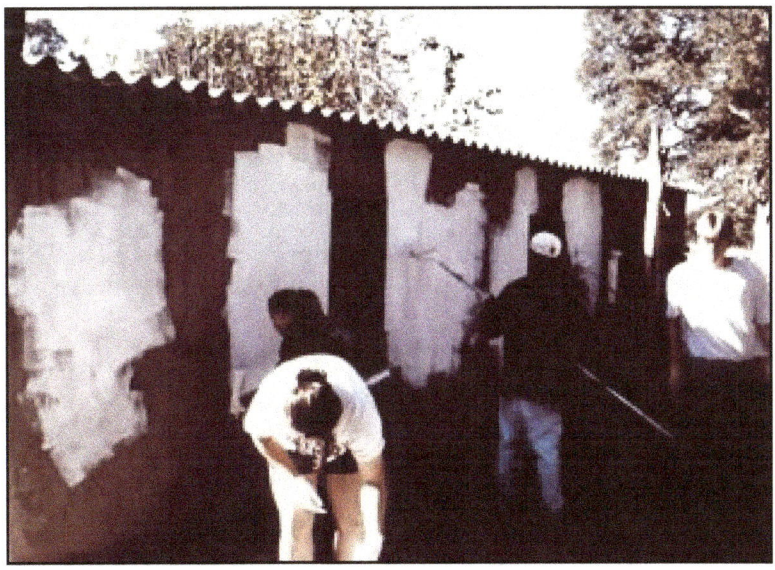

Mission youth painting Kandiana housing units

Salvador had suggested we bring soccer balls and soccer goals with us when we came as gifts from our youth to the village.

The village youth were quite good, and we had a number of youth who played in soccer leagues so both sides really enjoyed the competition. Bridget, one of the youth on the US side, was an exceptional player and the Lozi youth knew she was the best US player. The Lozi players kept teasing her and her teammates that they'd trade three cows for her if she'd stay and be on their team.

The daily games drew spectators from the village. They matches were always fun to watch and the youth from both sides really enjoyed the competition and camaraderie. The chief would occasionally come out of the palace to watch. We learned it was highly unusual for a chief to appear at such an event. His presence added to the rapport our group had developed with the village.

The church in the village was affiliated with the United Church of Mwandi. Several nights a week, the church choir would gather and rehearse. Their rehearsals were magnets for our youth and adults, many of whom were in their own church choirs. We were all mesmerized by the Mwandi choir. Often, they simply sang *a cappella*, and the rich, harmonic tones of their voices were truly glorious to hear. One Sunday while we were there, our group sang at the worship service and then the combined choirs together sang songs they had prepared for the service.

The chief supported the church and Christianity within the tribe, and we heard he was a frequent attendee on Sundays to indicate his personal support for the church and the mission. Two of our adult group members were ordained clergy and each had been asked to preach a Sunday service while we were in the village. The chief attended both of these services and he encouraged the village elders to come as well. I was sitting with Salvador and Irma one Sunday when the chief arrived; they both chuckled, noting that he had also arrived with three of his wives. "A bit of culture clash intrigue," Irma said laughingly.

Many evenings either before or after dinner, many of us would walk to the trading post, a little wooden shed-like building that sold sodas and a few snack items. The trading post was on the entry road into Mwandi near the tower. The tower was a popular place to climb up

The Mwandi Road

in the late afternoon and take pictures of the sun setting over the village, or later in the evening to stargaze at the clear African sky.

While our trip wasn't always idyllic, we did try to treat the trip as the adventure that it was. As such, the annoyances, missteps, and mishaps that occurred were viewed as obstacles to overcome and endure. Teenagers tend to pose their own special set of challenges. We had a few individuals who felt a little full of themselves and rebellious outside the jurisdiction of their parents' home; they didn't feel obliged to follow the rules when it didn't meet their purposes.

Smoking, non-conformity with dress codes, and laziness were the primary obstacles we encountered. Prior to the trip, all had concurred that this would be a non-smoking venture. Once we arrived in Mwandi, Irma asked that members of our group not smoke even though smoking was pervasive in the local culture. One of our oldest teenagers declared that she had been smoking for years, was 18, and therefore an adult; she didn't see why she couldn't smoke. She admitted her parents didn't let her smoke at home, but, "she wasn't at home." Peer pressure handled this obstacle pretty quickly; her roommates told her she couldn't stay in the room with them if she smoked, even if she smoked outside. *Touché!*

Peer pressure handled another obstacle as well when some of the teenaged girls were felt to be dressed in too provocative a fashion. Several of the adults had expressed concerns about the dress of one or two individuals specifically. Each evening after dinner, we met as a group for an evening devotional and to discuss any "concerns of the group." One of the adults brought up the issue and murmurs of "we didn't mean to be offensive" came from several of the young women. That was the end of that.

I found the resolution to the situation of laziness to be a little humorous. The largest and one of the older male teenagers was a football player at his local high school. Unfortunately, in his work group, he was slow, un-energetic, lacked initiative, and in general wasn't contributing much to the work effort. I noticed it and Bob Timberlake, one of the adults on the trip, noticed it as well. Bob was a good friend and colleague from Children's Hospital who had previously served as a Presbyterian minister. He had also been a starting quarterback for the Michigan Wolverines in the 1960s and had even secured a few votes in the Heisman Trophy balloting his senior year. He had played a year of professional football for the New York Giants.

Bob told me he'd handle the situation. One morning, I saw Bob drape his arm around the teen's shoulder and pull the young man aside. I watched Bob speaking softly to the teen, who almost immediately started nodding his head vigorously. Shortly thereafter, they parted ways. I walked up to Bob and asked, "What did you say to him?"

"I told him that several of us didn't think he was pulling his weight and that he should step it up—otherwise we'd kick his ass."

I couldn't help but laugh, and think how the kid must have been embarrassed by having the former quarterback pull him aside. Let's just say his productivity and enthusiasm improved markedly for the remainder of the mission!

Two of our youth, Abby and Charlotte, had birthdays while we were in Mwandi. Marlene made sure there was a large cake for them both as a surprise at dinner one evening.

On the 4th of July, we were all thrilled and amazed when Lontia surprised us with a lunch of hamburgers, hotdogs, French fries, and cupcakes with red, white, and blue icing.

We were taking the 4th off from our labors, and after lunch, Don took groups out on the Zambezi River in a small power boat.

The area of the Zambezi River around Mwandi is world-renowned for its tigerfish. Tigerfish are prized as a game fish and are distinguished by their large, razor-sharp, saber-like teeth. African tigerfish are very aggressive predators, and Salvador shared with us that the tigerish is the first freshwater fish to attack and catch birds in flight by leaping out of the water. During our time in Mwandi, several of the group caught tigerfish, but for us, it was a catch-and-release exercise. A professional fisherman would have paid a pretty penny to have caught a one of these fierce fish!

All of us grew to love this remote village and mission hospital. We certainly came to appreciate the ten years of self-sacrifice that Dr. Salvador de la Torre and Irma had committed to building not only a hospital, but a better environment medically, educationally, and economically for this village.

A highlight for our group was going on hospital rounds with Salvador. The day I rounded with him, we saw patients who were hospitalized because of accidents. We saw a patient suffering from syphilis and one who had fallen into a fire because he suffered from epilepsy and had lost an arm as a consequence of the severe burns. This same man had been rejected by his family because the village witch doctor had told the family he was possessed by evil spirits. And every day, both in and out of the hospital, we saw patients suffering from AIDS and malaria. Millions of Africans die each year from AIDS and malaria and Mwandi village had lost hundreds, Salvador said, many of whom they knew well.

As I followed Salvador around that day, I recalled that Irma had told me that Salvador had contracted malaria seven times that year and one of those times, he had to be evacuated to South Africa, where he spent several days in an intensive-care ward. I thought about how both Salvador and Irma were here delivering their skills and compassion to others with little concern for their own health and well-being. I admired how they had entered into solidarity with that humanity that so many turn their backs on. And I thought of the remarkable gift and blessing our group was receiving through their example of servant leadership and self-sacrifice.

The trip began to draw closer to an end, the sense of sadness was palpable within the youth in our group. They had really bonded with each other and with many of the village youth. A couple of nights before we were to depart, all 18 of the youth brought their sleeping bags to Simba House for a sleepover party. Lontia and Irma prepared pizzas for them and the US youth invited several of the youth from the village to come and share dinner.

The night before we were scheduled to leave, Don and Marlene hosted a dinner at their house for our group, Salvador and Irma, and members of Don's Lozi work group with whom we had toiled the previous two weeks. At the dinner, all of the female members of our group wore *chitenges* as a symbol of solidarity with our Lozi friends.

THROUGH THE LENS OF HUMANITY

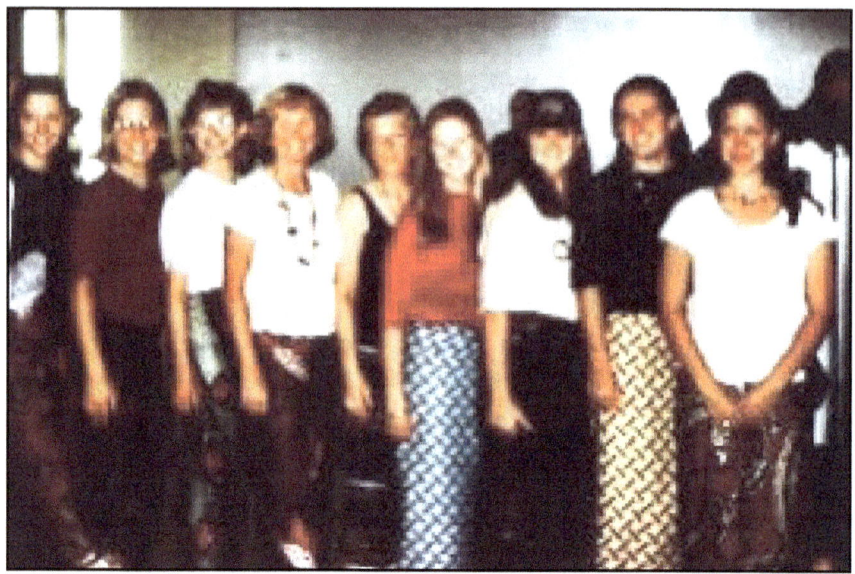

Female Mission Group members wearing their chitenges at farewell party

As we ate, we realized how much work we had actually completed—not only had we painted all the staff houses, Kandiana, Kalane, and portions of the hospital and clinic building, we are also laid a parquet floor in the church and varnished the church benches/pews. Some members of our group had worked in the primary school and helped in the teaching/learning center. Our youth had formed a choir and participated in the Sunday worship services singing special anthems and hymns. Two of our members had preached the sermons on Sundays and several of the youth had led morning devotionals held for the hospital staff.

As we reviewed all we had done, spontaneously youth members of our group started sharing how much the trip had meant to them personally. They thanked Salvador, Irma, Don, Marlene, Lontia, me and all the adult members for the opportunity to be part of remarkable experience. There was much laughter and many tears when it dawned on us how much Mwandi and the Lozi tribe had impacted our lives.

The next morning we prepared for our departure. Everyone in our group in their own way took the time to visit the hospital, the clinic, the school, and the village to see and say goodbye to new-found friends. As

THE MWANDI ROAD

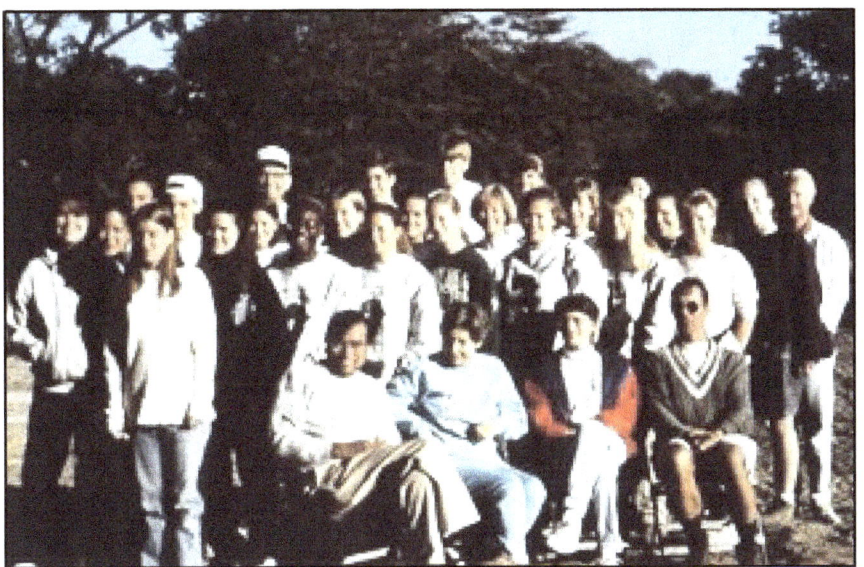

Milwaukee Presbytery's Mission group as we prepare to depart Mwandi
Seated in the front (L to R) Salvador de la Torre, Irma de la Torre,
Marlene Holmes, Don Holmes

they had throughout our visit, the young children of the village shouted, "*Mukuwa, mukuwa!*" as we gathered next to the bus Don had arranged for our departure. We didn't require the flatbed truck this time because we were donating the action backers to the mission station. All of our belongings fit into the bus.

In small groups, everyone climbed the tower for one more look and photo opportunity of the village and river before we left. It was a very emotional departure as we said goodbye to Salvador, Irma and Lontia. Don and Marlene Holmes were going with us. We were going from Mwandi to Chobe Game Park in Botswana for a couple of days before flying back to the United States. The Holmes were taking some R-and-R days at the game park with us, and then they were taking us back through customs at the border for our flight out of Victoria Falls, Zimbabwe.

As our bus pulled away, the village children followed us shouting, "*mukuwa!*" and clapping and singing. At the intersection with the Seskeke Road, the bus turned right and we headed back down the road toward Livingstone. At the Kazungula intersection, we turned right in the direction of the Botswana border. Shortly after the turnoff, we had to cross the river in a car/truck ferry to get into Botswana, and then about an hour's drive later, we reached Chobe Game Park.

Chobe Game Park is located within Chobe National Park and borders four countries: Botswana, Zimbabwe, Zambia, and Namibia. It is known for its elephant and zebra herds, and for lion prides and birdlife. We arrived at the game park in time for lunch. The lodge was situated on the banks of the Chobe River and was a thatched-roof, multi-story structure whose expansive patio overlooked the river. We checked into our rooms (we had 12 rooms, two travelers per room) and then returned to the patio, where a beautiful buffet had been set for us.

At lunch, many commented on their lodgings—clean rooms with electricity and hot running water with stunning views of the Chobe River and surrounding African landscape. After lunch, our entire group took an afternoon boat ride on the Chobe River (in several Chobe Park

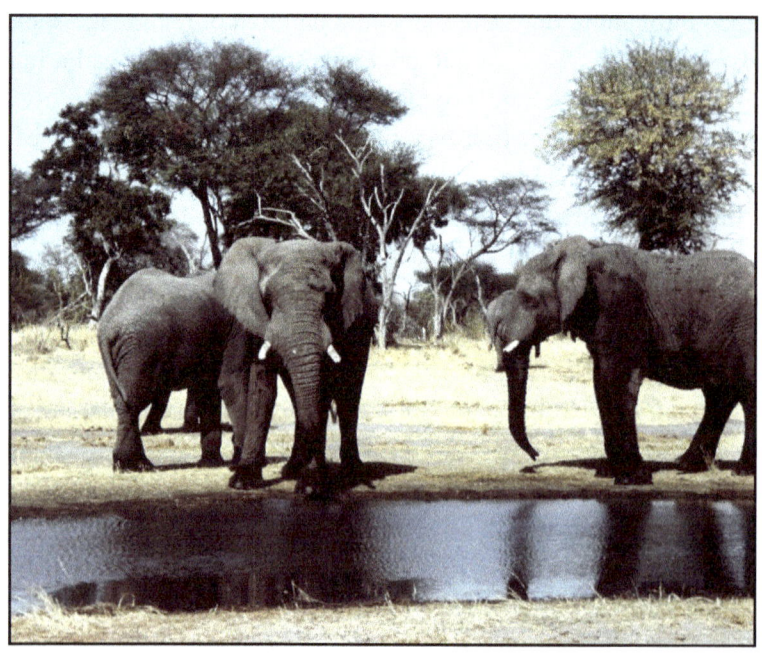

Thirsty elephants in Chobe Game Park, Botswana.

tour boats. The river was flush with hippos, crocodiles, and elephants, all bathing and cavorting in the water.

Early the next morning, we divided into four groups of six, took guided game drives through the park in Range Rovers, and returned to the lodge at noon for lunch. It was a relaxing morning and most of the group reported getting great photos. One group told excitedly about being charged by a huge, angry elephant. It brought back memories and a chuckle from my own experience with a charging elephant a few years earlier in Moremi Game Reserve, which is also in Botswana.

As we finished lunch, I think we were all bracing ourselves for the 24-plus-hour return flights to Milwaukee. We loaded up the bus and headed to Victoria Falls and the airport!

For weeks after our return, I heard comments from the parents of the youth on the trip and the pastors of the churches our travelers attended. The stories told by the volunteers brought the excitement and vibrancy of the trip to their local churches.

There is no doubt that this experience enriched not just the participant travelers but also their families and churches with whom they shared their stories. I believe the trip's travelers brought back a global perspective on the issues of faith, hope and justice. One of the youth, Bridget Salisbury from Immanuel Presbyterian Church said it well, "Mwandi in Zambia is a magical desert land full of exquisite beauty and warm-hearted citizens. The overall learning experience was so much more than us trying to improve the lives of the people of Mwandi. The people of Mwandi helped to open our eyes and realize that, what we take for granted, they can only pray for."

Listening to the youth I was reminded of the following phrase from the book *The Road Within*:

> Some journeys are destined to alter our lives irrevocably. Many of us have had experiences on the road which have changed our view of the world in ways we have difficulty articulating on our return home. We come back from travel changed, awareness broadened, consciousness clearer—a feeling of being closer to who we really are ....
> —Sean O'Reilly, James O'Reilly, and Tim O'Reilly

THROUGH THE LENS OF HUMANITY

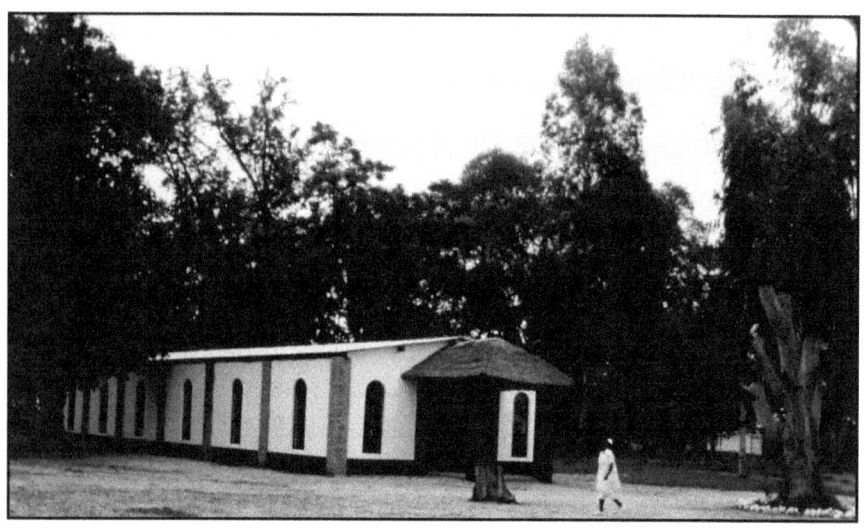

Mwandi's Bethel Chapel

There is no doubt that all 24 of us came back from Mwandi changed, our awareness broadened, our consciousnesses clearer, with a feeling of being who we really are and can be.

Returning to Milwaukee from our marvelous journey to Mwandi didn't spell the end of my, and Immanuel Presbyterian Church's relationship, with Mwandi and the de la Torres. Indeed, our journey together had only just begun.

One evening while we were in Mwandi, Irma and I spoke about her and Salvador's vision for the community. I keep a journal when I travel. Here is what Irma said to me:

> "Salvador and I have been in Mwandi almost 10 years. Life is hard here—the people are so poor and have little or no money. There is so much here that can cause harm, and what brings so many to the hospital is a hope that we can help.
> We help so many, but some we can't help..... Sometimes the best we can do is instill hope, the hope of God's presence, so that sorrow, despair, and even hatred have no soil in which to take root.

> I dream of a chapel for the staff and for patients and their families, and for the village that lets them know that God is in this place, and is with them no matter what. I think a chapel would complete the mission station - I want to have it right next to the mission hospital. I want the chapel to be named the "Bethel Chapel.""

Irma's desire to name the chapel Bethel Chapel stems from the famous biblical story in Genesis of Jacob's fleeing from the rage of his brother Esau and stopping for the night at the town of Bethel (formerly named Luz). Using a stone as a pillow, Jacob went to sleep and dreamed of a stairway to heaven, with angels ascending and descending on it, and the Lord standing above it (Genesis 28:10-22). In this vision, God made a promise to Jacob—that he and his children would someday own the land he was sleeping on. After Jacob awoke, he took the stone he had slept on and set it up as a monument, and he named the place where he had slept Bethel, which means "House of God."

In 1997, Immanuel Presbyterian Church contributed funding of $45,000 toward the construction of Irma's vision of a chapel in Mwandi adjacent to the mission hospital. Construction of the chapel began in 1998 and was fully completed in 1999. Services are held every morning for hospital staff, families of patients who are in the hospital, and for all who wish to attend.

Irma's vision of a Bethel Chapel is a reality now, and the chapel now stands, adjacent to the hospital as a symbol of God's presence and of God's mercy, comfort, compassion and love. It is a 'House of God' for the people of Mwandi.

The chapel was being constructed at the same time as a new 100-bed mission hospital. Medical Missions, Inc., was helping facilitate the construction projects, and Francis Burriss,, CEO of Medical Missions, was scheduling a dedication ceremony for both the hospital and the chapel for summer of 1998. Nine individuals from Immanuel, including myself, were designated to represent Immanuel at the dedication ceremony.

As we planned our trip, little did any of us realize how our ceremony would intertwine with a centuries-old traditional Lozi ceremony and celebration.

THROUGH THE LENS OF HUMANITY

For hundreds of years, the traditional ceremony of "Kuomboka," which in the Lozi language means "to move out of the water" has taken place annually. The ceremony marks the movement of the Lozi king (the *Litunga*) at the end of the rainy season from his compound at Lealui in the floodplains of the Zambezi River to Limulunga on higher ground. The Litunga travels on a large barge called the *Nalikwanda* ("the people's boat"), which is painted white. On the barge is a replica of an elephant, which is the insignia of the Litunga. The barge is large—it carries the Litunga, his attendants and musicians, and over 100 paddlers. Usually the date of the Litunga's departure is kept secret, but it is typically in late March or early April.

The dedication ceremonies for the chapel and the hospital were being planned for June and Chief Yeta of Mwandi indicated he'd inquire if the Litunga (who was his father) would come to Mwandi after the Kuomboka ceremony when he was in residence in Limulinga and participate in the hospital and chapel dedications.

When our travel group of nine arrived in Mwandi in early June, the villagers were all excited that their king would be visiting their village. Day by day, the village swelled as more and more Lozi flowed into the village in anticipation of the Litunga's arrival.

In the meantime, our group of nine, along with a group of ten from South Carolina, and a delegation of students from Davidson College in North Carolina led by Irma and Salvador's AnaRosa, spent our days preparing for the dedications.

For our group that meant painting and working on the chapel, which though constructed, had not yet been painted nor had a floor been laid inside. The South Carolina group took charge of painting the hospital and the landscaping around it.

Our group of nine was comprised of all adults; the youngest was college-aged and the daughter of one of our travelers. Our group knew each other as members of the same church, and we meshed well amongst ourselves and with the South Carolina group. The Davidson students were bright and enthusiastic and reminded me of Milwaukee's youth group of a few years previously.

THE MWANDI ROAD

The day of the dedication arrived to much fanfare. The drumming heralding the arrival of the Litunga early in the morning. The Maoma drums are the royal drums, made from trees at the base and the skins stretched over the drum's hollow mouth. Their sound is deep and powerful; the intent is to imitate the roar of the lion to instill fear among enemies and inspire courage within the Lozi.

The Lozi gathered by the hundreds to catch a glimpse of their Litunga. The women were wearing their colorful *chitenges,* ululating high-pitched sounds as the Litunga passed. The ululations were signs of acknowledgment and approval and spread throughout the crowd to proclaim their affection for the Litunga. The crowd swelled as the Litunga walked through the village and strolled toward the hospital and chapel where the dedications would take place.

The Litunga was a tall, slender man of perhaps 70 years with a regal bearing and an erect gait. He was bespectacled, and wore a brown

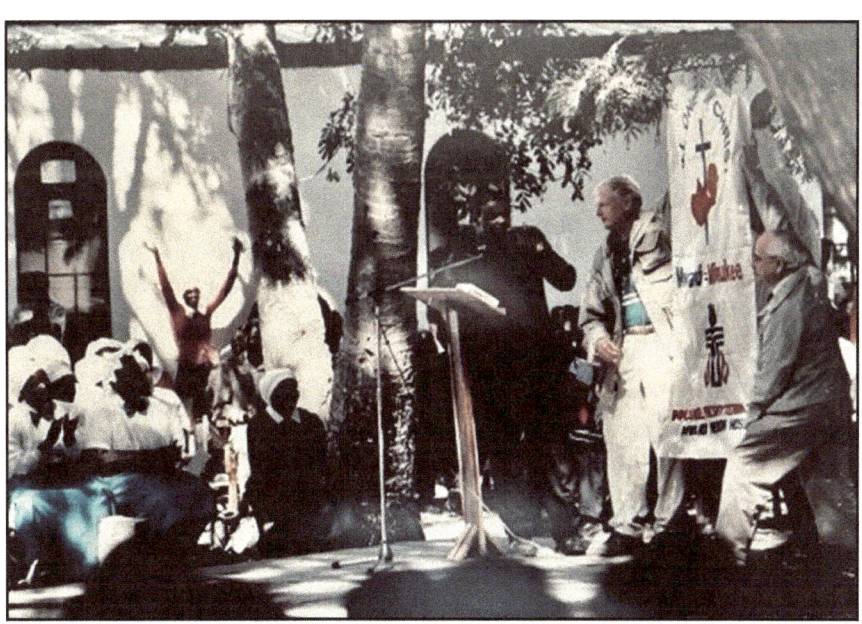

The Mwandi chapel and hospital dedication ceremony, June 1998.
At the podium is a United Church of Zambia clergyman. I am standing and holding a banner proclaiming the friendship between Mwandi and Milwaukee.
Charles Newsome from South Carolina is sitting and holding the banner

sport coat and tie and a butternut-colored beret. He was followed by his *indunas,* his tribal counselors. He nodded and smiled at his tribe and moved toward the stage where those participating in the festivities were already waiting.

The Master of Ceremonies for the event was Charles Newsome, who had had a multi-year relationship with Mwandi through his church in South Carolina. Charles was largely responsible for helping negotiate the provision of electricity for the mission compound and had also helped with fundraising for the hospital.

At the dedication ceremony, several individuals spoke, including me. I spoke relative to Immanuel's sponsorship of the chapel, while Charles, Francis Burriss, and Salvador spoke about the hospital. There were also dignitaries from the United Church of Zambia, and even a representative from the global mission office of the Presbyterian Church, USA.

Finally, the Litunga rose to speak and the crowd erupted again with ululating, shouts, singing, clapping and stomping of feet. This went on for at least ten minutes before the crowd quieted and the Litunga was able to speak. In a strong, deep, and rich voice, he spoke in Lozi with his son, the chief, translating his comments into English for those of from the US. He praised the work and Salvador and Irma and all those associated with the hospital. He thanked all from the US who had contributed to the development of the mission. He encouraged the continued friendship between the Lozis, particularly those in Mwandi and the peoples of the US.

When the Litunga finished speaking, the Lozis started clapping and singing. The Litunga stood for several moments before his adoring tribe, then turned, spoke with everyone on the stage and then with the chief and the indunas, slowly started walking back toward the village followed by the enormous crowd of Lozis.

The US delegations from Milwaukee and South Carolina, adjourned to the Simba House, where Lontia had prepared a luncheon buffet. Over the delicious food, we remarked what a historic event the Litunga's visit had been for the village and the dedication. His appearance at public gatherings is extremely rare, as are appearances in front of such a large contingent of his tribe. The fact that he had appeared reflected his support and appreciation for all the magnificent work that the mission had done for the Lozi tribe.

Our group from Immanuel stayed in Mwandi for several more days working to complete the chapel and make it operational. We departed with a sense of accomplishment and also with a sense of ongoing commitment to Mwandi. I for one knew I would be returning frequently to this very special and sacred place.

Tragedy on The Mwandi Road

I have met many incredible and wonderful people in my travels abroad. One of these people was Reverend Elizabeth Silishebo. I first met Elizabeth, as she permitted me to call her, in Mwandi in 1999. Elizabeth, a recent graduate of the United Church of Zambia's theological program, also had some training in accounting and business management and had been appointed by the United Church of Zambia to sit on the mission hospital's board.

At the time, I too was serving on the joint US–Zambia board that was overseeing the operations of the hospital. Over the course of several visits to Mwandi, I spent many hours with Elizabeth discussing the hospital's finances, personnel issues, how she should go about her role, in short, how could she ensure that the hospital best served the medical needs of the people as well as be a Christian beacon of hope and sustenance for the Lozi people.

Elizabeth was thoughtful, inquisitive, humble and determined to do her very best in her roles as a hospital board member and as a minister in the United Church of Zambia. She certainly had her hands full. In addition to her professional roles, Elizabeth was a widow, and the mother of nine children—eight girls and one boy. She was also taking care of her aging and disabled father. Nevertheless, she was always cheerful and quick to laugh and smile.

In 1999, a number of the Presbyterian Church USA's mission partners were invited to churches in various cities within the United States to provide an in-person perspective and witness from the Church's mission partners abroad. Elizabeth was selected to come to the United States. Her host church was Milwaukee's Immanuel Presbyterian Church.

I met Elizabeth at the Milwaukee airport the day of her arrival; she was exhausted but excited. It was trip of firsts for her: first time on a plane, first time out of Zambia, first time in Europe and America. I had volunteered to show Elizabeth around while she was in Milwaukee, and she marveled at the sights she saw in the city and along Lake Michigan.

Elizabeth preached at Immanuel the Sunday she was in town, and I know she was anxious, excited, and eager to represent Mwandi and share stories of the village and mission hospital and chapel with Immanuel's congregation. She spoke of the bonds of friendship and commitment between Mwandi and Milwaukee, and she noted the words of a well-known West African prayer: "Lord, we thank you that our churches are like big families…Lord, we thank you that we have brothers and sisters in all the world."

After the service, Elizabeth was feted at a welcoming luncheon and I saw her happiness reflected in her beaming smile.

Late that afternoon, I took Elizabeth to the airport for her return to Mwandi. She confessed she was quite nervous about getting lost in Pittsburgh, which was where she'd catch her connecting flight to Lusaka. I told her she would be fine, and before she left Milwaukee, we were able to identify which airline gate she'd be departing from in Pittsburgh. That relieved her a bit once she knew what gate to look for. Then I joked with her and said the most difficult part of the return trip will be the road from Livingstone to Mwandi. She agreed and we shared a laugh about "the road."

A week or so later, I received a wonderful letter from Elizabeth expressing her thanks for the trip to me, and Immanuel's clergy and membership for our kindnesses and hospitality to her during her visit to Milwaukee. She also shared her thoughts about my upcoming trip to Mwandi, which at the time was only months away. She also wrote in terms of additional collaborations Immanuel and Mwandi could consider. At the end, she added these lines about her travel home:

The Mwandi Road

> "I traveled well that day and reached Pittsburgh and I had no problem in finding my gate. We arrived in Lusaka after a nice trip. I did have a breakdown when traveling from Livingstone to Mwandi because of the bad road. I arrived in Mwandi and found my children in God's care and protection."

Every year between 1999 and 2002, I traveled to Mwandi and would always see and spend time with Elizabeth. It was a joy to see her grow into each of her roles and observe the confidence she had developed in herself and the obvious respect and affection all had for her.

In May of 2003, I received word that Elizabeth had been killed on May 7th in a car accident on the Mwandi Road. Elizabeth was riding in the passenger seat of the vehicle as she and a number of individuals from Mwandi were traveling to Livingstone. The front wheels of the vehicle bounced down into a bad pothole, and apparently the unexpected jolt caused a whiplash that fractured Elizabeth's neck. She died at the scene. No others in the vehicle were injured. Elizabeth was 51 years old.

I was told that the entire village turned out for Elizabeth's funeral. She was a beloved figure at the hospital and within the village community. Elizabeth is buried in the Mwandi mission station cemetery, near the hospital and chapel that she loved so much and so faithfully served.

> **Author's Note**: My own and Immanuel Presbyterian Church's involvement with the village of Mwandi and the Lozi people has continued through the years. Though the de la Torres have long since moved to other mission sites in Kenya and Malawi, members of Immanuel, including myself, continue to visit Mwandi periodically, and Immanuel and the Center for International Health have continued to provide financial support for Mwandi's schools and the chapel, as well as provide food relief for the village during times of drought. This tiny African village has touched and stirred the hearts of the hundreds of volunteers who have visited over the years. Irma de la Torre's desire to name the chapel Bethel was an appropriate acknowledgment of what so many have come to know: "Truly, God is in this place."

Part Four

Welcome to Hell

CHAPTER 8
WELCOME TO HELL

In the aftermath of World War II, boundaries, alliances, and the balance of power changed throughout the world. In Europe, the Balkan states of Bosnia-Herzegovina, Serbia, Montenegro, Croatia, Slovenia, and Macedonia became of part of the Federal People's Republic of Yugoslavia under the leadership of Josef Tito. Tito, from 1943 until his death in 1980 ruled with an iron fist and during his rule ensured that no ethnic group dominated the country. Following Tito's death, and the subsequent collapse of the Soviet Union and the post-1945 Communist order in Europe in 1991, the various ethnic groups and republics inside Yugoslavia, including Bosnia and Herzegovina sought independence.

These declarations of independence triggered a civil war that lasted from 1992 to 1995. At the time, Bosnia's population was a mix of Muslim Bosniaks (44%), Orthodox Serbs (32%), and Catholic Croats (17%). Slobodan Milosevic, who had come to power in 1987, fueled Serb nationalism and stoked tensions by convincing the Serbian population that the other ethnic groups posed a threat to their rights. Religion was also used to fuel animosity between the three parties.

The war was particularly vicious because one of the principal aims of the nationalistic leaders like Milosevic was to create ethnically "pure" states in areas where historically ethnic and religious groups had been intermingled in every way: as citizens, as neighbors and even as family members. Consequently, in order to create these pure states, this was a war where the nationalistic strategy was "ethnic cleansing"; the target of the military operations was directed toward specific ethnic and religious civilian populations with the intent to drive them from their homes.

Through the Lens of Humanity

In early April, 1992, Bosnian Serbs laid siege to the city of Sarajevo. For 44 months, Bosnian Serbs targeted mainly the Muslim Bosniaks, but also killed many other Bosnian Serbs and Croats with rocket, mortar, and sniper attacks. The siege of Sarajevo stands as the longest siege in modern history - a year longer than the siege of Leningrad during World War II.

As shells fell on Sarajevo, bitter fighting and indiscriminate shelling of cities and towns, horrific ethnic cleansing and systematic mass rape occurred throughout the countryside. The height of the killing and ethnic cleansing took place in July 1995 when 8,000 Bosniaks were killed in what has become known as the Srebrenica genocide, the largest massacre in Europe after the Holocaust.

Finally, in 1995, United Nations air strikes and United Nations' sanctions helped bring about a peace agreement. The war in Bosnia claimed the lives of an estimated 100,000 people and displaced more than two million. As of November, 2017, 161 people have been indicted for war crimes. Of those, 83 have been convicted, 37 proceedings have ended, 19 people have been acquitted, and 22 proceedings are ongoing.

"You must meet Jeanne McCue," Dr. John R. Petersen said to me in late 1995. "You must meet her and hear of her humanitarian trips to Sarajevo and Bosnia. She is doing incredible things there. You two should team up for a trip and do something together. I think you'll find that what you both can do there together could really be meaningful."

Dr. John Petersen—JR as he was known by many—was a slight, bespectacled man who had served for years as Milwaukee County's Medical Director, and for a period of time, as the Interim Administrator of Milwaukee County Hospital. No stranger himself to the international health field, Dr. Petersen had been at the forefront of the creation of the Milwaukee International Health Training Center, which was developed as a mechanism to provide health education and training to health professions primarily in emerging and developing countries.

My meeting with him this day was serendipitous. I was having a late lunch in the Children's Hospital of Wisconsin cafeteria on the Milwaukee Regional Medical Center campus, when JR came in, also alone, and joined me at my table in the sparsely filled cafeteria.

After being with JR for a moment or two, you always knew what was on his mind, and invariably, he was very knowledgeable on the topic and very intense in his opinions. Today, he was very excited about the work that Jeanne was doing in Bosnia. Jeanne was a nurse who had worked at Milwaukee County Hospital for years and was a close friend of Dr. Petersen's. As I listened, Dr. Petersen told me about the trips Jeanne had made to Bosnia, even during the midst of the war. "I've helped her get used medical equipment from Milwaukee County Hospital," he said. "She's told me of her incredible experiences and I know the medical supplies and equipment that she has taken into the area is a godsend," he continued.

JR knew of my own international travels to India and Africa, and with a twinkle in his eye, he asked: "What are the chances that you might be persuaded to go on a trip with Jeanne to Bosnia."

I didn't tell him that I already felt an irresistible urge to go, but I had only recently returned from a several-week-long trip to Africa as a chaperon for a Presbytery of Milwaukee mission trip to a remote village in Zambia and wasn't sure about going off on a new adventure so soon. So I told him I'd love to meet with Jeanne and learn more about what she was doing. In JR's typical persuasive fashion, he immediately pulled out his address book and gave me Jeanne's phone number; I promised him I'd give her a call.

Though I had never officially met her, Jeanne was quite well known around Milwaukee's Regional Medical Center Campus. I gave her a call, explained who I was, and told her that Dr. Petersen was adamant that I should talk with her about her humanitarian work in Sarajevo and cities throughout Bosnia. She laughed and said that Dr. Petersen had told her about my work overseas and suggested she get in touch with me! We agreed to meet at a local Milwaukee restaurant the following week.

I recognized Jeanne immediately from having seen her around the campus. She was a petite, blonde woman in her mid-fifties with a beaming smile and engaging manner. And without much ado, we dove into each others international experiences and the motivations that drove us in our desire to help others abroad.

Jeanne told me that in many ways, it was her son Daniel's untimely death at 27 that had impelled her to look for ways to honor his memory. Shortly after Daniel's death in 1990, Jeanne, a devout Catholic, took a pilgrimage to the city of Medjugorje in Bosnia-Herzegovina with members of her parish. Returning from this life-altering pilgrimage, Jeanne knew her calling was to render humanitarian aid to the people of Bosnia.

Within a year of her pilgrimage to Bosnia, war broke out in the Balkans as Yugoslavia began to unravel. This provided further impetus for Jeanne to initiate her humanitarian relief activities. Having already seen dismal living conditions in Bosnia prior to the war, she knew the situation would rapidly spiral down even further.

Jeanne told me that from June of 1992 until our dinner together in January of 1996, she had made ten mission trips to Bosnia. Working essentially as a one-woman humanitarian aid organization, Jeanne, through the support of friends, co-workers, local Milwaukee hospitals and clinics, and her parish, had been able to collect and personally deliver over 15 tons of donated medical and refugee supplies directly to people in Sarajevo and refugee villages in Bosnia-Herzegovina. Perhaps the most remarkable aspect of her stories was the fact that she was delivering these provisions in the midst of a war zone, putting her own safety and well-being in harm's way. The more she told me, the more compelled I was to go on her next mission visit.

As we continued to share our international experiences, hers from Bosnia and mine from my travels to India and Africa, I realized what an incredible person Jeanne was to devote herself to this particular cause. As our dinner drew to a close, she asked if I would be interested in participating in her 11th mission to Bosnia, which she had planned for

WELCOME TO HELL

either late April or early May. When I indicated I was interested, she said she'd send me some information on the Bosnian conflict, information on Refugee Trust, an entity she worked with to get her donated supplies into the area, and more background information on her previous trips.

True to her word, in a few days, Jeanne delivered a packet of information to my office in Children's Hospital, along with prospective dates for the trip: May 3rd to May 12th. I eagerly read the information Jeanne had provided and was particularly captivated by a letter Jeanne had written to her donors after her 8th mission trip in 1995, a time when the war continued to rage on. Her words brought to life the depth of the impact she was making, as well as the breadth of her humanitarian spirit and generosity:

> It was truly a blessing for me to be able to bring aid to the people of Sarajevo. They have been under siege for well over 1,000 days. With the help of Brother Thomas O'Grady of Refugee Trust/Sarajevo, I was able to obtain UN clearance and fly to Sarajevo abroad a UN transport plane. The cargo was transported by truck via the Blue Road through the mountains. While in Sarajevo, I made home visits to the blind, deaf, elderly and handicapped who live in unheated and damaged apartments without adequate food, medicine, and electricity. Many have not been out of their dwellings in the three years since the start of the war due to sniper fire and their physical disabilities. I lived with a wonderful Sarajevo family and was deeply moved by their heart-wrenching stories of suffering and survival—and so impressed by their courage.

As I read the her words, *"and so impressed by their courage,"* I was in awe of Jeanne's courage.

I confirmed with Jeanne my intent to be a part of her 11th mission to Bosnia and within days, we had booked our tickets, departing on May 3rd from Chicago to Frankfurt on Lufthansa Airlines and then nonstop from Frankfurt to Split, Croatia, on Croatian Airlines. We'd return on May 12th simply reversing our route. Drivers from Refugee Trust would take us to our destinations during our time on the ground. Our in-country itinerary included Medjugorje, and then Mostar, Sarajevo, and Gorazde—cities where some of the most intense fighting took place during the war.

PREPARATION

Between January and late April, donated medical and dental supplies and equipment and refugee packets were collected and sorted. In late February, Jeanne advised me that she already had 30 boxes packed and ready to go that included mainly clothing for the elderly and school supplies for children. In addition, a local dental supply company donated a comprehensive array of dental equipment and supplies for the dental clinic in Sarajevo. A Medical College of Wisconsin faculty allergist donated several cases of allergy/asthma medications. Children's Hospital donated pediatric medications, medical supplies,

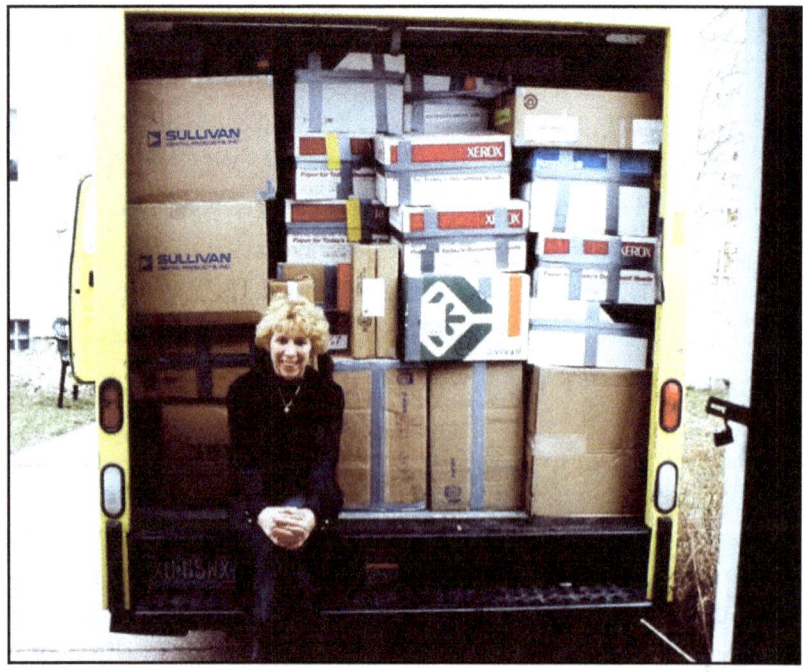

Jeanne McCue with our collected medical supplies for Sarajevo

and computer equipment, and other medical institutions donated varieties of small medical equipment and supplies.

All these items and others collected prior to our journey were stored in a warehouse on the Milwaukee County Regional Medical Center grounds. In late April, two Saturdays before our departure, Jeanne and I took all these donated items in a rented van to the Luftansa Cargo storage area at Chicago O'Hare airport to ensure that all these items would be in Split, Croatia, at the time of our arrival in May. This was old hat to Jeanne. Having made ten previous trips, she was familiar with where to take the cargo and she even knew the workers at the Luftansa storage area!

On the morning of Friday, May 3rd, Jeanne and I took a limo bus from Milwaukee's Amtrack Station to Chicago's O'Hare airport. We flew uneventfully from Chicago to Frankfurt, where, after a six-hour layover, we boarded our Croatian Airlines flight to Split.

We arrived in Split at 4:30 p.m. May 4th at the tail end of a glorious afternoon. The temperature was about 70 degrees with bright blue skies. We soon learned that our pre-sent cargo had arrived okay, but one of Jeanne's checked bags had not made the connection from Frankfurt to Split. Fortunately, all my items arrived in good order. I had brought with me a computer that I was going to donate and I was particularly glad that it, with all its accessories, had arrived with the rest of my checked luggage.

Brother Thomas O'Grady, based in Sarajevo with the Irish aid agency Refugee Trust, was Jeanne's primary contact in the region. The Refugee Trust initiated activities in Bosnia in 1990 and engaged in emergency aid and finances to the people of Bosnia. Additionally, Refugee Trust acted as a conduit for organizing conveys of food and other medical and social services for displaced persons, specifically focusing on the elderly, children, the blind, and mentally disabled. Jeanne had worked with the Trust on a number of her previous visits and their help had been invaluable in enabling Jeanne to coordinate her efforts in Bosnia.

We were met in Split by Admir, a worker for the Refugee Trust whom Brother O'Grady had dispatched to pick us up and assist us throughout our visit. As we moved toward the car, Admir assured us that our pre-shipped cargo had already been transported to Sarajevo and he suggested that since it was still daylight on a beautiful afternoon, we take a few moments to take in Split before heading for Medjugorje, where we would be staying our first evening. After our long flights, Jeanne and I were both up for that.

Split is a beautiful port-city on the Adriatic Sea at the base of the Dinaric Alps. On the drive from the airport into Split, I saw luscious green fields, many vineyards, glorious blue skies, and scenic mountain ranges in the distance. As we pulled into the city, by all indications, it was a sleepy Saturday afternoon in Split.

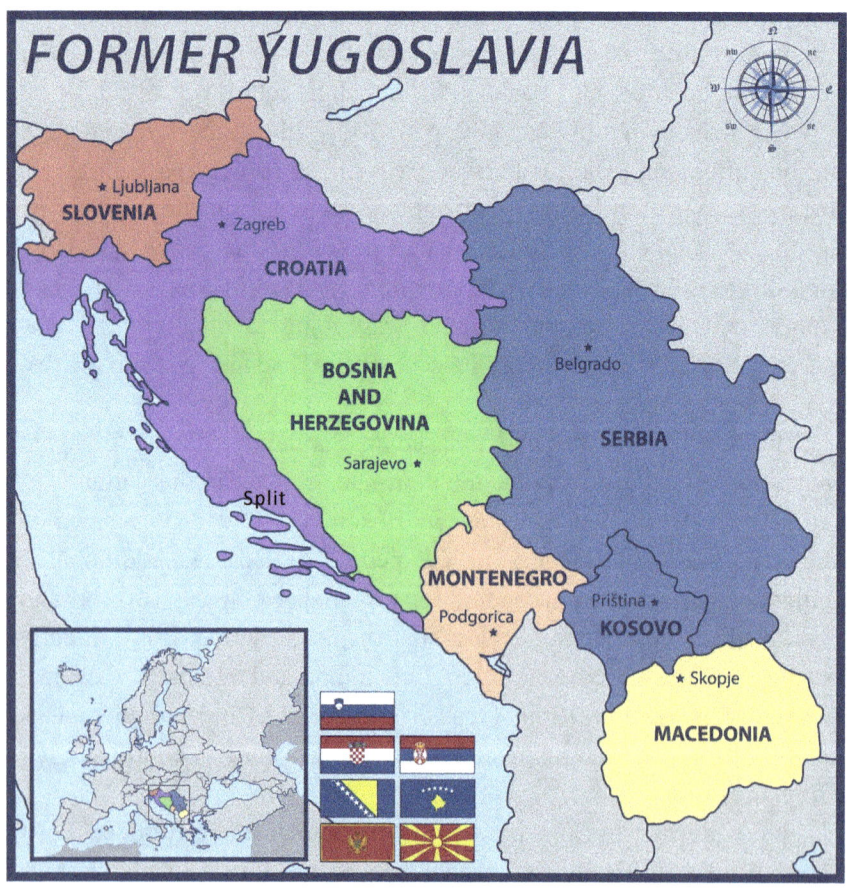

Map of the former Yugoslavia

WELCOME TO HELL

Admir parked along the seaport's docks and Jeanne and I strolled through parts of the city for about an hour. We were in the Old City, built in medieval times and as we passed the Cathedral of St. Domino, a wedding party spilled out of the church in noisy celebration. We walked a little further and out of St. Anthony's church, another wedding party was just exiting. Many of the guests were waving Croatian flags, an apparent sign of the new nationalism that had swept the area.

We returned to the car and began our journey to Medjugorje. Initially our drive took us along the coast of the Adriatic Sea; the scenery was simply stunning. Gradually our road narrowed and became a winding road up through the mountains. About three hours later, in what for me was a very harrowing drive along narrow roads with no guard rails, we arrived in Medjugorje and checked into our rooms at the Pax Hotel (Peace Hotel), aptly named I thought for the purpose of our trip to Bosnia.

MEDJUGORJE

Medjugorje is a small town located about 16 miles from Mostar. It gained international recognition in 1981 when six local children (now adults) alleged a series of visions of the Virgin Mary which they say continue to this day. As a consequence, Medjugorje became a popular Catholic pilgrimage site that through the years has experienced millions of pilgrims.

Jeanne indicated to me that she has visited Medjugorje several times on her previous mission trips to Bosnia, and I was interested in sharing the experience of Medjugorje with her.

We started the day by climbing Mount Krizevac (Cross Mountain). In 1933, a cross was erected on the mountain to commemorate the 1900th anniversary of Jesus' passion and death on the Cross. The route up the mountains is very winding and steep and was about a two-mile journey. It is alleged that in one of the visions of Mary, she admonished people to go there "often and pray." On this Sunday in May, thousands of pilgrims crowded the trail up and at the foot of the Cross.

After visiting Mt. Krizevac, I joined Jeanne at Mass in the Catholic church near our hotel. During the service, we saw four US soldiers.

After the service, we spoke briefly to them. They were from Rhode Island, Connecticut, Pennsylvania, and New York and were based in Sarajevo as part of the Implementation Force (IFOR), a NATO-led multinational peace enforcement force in Bosnia and Herzegovina. They too were just visiting Medjugorje for a day and told us that Sarajevo was a safer place, but that we should still be very careful due to the persistence of snipers in some parts of the city and the presence of land mines still uncovered in various parts of the city.

Late in the afternoon, Jeanne and I undertook our second climb of the day—Mount Podbrdo—otherwise known as Apparitions Mountain. It is on this mountain that the first visions of the Virgin Mary are reputed to have occurred. The path to the top of the mountain was steep and rock-strewn, but a shorter distance than the climb up Mt. Krizevac. Once again, thousands of pilgrims from all parts of the world were on the trail.

After my day in Medjugorje, there is no doubt in my mind that for many of the millions of people who have pilgrimaged to Medjugorje since 1981, their experiences there were deeply personal, moving, intimate, and for many, including Jeanne, life-changing.

Mostar

Mostar is one of the largest cities in Bosnia/Herzegovina with a population at the time of our visit of approximately 100,000 people. It is located about 18 miles from Medjugorye. Admir picked Jeanne and me up early Monday morning; it took about an hour for us to reach Mostar. Once we arrived, Admir drove us through the main area of the city and I saw that virtually all the buildings were scarred in some manner by bullet and shrapnel holes. Admir pulled over on a hilltop and showed us parts of the city that were the most devastated by the shelling and fighting. Admir mentioned that it was in East Mostar where the damage was most intense. We were able to see many homes where the roofs had been blown off or had collapsed due to heavy mortar fire and shelling.

Brother O'Grady had traveled from Sarajevo to meet us in Mostar, and we met with him and one of his project managers, Mark Sheppard, in the East Mostar Refugee Trust office. Brother O'Grady was a gregarious, portly, silver-haired Irishman likely in his early sixties with an easy smile and Irish brogue. He hugged Jeanne like a long-lost sister and bear-hugged me as if he had known me forever. He then thanked us profusely for the supplies that we had brought on this trip. After that, he proceeded to brief us on current conditions in Bosnia.

He stated that though open hostilities had ended months earlier, there were ongoing undercurrents of strife and conflict that were still very deeply seated and constantly simmering. "You will see a veneer of normalcy" he said, "but you will notice the strain and despair on people's faces which reflects deep traumatic and emotional disability."

Looking at me, he said, "You must understand that the nationalism and ethnic discord that occurred during the Bosnian war has its historical roots dating to medieval times. The Bosnian war reflected the desire of Serbia and Croatia to re-establish their ancient frontiers after the collapse of the Soviet Union and the end of the Cold War, and they were willing to use modern weaponry to do so. This is not new. For generations, there has been distrust and animosity between the ethnic groups and these ancient animosities boiled over in the Bosnian war, often in unspeakable ways."

As I listened to Brother Thomas, I couldn't help but think of the proverb: "Old sins cast long shadows." In the Bosnian war, the memories of long-held injustices and unhealed wounds rooted in centuries-old animosity were revived in an aggrieved historical emotion that had led to the deaths of thousands and displaced millions of people. And sadly, though peace has been declared, the shadow remains long and dark.

Part of Brother O'Grady's purpose in coming to Mostar was to attend a meeting of humanitarian organizations working in Bosnia, and as he departed for his meeting, he asked Mark Sheppard and members of Mark's staff to take us to some of the ongoing Refugee Trust projects in Mostar. This gave Jeanne and me the opportunity to visit some of the areas where our donated cargo had been recently delivered by Admir and other Refugee Trust staff.

Through the Lens of Humanity

The next several hours were a whirlwind of activity as we visited hospitals, schools, a pediatric clinic and homes for the elderly and the blind. For me, the most unforgettable part our time in Mostar was listening as Mark and his staff gave voice to what it had been like living through the war and its immediate aftermath.

Mark Sheppard was from Wales and served as the manager of Refugee Trust's projects in Mostar. He was 27 years old, an attorney, and had been in-country for several months. Sanela Balta was 21, was studying business in school, was a Muslim and had grown up in Sarajevo and Mostar. She was a translator and helped with various Refugee Trust projects. Maryjo Sidika was a social worker who had grown up in Mostar and who worked primarily with projects directed at the elderly and disabled.

En route to the different projects, Mark filled us in on the situation in Mostar. Basically, he said, Mostar was divided into East Mostar, which was predominantly Muslim, and West Mostar, which was mostly Croat Christian. Mostar's pre-war population was estimated to be 130,000, but post-war, it had dropped to around 100,000 with 60,000 of this number being Mostar inhabitants prior to the war. The remaining 40,000 were classified as refugees. Many people, he said, but mostly Muslims, had been displaced from one part of the city to another. And, as the conflict started, academics and professionals were deliberately harassed, with some even killed, to deter the possibility of organized resistance to the targeted displacement strategy.

We visited a field hospital in East Mostar, which was essentially a MASH-style hospital with 91 beds/cots for patients. Mark said it was the only hospital in East Mostar. It had limited surgical capacity, but no trained anesthesiologists and no general surgeons. All of the supplies of the hospital were from donated humanitarian supplies from relief organizations. There was some food product with UNICEF and NATO markings. At the time of our visit, the hospital had a very limited supply of drugs and medications. Remarkably, Mark said that many of the hospital staff were volunteers, the main staff were very poorly and apparently irregularly paid.

WELCOME TO HELL

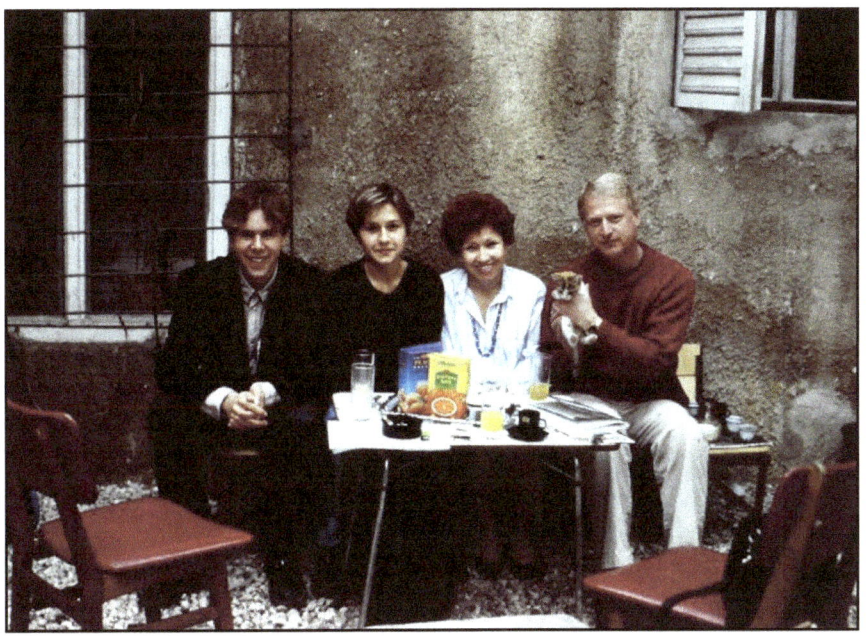

Having lunch with the Refugee Trust staff in Mostar
Left to Right: Mark Sheppard, Sanela Balta, Maryjo Sidika, Mark Anderson

In the morning, we also visited schools and gave school supplies and Teddy bears to children. At a home for elderly patients, we left clothing and other donated items.

As the noon hour approached, Mark recommended that we walk to a nearby restaurant that was quite nice and featured the traditional foods of the region. As we walked, Mark cautioned Jeanne and me to walk only on the pavement. He mentioned that land mines were still present around the city in grassy areas and parks, and were still killing or maiming many; far too often the victims were children at play.

As Mark, Sanela, Jeanne, and I sat down for lunch (Marygo had left for another meeting), I asked Sanela if she'd mind sharing some of her personal experiences during the war. She agreed, and quietly began to speak.

"I live with my mother," she began, "in a high-rise building."

Through the Lens of Humanity

Near the beginning of the fighting, her mother was injured in a shelling attack and incurred wounds to her back, leg, and head. She said because of conditions in the hospital, including a lack of staff and supplies, and the high number of injured people, her mother lay on the hospital floor for three days before she was operated on to remove the shrapnel. While her mother survived, she continues to have difficulty moving because of her injuries. Sanela continues to be the primary caregiver for her mother.

In addition to her mother's injuries, Sanela said during the war their building had been without electricity and water for three years. Because of the threat of snipers, she stayed inside her building until evening, then she'd creep down the stairs and run from building to building to get water and groceries. Often, she said, she'd crouch under cover for hours because she heard sniper fire in the area. She mentioned it could take hours to get food and water because of her fear of snipers, and her long absences caused great stress and worry for her mother.

As she spoke, tears filled her eyes. Nevertheless, she continued to speak softly. She said occasionally, she would go downstairs at night and run to buildings where her friends lived. She mentioned that she continues to have nightmares about the shelling and gunfire.

While we ate, I noticed she ate everything on her plate. I encouraged her to order more for herself and happily she did. It was clear she didn't have the opportunity to partake in many meals like this. Jeanne and I also made sure she ordered food to take home with her. She was tearful and very appreciative; we thanked her for her willingness to share her experiences.

After lunch in the Old Town of Mostar, Mark suggested we continue to walk through this area for a while. We quickly came upon the Stari Most (Old Bridge), which had been built by the Ottomans in the 16th century. The bridge was one of the iconic landmarks of Bosnia, but had been damaged from shelling during the war. The bridge spans the Neretva River and is a primary connection between East and West Mostar. The bridge, even damaged, was truly a magnificent structure, and the river water possessed a greenish hue. Despite the damage sustained by the city during the war, Mostar clearly remains a very picturesque city.

As I was taking in the beauty of the city, Mark reiterated Brother O'Grady's earlier comments about the "veneer of normalcy." He mentioned that the day before, he had witnessed a brutal public fight between a Serb and a Croat, and noted that tension between "East" and "West" was omnipresent. He pointed to several churches and mosques in the vicinity and observed that they were flying nationalistic flags from atop their buildings. And, he shared the story of a woman the Refugee Trust had recently assisted who was literally living next door to the couple that had killed her husband.

"Can you even imagine that?" Mark asked. "But it is more common than you'd believe. During the war, neighbor turned on neighbor. Even worse, in inter-ethnic marriages, families turned on families. And the impact of these conflicts didn't go away with the peace agreement," Mark said.

In Mostar, it was obvious that though the war was over, peace was tentative and still elusive, and healing was still a long way away.

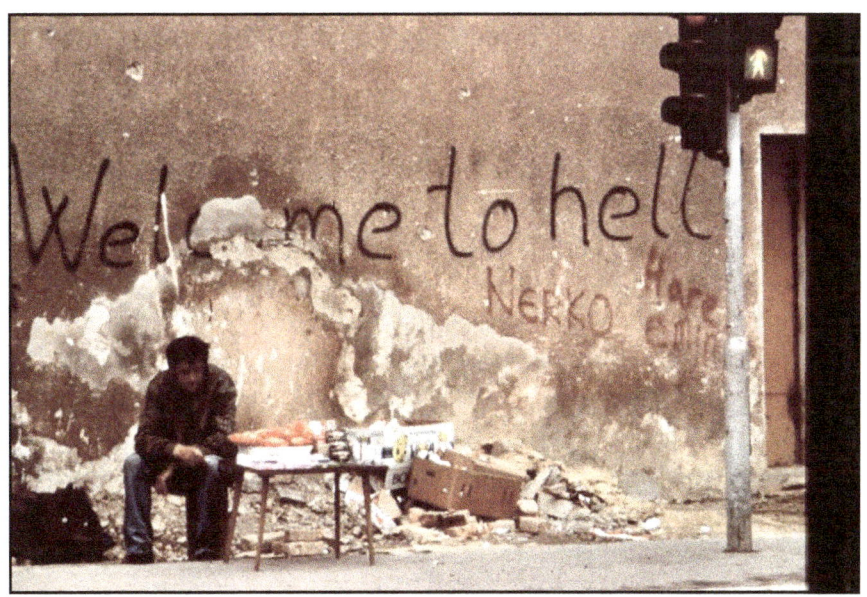

A street vendor in bombed-out Sarajevo—*Welcome to Hell*

Through the Lens of Humanity

Sarajevo

After Jeanne's and my full day in Mostar, late in the afternoon, Admir picked us up at the Refugee Trust offices to take us to Sarajevo. Our trip to Sarajevo was a two-hour beautiful drive through the stunning countryside. Along the way, Jeanne and I recapped our experiences in Mostar and planned activities for our next several days.

When we reached the outskirts of Sarajevo, we started to pass many bombed-out buildings that used to be people's homes. Everywhere, buildings were riddled with bullet and shrapnel holes, including high-rise buildings. The devastation was severe, streets were potholed where they'd been hit by artillery fire. In some areas, destroyed buses or burned-out cars remained on the streets. Despite the surroundings, many people were out on the street, I could hear the hustle and bustle of street life.

I'll never forget as we turned one corner seeing a disheveled, middle-aged man looking desolate and destitute sitting at what appeared to be his fruit and vegetable stand. Behind him was a concrete wall marred by bullet and shrapnel holes with the words WELCOME TO HELL scratched in the wall. At that moment, this image seemed to encapsulate and summarize the entirety of the Bosnian War: *Welcome to hell.*

How does one make a home in hell, I wondered. As we drove further into Sarajevo, I asked Admir, who was from that city, if he would describe conditions in Sarajevo during the siege.

"Sarajevo is a beautiful city," he began. "We had the Olympics here in 1984. Everyone talked about our beautiful city. As you see, Sarajevo is surrounded by mountains, it is like Sarajevo is the bottom of a saucer surrounded by all the mountains. During the war, the Serbs surrounded the city and controlled things by occupying the mountains. The Serbs pointed and fired their artillery down on the city. Sarajevo was under siege by the Serbs for over three years. For three years, we were without lights and electricity, without running water, without the garbage being collected. People were distrustful and didn't interact.

WELCOME TO HELL

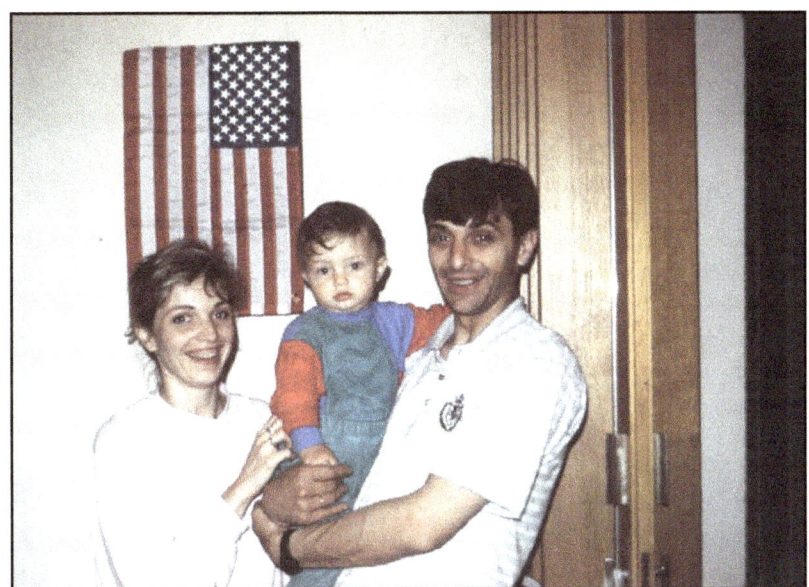

Dino, Samra and their infant son—my hosts in Sarajevo

Every morning, you would see silent figures going to collect water and food. There were no smiles and no real greetings among people.

"In many areas there were land mines, and there is an area we called 'sniper alley' because so many people were killed by snipers there.

"Every day, there was artillery shelling, usually hundreds of shells a day fell on the city.

"The Serbs also used to take the big truck tires and fill them with dynamite and then rolled the tires down the mountains and hills so they would explode in the city or on people's roofs and homes.

"We were not able to live normally. Everyone was always on guard. I thought the daily shelling was the worst—we wanted to go to work, but the shelling disrupted everything.

"Everyone just wanted peace, I am happy the fighting stopped. It was time for peace."

As Admir was talking, we pulled into the offices of Refugee Trust Sarajevo. I was picked up by Dino Mahgafic; I was going to be Dino and his family's guest while we were in Sarajevo. Jeanne was staying at one of the guest houses where she had resided during prior visits.

Dino and his wife Samra were a young Muslim couple in their late twenties with a young baby son. They lived on the 15th floor of a high-rise apartment building with Samra's father Hazim. Dino had been a soldier during the war and was currently a driver for Refugee Trust. Samra was a physician, and our driver Admir was her brother and Dino's brother-in-law. Their apartment was quite nice. During my stay, it didn't have running water, but the small elevator was working, which had not been the case during the war.

Samra told me she had worked at the city hospital during the near and had seen some of the horrific injuries caused by snipers and mortar shells. Now she said she worked primarily as a pediatrician at the hospital. Samra also shared some experiences of the war that her brother Admir had not mentioned.

Their mother had died in 1992 from an asthma attack. They were not able to get her to the hospital because barricades had been set up preventing passage into certain areas of the city. Samra became emotional as she told this story. She felt her mother would have survived had the barricades not prevented them from getting to the hospital.

She told me that both Admir and his wife had been shot at by snipers but fortunately neither had been hit. During the worst of the siege, when food was very scarce, she stated that everyone took more risks to try and get food for their families and the likelihood of being a sniper's target increased. Similar to Sanela's story in Mostar, she spoke of how they would wait until dark to get water to better avoid being spotted by snipers, and then having to carry ten liters or more of water up 15 flights of stairs.

The next several days in Sarajevo were a flurry of activity. Early our first morning in Sarajevo, we went to the customs area at the airport to retrieve our full pre-shipped cargo. After a brief delay, we claimed our items and proceeded to visit various project sites.

One of our first stops included a children's hospital. Given my background in children's medical facilities, I was particularly interested

WELCOME TO HELL

in visiting this facility and delivering a variety of donated equipment and supplies provided by Children's Hospital of Wisconsin. I was told that the hospital currently operated 50 beds; prior to the war, the hospital was operating 200 beds. The hospital was located near the front lines of the fighting and the mortar shelling, and the children were routinely evacuated to the basement to try and provide a safer environment. The hospital was receiving some assistance from UNICEF, but that assistance had become more erratic. The hospital was in dire need of drugs and medications and very basic supplies.

We also visited the city hospital, which had incurred significant damage during the war. We were told that both the children's hospital and the city hospital had been specifically targeted numerous times during the war by Serbian artillery fire. The capacity of all the hospitals in the city had been reduced as a consequence of the war and many were only open due to donations from humanitarian organizations. As a consequence of the reduction in capacity, Samra had shared that most hospitals were overwhelmed with patients and many patients were simply not being seen or treated.

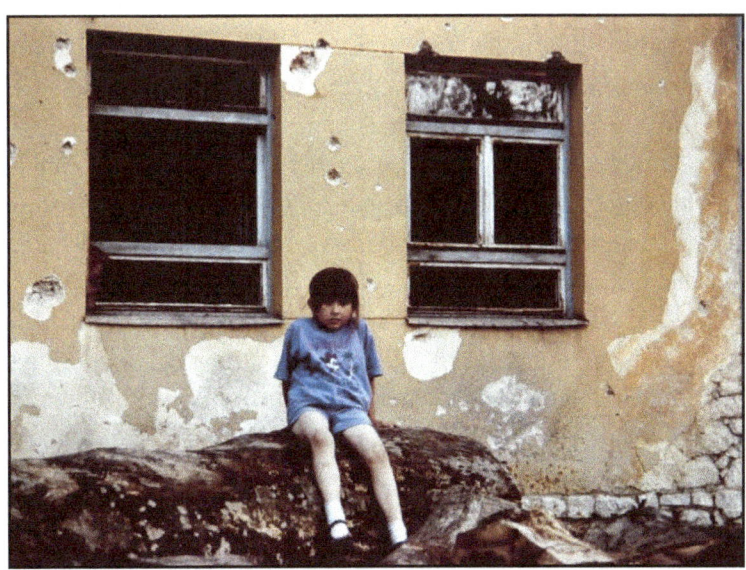
Young village girl in Goradze sitting in front of her bullet-riddled school

THROUGH THE LENS OF HUMANITY

The first home for orphans in Bosnia-Herzegovina was EGYPT orphanage, which was established in 1894. Over the years, thousands of children had been raised there, but the orphanage was heavily damaged during the war. As with hospitals, it was claimed that orphanages and schools were specific targets during the war.

Grbavia is one of the largest districts of Sarajevo reputed to be an area that the Chetniks (a derogatory term used by Bosnian Muslims and Croats for the Serb troops) raped and humiliated hundreds of women during the war. As we toured this area one afternoon, Brother O'Grady talked about the many Muslim and Croat women who were raped in prisoner camps and then forced by the Serbs to deliver the child. Refugee Trust was helping the women (and children) deal with the emotional trauma of not just the rape itself, but then the aftermath of the woman raising a child from a different ethnicity. Brother O'Grady mentioned that for him, this was one of the most painful aftermaths of the war to deal with. He also noted this was an area of Sarajevo where many professional people were imprisoned and forced to do manual labor as a means of humiliating the prisoners.

Goradze is a town about 35 miles from Sarajevo. Early one morning, Brother O'Grady arranged for us to drive out to this area. It had been an area of intense fighting and the town's buildings reflected the hostilities—bullet holes were present in the building structures that were still standing. As we walked through the city, we distributed refugee packets to people and visited some of the bazaars in the area. A wizened, stooped woman who appeared to be in her 70s, but might actually have been closer to 50, began following our group, seeking to sell her knitting. I bought a gray wool sweater from her that became one of my valued treasures of the trip.

Children came up to our group as well and we distributed teddy bears and some clothing items to them. I found myself wondering what their futures held as they posed for our pictures in front of their school that was riddled with bullet holes. Brother O'Grady spoke about the massive unemployment of people in Bosnia. For example, in Goradze, he said, there used to be a cement factory, but the war had completely destroyed the facility.

WELCOME TO HELL

We had planned to drive to Srebrenica, about 100 miles from Sarajevo, but timing didn't permit our getting there. Our intent had been to distribute refugee packets and visit the facilities housing the elderly and the blind.

Srebrencia had made international news during the war when it was discovered that mass executions had taken place there as part of an "ethnic cleansing" strategy. In July 1995, more than 8,000 Muslim Bosniaks, mainly men and boys from in and around Srebrenica, were killed and buried in mass graves during what has become known as the Srebrenica Massacre. This massacre was subsequently designated an act of genocide by the International Court of Justice in The Hague. Brother O'Grady told us that with the war's end, thousands of refugees are seeking to return to Srebrenica and Goradze and other areas in East Bosnia where so many were displaced. Sadly, Brother O'Grady lamented, the sheer volume of refugees is overwhelming the system and those organizations seeking to help resettle them.

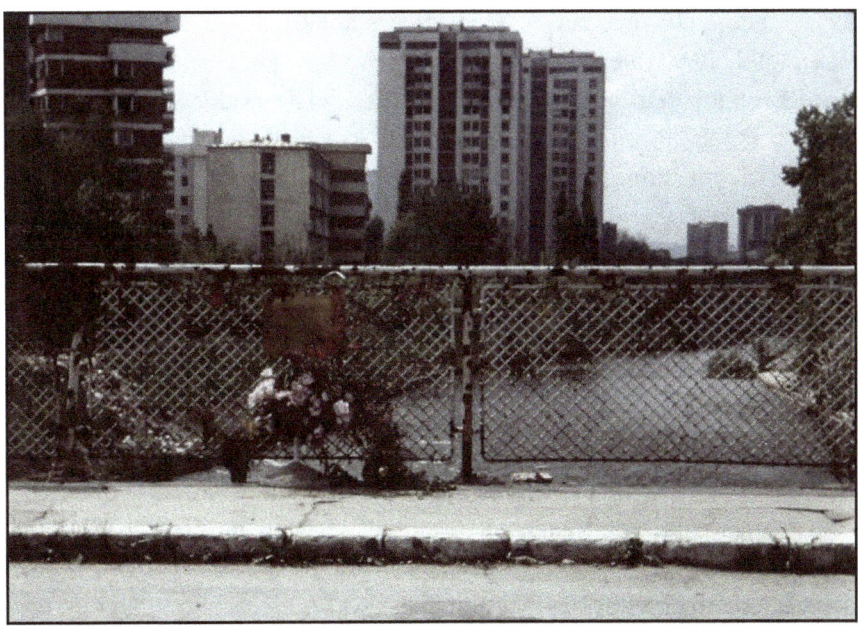

The "Romeo and Juliet Bridge" in Sarajevo where a young Bosniak/Muslim woman and a young Christian Bosnian Serb were killed by sniper fire

Through the Lens of Humanity

Returning from our visit to Goradze, we stopped at three schools in Sarajevo, one Catholic and two "public schools." We distributed various school supplies and talked with the students and teachers. The schoolmaster at one of the public schools said that school continued through much of the war for many students because of the dedication of the teachers, who did everything possible to stay in communication with the students. At one of the schools we visited, Muslims, Croats, and Serbian students all attended the same school. Remarkably, that was true even during the height of the siege. Sadly though, often schools were target of shelling attacks. One young teacher recalled the day she counted 39 mortar explosions around the grounds of the school. She noted that many times, students were injured during these attacks.

After visiting the schools, Brother O'Grady took us to several notable sites from the siege. The most poignant site was the Vrbanja Bridge. Located in the area that became known as Sniper Alley, the bridge was where two young women were killed by snipers while attending a peace rally in April 1992. Suada Dilberovic and Olga Sucic—one a Serb, one a Muslim—were amongst the protestors on the bridge and were fired on by Serb snipers holed up in a nearby Holiday Inn Hotel. In Sarajevo, the bridge is primarily known as the Vrbanja Bridge or the "Bridge of Suada and Olga." The bridge is also locally known as the "Romeo and Juliet Bridge" because a young couple—she a Bosniak Muslim and he a Bosnian Serb (Orthodox Christian)—were killed near the bridge while trying to cross into the Serb-occupied territory of Grbavia.

As we stood on the bridge, it was hard not to think of the terror that people must have felt knowing that they couldn't go about their normal lives with the fear of being in a sniper's crosshairs. I thought again of Sanela's words and better understood her terror as she crouched for hours in the dark until she could run to get food and water. And, it was hard to imagine the mindset of a sniper, hidden in safety and being willing and capable of ambushing and murdering a fellow human being. Even as we stood on the bridge almost a year after the Peace Accords had been signed, it was still disconcerting knowing that sniper attacks were still occurring in Sarajevo.

Welcome to Hell

As we walked off the bridge, we passed a small bazaar where I noticed a vendor was selling spent sniper shell casings. Carved into the shell casing were roses and the word "Sarajevo." The casing was being used as a vase and a single red rose had been placed in the casing in memory of a sniper victim. I solemnly bought one of the casings and even today, display the casing in my home study.

The night before our departure, Jeanne, Dino, Samra, Brother O'Grady, and I had dinner at the Red Goose restaurant in central Sarajevo. It was a beautiful location overlooking the city, and a wonderful locale for a farewell dinner. We discussed the various experiences of the week and Brother O'Grady talked of the many, many challenges ahead. Things such as electing new leaders willing to continue to support the new peace accords; how to handle and process the overwhelming numbers of refugees flowing back into Bosnian cities; how to address massive unemployment; how to morally and politically deal with the issue of war crimes and war criminals; how to secure international funding and support necessary to rebuild Bosnia and Herzegovina; and what to do with the NATO peace forces (IFOR) and what will their role be going forward.

It was a sobering discussion. So much still needed to be done. I looked over at Jeanne during dinner and realized just how much she had done herself over the course of 11 missions. After dinner to begin to prepare for our journey home, it was comforting to know that this persistent angel would continue her work of comfort and peace for the people of Bosnia.

After Jeanne and I returned home to the normalcy of our lives, I continued to reflect on all we had seen and experienced. I remembered the many people we had met who had shared with us the most shattering and devastating moments of their lives—yet their hope and dreams for rebuilding their lives and their country remained alive. Their human dignity and our shared humanity calls for our ongoing concern in building peace there and throughout the world.

Shortly after we got back to Milwaukee, I received Jeanne's letter to her "supporters and donors" regarding her 11th mission to Bosnia:

> With your help we collected and transported over 2 tons of medical, dental and refugee supplies to Sarajevo and surrounding villages......
>
> Humanitarian aid is still desperately needed. Many organizations have stopped sending aid, jobs are non-existent, homes and families have been destroyed. Many villages like Goradze are still without electricity. Your wonderful refugee packs, school supplies, letters of friendship, soccer balls and Teddy Bears delighted children in schools, hospitals, and orphanages......
>
> Funds were donated to repair EGYPT, an historic orphanage in downtown Sarajevo, heavily damaged during the war. Floorboards were missing—used as fuel for heat in the bitter cold winters......
>
> Dental supplies were given to Refugee Trust Dental Help for the Blind. A young dentist told of providing services under the most difficult circumstances during the war without water, electricity or basic materials. Thanks to Sullivan Dental Products, we can continue to support this worthy program which serves the poor in Sarajevo.
>
> Our cargo also included 5,000 packs of seeds - just in time for spring planting and of course, life-saving medical supplies distributed to the Children's and TB Hospitals in Sarajevo and Refugee Trust's clinics for the elderly and handicapped...

The last paragraph of Jeanne's letter stated, "I thank God for his love and protections and for your generous hearts! I remain deeply committed to continue these missions and will return again in November. Please pray for a lasting peace in Bosnia and let me know if you would like to help!"

I thank God for Jeanne McCue, and for letting me share a part of her life's calling with her!

> Author's note: In 2016 Jeanne McCue published a book entitled: *Transport of Hope: How One Humanitarian Made a Difference in the Balkan Conflict*. The book details Jeanne's experiences in the Balkans over 24 years and 40 mission trips.

CHAPTER 9
"Where God Goes to Weep"

The Center for International Health (CIH) is a consortium of prominent academic and medical centers located in Milwaukee, Wisconsin. Its mission is to provide health education and training services to health professionals and health delivery systems in emerging and developing countries worldwide. Children's Hospital of Wisconsin (CHW) was one of CIH's consortium members, and during my tenure as Executive Vice President of CHW, I had served for a number of year's on CIH's Board of Directors. In September of 2000, I resigned from CHW to assume a senior administrative role with the renowned international health organization Project HOPE, noting at the time that I felt compelled to explore full-time international health work; otherwise, I'd regret not doing so years later. After serving two and a half years in a variety of senior roles at Project HOPE, I was recruited by CIH and returned to Milwaukee in March 2003 as CIH's President and Chief Executive Officer.

Following the September 11, 2001 attacks on New York City, the United States military launched strikes against Al Qaeda in Afghanistan and Iraq. In 2004, as the hostilities began to subside in Afghanistan, CIH, in collaboration with the International Medical Corps (IMC), a non-governmental organization (NGO) with deep ties in Afghanistan, applied for and received a United States Agency for International Development (USAID) grant to assist in rebuilding Afghanistan's maternal and child healthcare delivery system. After years of Taliban rule and oppression, Afghanistan's maternal and infant mortality rates were the highest in the world. The following is the story of CIH's involvement in Kabul, Afghanistan in 2005 to 2006.

Through the Lens of Humanity

At 9 a.m. on Sunday, February 13, 2005, I boarded a United Nations aircraft in Dubai, United Arab Emirates, along with five other healthcare professionals and colleagues from Wisconsin for a three-hour flight to Kabul, Afghanistan. We were on the last leg of our journey from Milwaukee to participate in a project designed to improve the quality of maternal and neonatal care at Kabul's Rabia Balki Hospital (RBH). As our jet streaked northeast above Iran toward Kabul, I sat in the austere, no-frills airplane cabin and reflected on the world events that had occurred in the previous few years that had contributed to this expedition.

Forty months earlier, after the terrorist attacks on the United States on September 11, 2001, laser-focus had been turned toward the hunt for the terrorist leader and mastermind of the attacks, al Qaeda's Osama bin Laden. Afghanistan and Pakistan were viewed as the primary sites where bin Laden would seek sanctuary and refuge.

Within a month of the terrorists attacks, on October 7, 2001, Operation Enduring Freedom (the official name used by the U.S. government for the Global War on Terrorism) was launched with airstrikes on Taliban and al Qaeda targets in Afghanistan. Al Qaeda had been linked to the September 11 attacks, and was operating in Afghanistan under the Taliban's protection. The purpose of the attacks was to impede the Taliban's ability to give safe haven to al Qaeda and to stop al Qaeda's use of Afghanistan as a base of operations from which to launch their terrorist activities.

As US military initiatives expanded into Afghanistan, so too did US humanitarian and development efforts. With the forced departure of the Taliban regime in 2001 and 2002, the desire to restore human rights and help establish a new, democratic Afghan government, led the US government to turn its efforts toward assisting in rebuilding Afghanistan's governmental and civil infrastructures.

Following decades of war and years of harsh rule by the Taliban, which included serious violations of human rights, including massacres of Afghan citizens and especially brutal treatment of women via rigid interpretation and enforcement of Islamic Sharia law, women and children, more than any other sector of the Afghan population had suffered the most devastating effects of the tragic mix of war, culture, politics and religion that had descended upon Afghanistan.

As the years of war and conflict continued, Afghanistan's healthcare delivery system, including its medical education infrastructure, disintegrated, with an especially disastrous impact upon the country's maternal and child morbidity and mortality. As the years of conflict continued, Afghanistan achieved the dubious distinction of possessing the highest rates of maternal and perinatal mortality in the world.

With US involvement in Afghanistan increasing, Secretary Tommy Thompson of the US Department of Health and Human Services (HHS) visited Afghanistan in October 2002. Shocked at the state of women's healthcare in Afghanistan, Secretary Thompson partnered with US Secretary of Defense Donald Rumsfeld and together, their combined departments committed to help rebuild and refurbish the Rabia Balkhi Women's Hospital in Kabul, the only tertiary women's hospital in Afghanistan. As the Department of Defense rehabilitated the physical structure of the hospital, HHS developed post-graduate training programs in obstetrics and gynecology, with training also to occur in the areas of anesthesiology, pediatrics, and midwifery.

On April 21, 2003, Afghan health officials, along with HHS Secretary Thompson and Department of Defense officials, dedicated the hospital as part of the US commitment to help rebuild Afghanistan's public health infrastructure and to specifically work toward reducing Afghanistan's maternal and perinatal morbidity and mortality rates.

To work with the US government in these initiatives, International Medical Corps (IMC) an NGO, was initially established in Afghanistan in 1984 to address medical care needs as a consequence of the Soviet–Afghan war. IMC had a significant organizational structure in Afghanistan and the surrounding region and was awarded funding by HHS to develop a physician training and support program. The goal of the program was to reduce the maternal and infant mortality rates in Afghanistan through the training of OB-GYNs and other health workers at the Rabia Balkhi Hospital (RBH) in Kabul.

THROUGH THE LENS OF HUMANITY

In 2004, as the IMC continued to roll out its program, the Center for International Health (CIH), the NGO where I served as president, subcontracted with IMC to assist in achieving the program's efforts to improve the capacity and capability of RBH's existing staff, to improve RBH's quality of care, and to work toward obtaining a substantial reduction in maternal and child illness and deaths at RBH.

It was these series of events that led to the composition of a CIH medical team to travel to Kabul, Afghanistan, and work for 12 days within Rabia Balkhi Hospital. Our five-person team was led by Dr. Doug Laube, Chair of the Obstetric and Gynecological department at the University of Wisconsin–Madison, and also included Dr. James Sanders, a Family Medicine physician from the Medical College of Wisconsin; Donna Harris, RN and Chris Gall, RN, nurses from Children's Hospital of Wisconsin, and myself. All of us were "veterans" of medical missions of one type or another. Dr. Laube, for

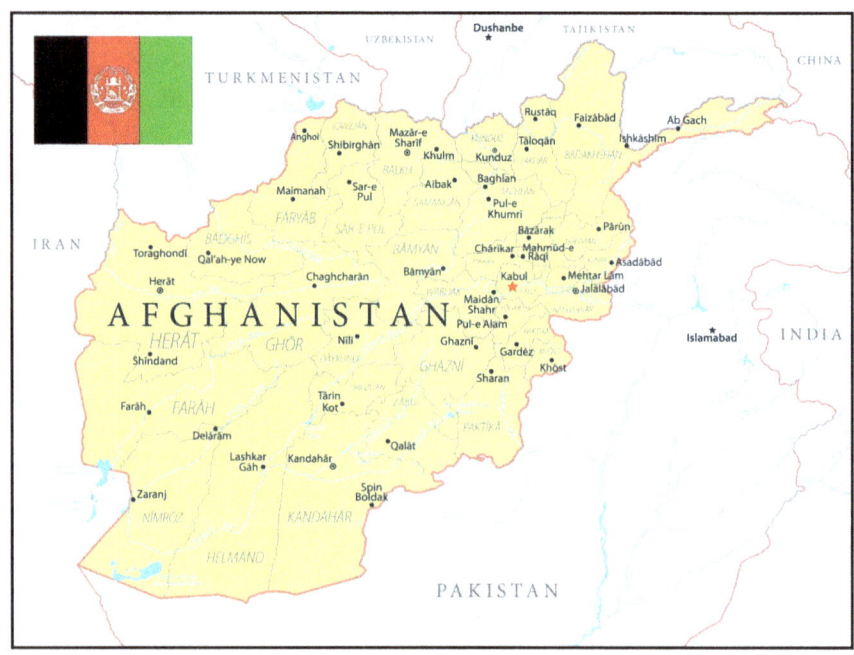

Map of Afghanistan

Welcome to Hell

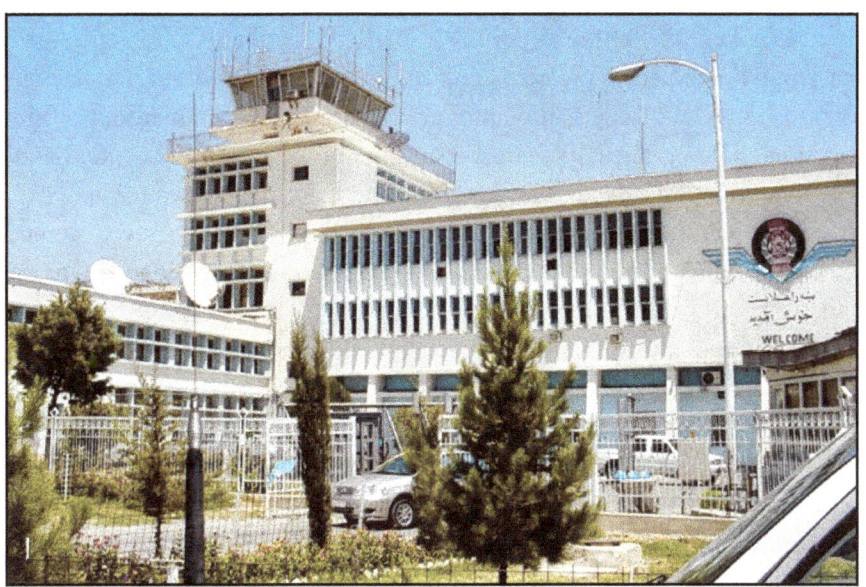

Kabul, Afghanistan Airport

example, had recently volunteered in Afghanistan at the behest of HHS Secretary Thompson, and Dr. Sanders had previously worked for Medecins Sans Frontieres, the international medical humanitarian organization, also known as Doctors Without Borders. Both Donna Harris and Chris Gall had participated in overseas medically oriented volunteer experiences. None of us however, had ever been embedded in a still-simmering conflict zone like Kabul, Afghanistan, where bombings, kidnappings, sniping, and shootings were constant risks and daily occurrences.

As we disembarked from the UN aircraft and walked toward the airport buildings, we were greeted by blinding sunlight and a dazzlingly blue and cloudless sky. A picturesque view of snow-capped mountain ranges was showcased in the distance. A brutally cold wind sucked the breath out of us, which changed our gait from a walk to almost a jog to the airport terminal building. We cleared customs in an area that didn't seem much warmer than outside, but at least the building offered protection from the damp, windy breeze.

Through the Lens of Humanity

We were met at the airport by a small delegation of IMC representatives, who helped us clear customs and collect and load our luggage on mobile carts. We braved the bitter cold and quickly streamed out of the terminal into a virtually empty parking lot where three white Land Rovers with IMC decals displayed on the front doors awaited us. The vehicles were smudged with dirt from Kabul's slushy, snowy streets and each had a prominent antenna affixed on its roof. We loaded Donna and Chris and their belongings in one Land Rover, and Doug, Jim, and I and our possessions in another. Each vehicle had a driver and a security person and once we were all loaded up, our two Rovers followed the third Rover, which was essentially a security escort vehicle, out of the airport. We headed toward town where we'd all be staying in a secured compound operated and maintained by IMC for its own personnel, as well as visitors and guests such as ourselves.

As our small convoy pulled out of the airport onto a two-lane road, my attention was again drawn toward the horizon and the beauty of the snow-capped peaks nearby. I recalled from studying the history of Kabul and Afghanistan prior to our visit that Kabul had existed in some form for over 3,500 years. However, it wasn't until the early 20th century that Kabul had emerged as Afghanistan's largest urban area. At an elevation of approximately 5,900 feet above sea level, Kabul sits in a valley between the Asamai and Sherdawaza mountain ranges in the east-central part of Afghanistan. The Kabul River flows through the city and the natural environment of the mountain ranges combined with the river provides a striking and scenic aspect to the city.

As we inched along the road toward our compound, we passed evidence of the decades of conflict and fighting within the city. The carcasses of abandoned and destroyed trucks and vehicles and even a Russian tank that still lay sprawled in the muddy snowbanks along the roadside, all gave witness to the fighting that had been waged around and within the city. We saw boarded-up buildings and the shattered ruins of businesses and homes—evidence too, of years of past bombardments. Many of the roads and side streets were potholed from multiple shellings and the absence of upkeep. The sparsely trafficked road let us see and sense some of the natural beauty and cultural heritage of Kabul. We also knew, however, that even though the

Welcome to Hell

Taliban had been driven from the city, tensions in the city remained high. Our little group had just landed in one of the most hazardous and dangerous locations on earth.

The route to our compound had us skirting around the edges of Kabul and after about 30 minutes, we turned down a side street lined with a number of buildings, each protected by solid metal, stone reinforced walls, and gated entrances. As we approached one building, the gate swung open, we drove into a driveway, and parked in front of a three-story building. We had arrived at one of the IMC guest houses. The building had a greenish-grayish hue, and as we disembarked from the Land Rovers, I could see that the building was completely enclosed by a ten- to twelve-foot-high wall. The entrance to the building had a couple of small steps leading into a rather uninviting entrance and a lobby that was poorly lit, with grayish-green walls that matched the external building façade. We immediately ascertained that the building was without a well-functioning heating system.

We unloaded our belongings and took them into the lobby. Then, prior to being shown to our respective rooms, we were directed to a sitting room and given briefings about the building, as well as the security precautions we were expected to follow during our stay in Kabul.

The first order of business was assigning each of us with a two-way radio with the mandatory instruction that we were each to check in twice a day at designated times, indicate where we were, and that we were safe and secure. We were told that the IMC vehicles would transport us back and forth to Rabia Balkhi Hospital every day, but the vehicles and drivers were also available to take us to various areas around the city as long as we were traveling at least minimally in pairs, and as long as the areas we wanted to visit were in designated "safe zones" as defined by daily updated US military reports. A mandatory curfew of 9 p.m. was in place each evening.

There was good news and bad news related to our guest house accommodations. The good news was we had a roof over our heads in a "safe" zone of the city. The bad news was that electrical service in the guest house was erratic. While the building possessed a generator, the latter's functionality was only marginal. The city imposed planned electrical outages during the day for conservation purposes. Unfortunately, there were also many unplanned outages, so power was at best unpredictable.

Our rooms were heated with kerosene-fueled heaters, which we were tasked with keeping functional, i.e., fueled up and lit. The entire building reeked of kerosene fumes and for allergy sufferers—which included me—this was particularly uncomfortable. Whether you were an allergy sufferer or not, the atmosphere was highly unpleasant as the fumes soon permeated our clothing, hair, blankets, bedding, etc.

The water in the communal bathrooms and showers worked—the cold water, that is. Water temperature rarely reached what might even be considered lukewarm. This certainly encouraged efficient and short showers, as well as sponge baths and the occasional pouring of water over one's head for hair washing.

Internet service was available, but it too was unpredictable. It did afford at least a sense of connectivity with our friends, families, and colleagues back home.

After our "orientation session," we deposited our belongings in our respective rooms and reconvened downstairs in a common room for an early dinner. We dined on a delicious meal featuring local Afghan dishes. Though our living conditions were challenging, we all were encouraged by this wonderful meal cooked for us by a pleasant Afghan woman of indeterminate age. As would become the norm, we ate bundled in our heavy winter coats and clothing, seeing our breath as we ate and exhaled.

We were all tired after our journey and shortly after dinner, we all adjourned to our rooms. My room was on a third-floor corner of the building with a window through which I had a view of the barbed-wire-adorned compound wall. Luckily, I also had a view of the street and the snow-covered mountaintops in the distance. The room had a tiny closet, a small metal table and lamp, and a bed that was more of a cot that sagged in the middle and was covered with several thin, multi-colored blankets. The most important item—the kerosene heater—occupied an important place in the room.

Welcome to Hell

IMC had provided us with a list of recommended items to bring along on our trip, and per their recommendation, I had brought an industrial-strength flashlight, which was clearly going to be useful given the unpredictability of electrical service. My room was freezing and it seemed to me the kerosene heater was doing little to combat the chill in the room. Also on the IMC list of recommended items was a sleeping bag, which I had also brought, and never been so glad to have in my life!

That first night, a little to my surprise, I was able to access the internet, and after notifying friends and colleagues in the States that we had arrived safely, I climbed fully dressed into my sleeping bag and tried to get some sleep. I repositioned my bed to get closer to the heater. Despite the frigid room, I soon fell fast asleep.

Dawn arrived in Kabul with the muezzins intoning the call summoning the Muslims to prayer. From my guest room, I could hear the call spread across the city from mosque to mosque. As I lay in bed listening, it was amazing and beautiful to hear the call ebbing and flowing from one part of the city to another.

Despite having turned in "fully clothed" and tucked into a Northern Face sleeping bag, as I lay listening to the call to prayer at dawn, it seemed that every inch of my body was chilled to the bone. I moved toward the showers, hoping for a warming wash before breakfast, but quickly discovered the sad state of the buildings plumbing. While the water flowed, the water was so cold I was actually surprised the pipes weren't frozen, and unbelievably, I left the showers far colder than when I entered. Sadly, I was destined to learn that this was to be my early-morning experience every day of the coming fortnight.

At breakfast, our contingent met Suzanne Griffin, the IMC administrative staff member in charge of the project, and Linda Barnes, a nurse midwife consultant employed by IMC and deployed to RBH to provide professional and clinical training to the midwives at the hospital. Also, our visit coincided with the visit of Jeanine Greenfield, PhD, RN, head of the Office of Global Health for the Department of Health and Human Services (DHHS), who was there to monitor progress of HHS's efforts to enhance maternal and infant care at the hospital.

Our convoy of IMC vehicles pulled out of the compound around 8:30 a.m. and began a slow, leisurely trek toward Rabia Balkhi Hospital. Linda Barnes was in my vehicle and as we drove, she reminded us that Afghanistan is a multi-ethnic and very tribal society. She noted that the Pastuns, Tajiks, and Hazara tribes were the most prominent tribes, and women from these tribes made up the bulk of the hospital's patients.

"Afghans," Linda said, "are governed by a set of cultural norms called the *pushtunwali,* 'the way of the Afghan.' This is their traditional lifestyle, their code of honor."

She continued to explain that basically at the heart of this tribal code are honor and revenge. And it is the rigid adherence to these elements of tradition and tribal-oriented code that has often created strife within Afghan society; over the centuries, compliance with the code has at times pitted brother against brother, tribe against tribe, Afghan against Afghan, and Afghan against external invaders. As she spoke, I recalled a comment I had read about Afghanistan: "It is a country mired in medievalism where terrible things happen to people." It is said that Afghanistan is "where God goes to weep."

It is important to understand the 'way of the Afghan' she went on, because you will see the impact of the tribal code behavior play out in all manner within the the hospital—between patients and staff, patients and patients, and staff and staff.

As we continued to move into the city and toward the hospital, we noticed the business and commerce occurring along the streets. There were busy bazaars with collections of items displayed: carpets, jewelry, live poultry, dead parts of animals, spices, clothing. The hectic scene took place under the high-pitched cacophony of honking horns, street noise from cars, trucks and motorized rickshaws, and the barter and negotiation between buyer and seller.

When we approached Kabul's central city, we began to see more and more traffic, including military vehicles from the US and other countries. Even here, we saw the remnants of disabled and discarded

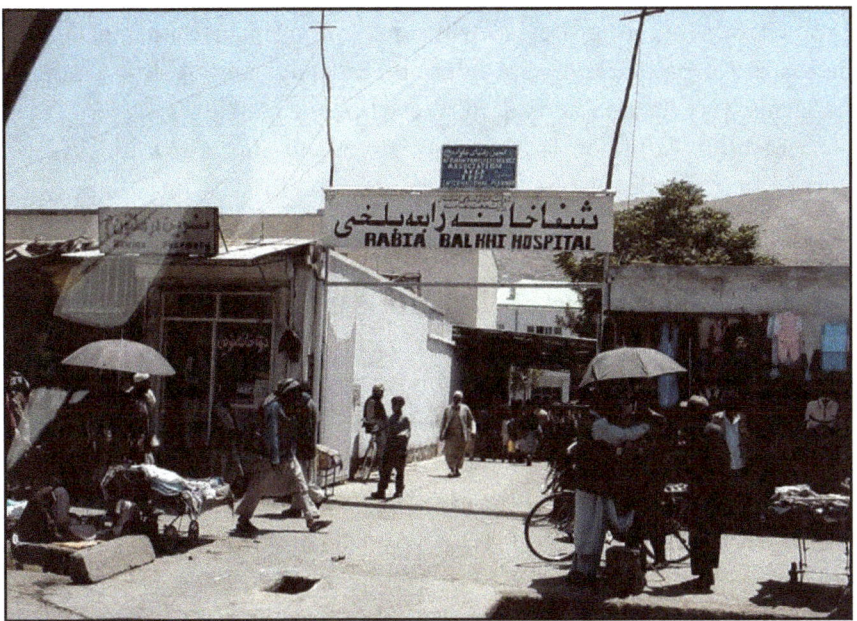

The main entrance to Rabia Balkhi Hospital

military equipment—heavy trucks and a few tanks. Linda also pointed out a building where just a day or two prior to our arrival, a suicide bomber had detonated his device near a crowded street corner during the middle of the afternoon.

"Death these days seems just around the corner for Afghans," Linda said.

The distant backdrop to the city and buildings we passed were the picturesque mountain ranges, and I sensed that Kabul, before recent wars and conflicts had marred its appearance, had been a vibrant and beautiful capital city brimming with centuries of culture and history. In many ways, I felt that I was seeing Kabul as it must have looked as a nineteenth or early twentieth century city.

Pedestrian traffic grew heavier as we moved further into the city proper. Many of the men were wearing round, flat caps or turbans and *kameez* (long shirts or tunics) and cuffed trousers. I saw several women wearing *burkas* (opaque veils and full-body covering), but many more women were wearing dresses with loose-fitting pants underneath and headscarves or *hijabs* to cover their head and hair. A few younger Afghans were dressed in modern, Western-style clothing.

Finally, we turned onto a major street and after a few blocks, we turned into an alleyway wedged between storefronts with a large sign above the alleyway indicating that we had arrived at Rabia Balkhi Hospital. The narrow alleyway funneled us toward the entrance of the hospital, which was packed with dozens of people—more men than women. Our Land Rovers slowed to a crawl due to the crowd milling around in the alley. Only through constant honking and some shouting and gesturing by our drivers were we able to inch forward to the entry gate.

Peering out the window as we threaded our way through the crowd, I noticed that both men and women were squatting and sitting on the ground around the gate. Some of the men were smoking and drinking—presumably tea, since alcohol is prohibited. As we got nearer the gate, I heard a clamor of angry voices speaking and shouting at a figure standing by the gate entrance.

Similar to our guest house, the hospital entrance was accessed via a solid metal gate that was approximately ten to twelve feet high. The gate permitted pedestrian and vehicular entry into the hospital courtyard. The agitated shouting we were hearing was directed at the hospital's gatekeeper, though from her own shouts, finger pointing and fist waving, she was clearly returning the retorts as well or better than she was receiving! From my perch in the Land Rover, it was abundantly clear she was a woman to be reckoned with. Her demeanor indicated that she was the gatekeeper and she was the one to determine who would be granted admission into the hospital's inner sanctum. Woe be it to anyone who doubted otherwise!

Our delegation came to know the gatekeeper well during the course of our visit. She was a tall, angularly faced woman of indeterminate age dressed this day, and in all subsequent times we saw her, completely in black from hijab to shoes. We learned from Linda that she ruled the gate with an iron fist, screening all who wished to enter. Traditional Afghan society dictates that only women care for women

Welcome to Hell

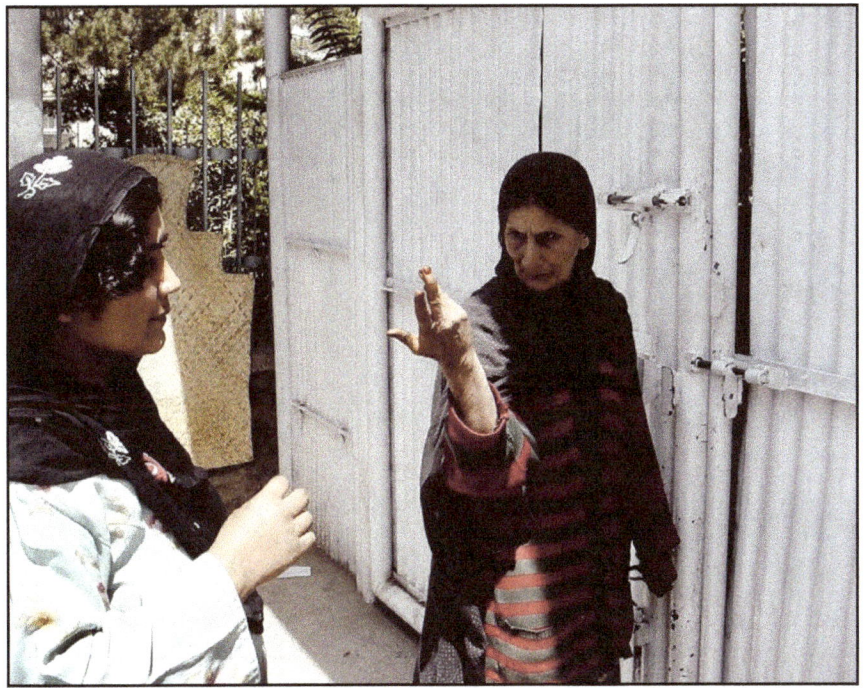

Rabia Balkhi gatekeeper, a.k.a. "The Gate Nazi"

and since Rabia Balkhi was a hospital exclusively for women, the gatekeeper's screening process primarily dealt with enabling female relatives of hospital patients into the hospital, as well as appropriate caregivers. Male family members or visitors were not permitted within the hospital.

The gatekeeper was a sight to behold. She paced around the gate area guarding her domain with a vengeance. She shrieked at those who challenged her, and was absolutely fearless, and even resorted to physical force in enforcing her decisions about who was going to obtain entry into the hospital. Swirling around her feet were several cats, some of them as black as her clothing as if they were her very own witches familiars.

I suspect because we were in a marked IMC vehicle, the gatekeeper waved us on through gate dismissively and the gate closed decisively

Through the Lens of Humanity

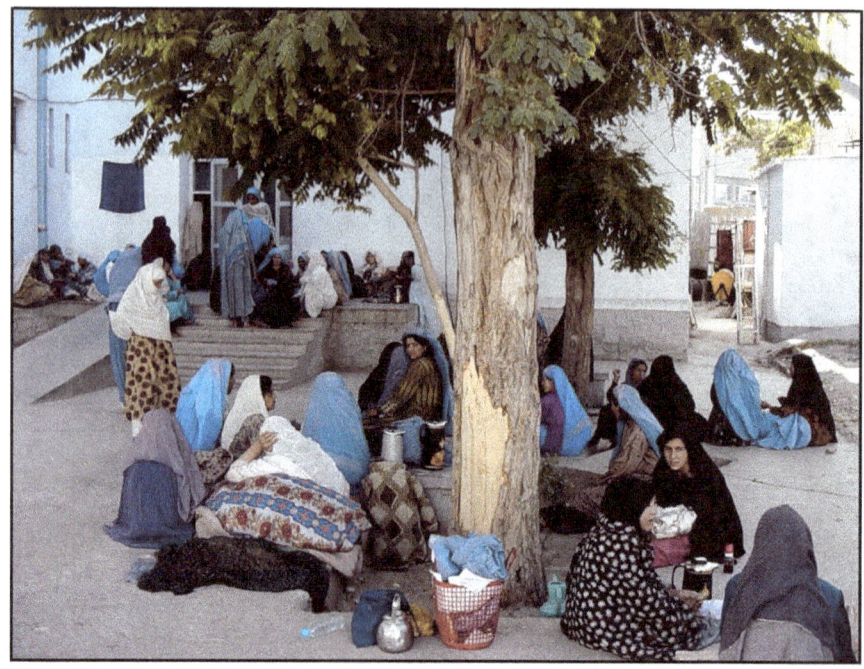

Afghani women waiting at the front door of the hospital to be seen or to receive word of their relatives

and immediately after our entry. Over the next two weeks, day or night, whenever we approached the entrance, this same gatekeeper was always present keeping vigil at her post.

Chris Gall in our delegation called her the "Admitting Department," Donna Harris called her the "Gate Nazi." As for me, I think she was perfectly cast as the Wicked Witch of the West from *The Wizard of Oz!* We learned during that our stay that there were other gatekeepers and that it was common for all gatekeepers to accept bribes from patient's family members to gain entry into the hospital.

We drove through the gate into the hospital's small central courtyard. A newly paved circular drive led to the front door. A cadre of workers was planting trees and others worked on leaks and water apparently flowing from a faulty septic system.

As we piled out of the Land Rovers, we were met by IMC staff, who indicated that our first order of business would be a tour of the

WELCOME TO HELL

hospital and the hospital grounds. We walked into the lobby and immediately saw a memorial to the hospital's namesake.

Rabia Balkhi is one of Afghanistan's most respected women. She was a well-known 10th-century Persian writer and poet whose poetry is said to match the level of the Persian poet Jalalad ad-Din Muhammad Rumi, more popularly known simply as Rumi. Her writings remain popular in Afghanistan even today and she is revered and celebrated as the symbol and voice of Afghan women. A bust and plaque honoring Rabia Balkhi stand in the stairwell of the hospital lobby; fresh flowers were strewn at the base of the bust.

Our presence was drawing attention even as we stood in the lobby. Dozens of women were walking around in the lobby and the adjacent hallways, many wearing *burkhas*, all wearing some form of head covering. Many were visibly pregnant and some were literally in the early stages of labor. When they saw us, most of the women hid their faces from us, stooping and turning to the walls to avoid eye contact, and drawing their headscarves over their faces. Part of this behavior, I'm sure, was due to the presence of the men in our small group, but we were told it was also due to our delegation's distinctly Western appearance.

All of our team were eager to see firsthand this hospital that had been designated as an important part of the solution for elevating the quality of care given to Afghanistan's women and children. We were all familiar with Afghanistan's infant, maternal, and childcare statistics. At the time of our visit, Afghanistan was one of the most dangerous places in the world to be either a pregnant woman or an infant or young child. Infant mortality in Afghanistan was arguably the highest in the world and about 25 percent of Afghan children died before their fifth birthday. An Afghan child had approximately a 1:7 chance of dying before its first birthday.

Maternal mortality in Afghanistan was among the highest in the world, with an estimated 17,000 women dying annually from pregnancy-related complications. Forty percent of deaths among women of childbearing age in Afghanistan were from preventable complications related to childbirth.

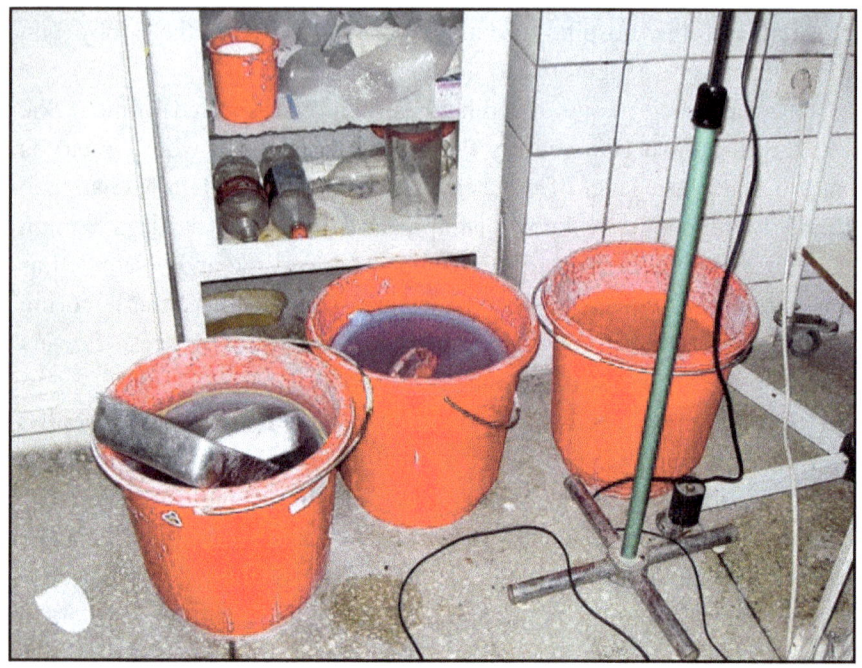

The "three-bucket" cleaning system for laundry and medical equipment

Bearing this information in mind, we started our tour. We were quickly stunned and heartbroken when we viewed the primitive conditions of the hospital. Sadly, what we saw was a hospital in disarray. Critical equipment necessary for surgery, anesthesia, lab assessments, instrument sterilization were obsolete, inadequate, or nonexistent. Basic surgical and medical instruments and standard medical items such as thermometers and blood pressure cuffs were insufficient to handle the needs of patients. Sanitation was poor due to the problematic and unpredictable building systems, such as plumbing and septic systems and inconsistent electrical services and utilities. Sewage from toilets seeped into the hallways in many areas. Soap and water were lacking in patient-care areas. We were told there was only one functional washing machine for the entire hospital. Sheets and patient gowns were washed in a three-bucket system of soak, wash, and rinse, or on the floor using a hose. Laundry and linens were drying on tables and chairs.

WELCOME TO HELL

Due to the cultural norm barring men from participating in women's care, the men participating in the tour were prohibited from viewing or touring some patient-care areas. Donna Harris shared that the number of hospital beds was insufficient in certain areas of the hospital and that she had observed two women recovering from deliveries sharing the same bed. She noted that there was no privacy in the delivery area; there were no curtains separating the delivery tables, which were just lined up in several rooms. As a pediatric nurse, one of Donna's immediate concerns was the absence of adequate bassinets, cribs, and incubators for infants. Given the brutally cold weather, the lack of blankets and quilts for mother and baby after delivery and recovery were also a great source of disquiet.

Outside, in an area of the hospital's courtyard, we saw a small structure that housed the OB-GYN clinic. Inside were an exam table and several chairs. We were told that daily dozens of patients came to the clinic and would wait outside for hours for an exam.

As our group debriefed after the hospital tour, the enormity of the challenge to raise the standards of maternal, child and infant care in Afghanistan was beginning to sink deeper and deeper into our consciousness. Horrified, we realized we had just viewed the best maternal care available in Afghanistan!

As I contemplated the myriad horrors we saw on our tour, coupled with the statistics denoting the reality of women's and children's care in Afghanistan, I was reminded of Shakespeare's phrase from *The Tempest*: "Hell is empty, and all the devils are here." It seemed to me that every demon, every conceivable variable that could adversely impact the delivery of quality care to Afghanistan's women and children, was present and conspiring against the Afghanis. While our role was to help upgrade the capabilities of Rabia Balkhi's health professionals and through the processes of education and experiential learning, to positively influence those determinants that impacted the quality of care provided at the Rabia Balkhi maternity hospital, it appeared that our efforts to do so would be in constant and direct conflict with the historic and traditional bedrock elements of Afghan societal culture.

Through the Lens of Humanity

After our first day at the hospital, each of us struggled to envision how our efforts could help bring successful change to the hospital. The realization of the extent and effect that decades of conflict and war had had on destabilizing and destroying the Afghani health system was disheartening as we reviewed our first day. Nevertheless, we all retained an enthusiast attitude that perhaps our efforts could be pivotal in contributing toward the developmental of a culture of care that enabled advances in the quality of care available to Afghanistan's women and children.

At breakfast the next morning, Dr. Greenfield advised me that she and Suzanne Griffin were going to meet with the Minister of Health to update him on the status of the project. I was invited to attend as well.

We drove to the offices of the Ministry of Health and presented ourselves at the minister's office. After a few moments, we were ushered in to meet Dr. Sayed Mohammad Amin Fatimi, Afghanistan's newly appointed Minister of Health. Dr. Fatimi, a tall, distinguished, bearded man with graying black hair and dressed all in black, greeted us in English with a lilting British accent. He greeted both Suzanne and Dr. Greenfield, whom he knew from previous contact, and then greeted me warmly with questions about where was I from and what did I think of Afghanistan so far. I shared with him who I was and how our team from Milwaukee fit into the overall strategy for the Rabia Balkhi project.

For the next hour over tea, Dr. Greenfield and Suzanne briefed him on the status of the hospital. It was clear from the conversation how sparse the resources of the Ministry were, and how dependent the Ministry was on NGOs like IMC for the provision of health services within the country. Dr. Fatimi expressed his enthusiastic support for the work of the project and constantly expressed hope that additional resources from the US Department of Health and Human Services and the US Department of Defense, would continue to be available.

The meeting came to a bit of an abrupt halt when Dr. Fatimi was summoned to a cabinet meeting by President Karzai. As we drove back to Rabia Balkhi, Suzanne, Dr. Greenfield, and I discussed how desperate the country was for resources of all types, and how fragile and perilous the country's entire health system was.

Our team's daily Kabul routine quickly became very basic and predictable over the remainder of our trip. I myself would get up as the *muezzin* began the call to prayer and head toward the showers on my floor. The water was always frigid; never once do I believe the water even reached lukewarm status. Hence, my showers, as well as those of everyone else, were brief events. Afterwards, I would dress, try and do a few emails if the internet was working, and then head downstairs and join the other team members for breakfast.

Typically, we'd all do our radio check-in together during breakfast, discuss our planned activities for the day, and then around 8 a.m, begin our journey to the hospital. Once at the hospital, we'd adjourn to our separate tasks and then reconvene between 5 and 5:30 p.m. for our travel back to the visitor's compound. We'd gather for dinner, do our radio check-ins and debrief each other on our day's activities. Then each of us would head to our respective rooms and our kerosene heaters; it was far warmer in our individual rooms with the smelly heaters than in the common areas of the compound.

It was at our dinner debriefing where our understanding of the reality of women's healthcare in Afghanistan most penetrated our consciousnesses. Many of our discussions focused on the observations of our nursing team members—Donna and Chris, and IMC's Linda Barnes—due to their more comprehensive access to the entire hospital than our male members, plus their intimate involvement with the educational and training processes associated with the nurse midwifery programs.

Despite the conditions we'd seen, in fairness, there were a number of encouraging signs. Under the Taliban regime, women were prohibited from attending schools and universities and as a consequence, created severe shortages of female healthcare providers, i.e., physicians and midwives to care for women of reproductive age.

With the fall of the Taliban in 2002, a critical strategy to reduce Afghanistan's maternal and infant mortality rates was to re-establish nurse midwifery training programs and physician residency programs in

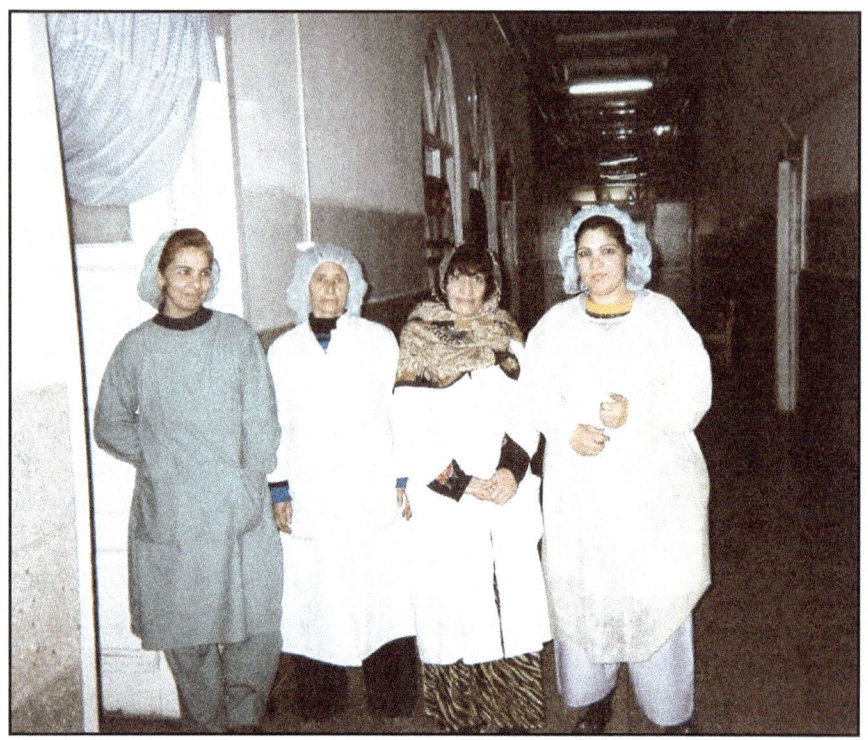
Afghani physician and midwife trainees

obstetrics and gynecology. This led to an influx of many Afghani women being admitted to Kabul Medical University, with which Rabia Balkhi Hospital had a relationship. Additionally, many women were now being enrolled in midwifery training programs and schools. Our team's function was to assist in the development and implementation of training curriculum and modules for both the midwifery and residency training programs.

What was quickly obvious to our team was the lack of basic nursing skills among the midwife trainees. While many had attended some formal education, basic nursing-skill training did not seem integrated into the midwifery training program. For example, when dealing with patients, the midwives did not wash their hands, consistently take a patient's vital signs, or interact meaningfully with the patients. Patient records didn't exist nor was there discharge planning for patients who had just delivered.

Linda, the IMC nurse educator, shared that she had previously served for three months at the hospital and provided clinical practice training for the midwives, but upon returning for a second three-month assignment, she found the skills she had initiated in her first visit had almost completely disappeared. Indeed, she said, many of the trainees she had previously taught were no longer at the hospital.

Nepotism, cronyism, and corruption also permeated both the midwife and physician staffs. We had several meetings as a team with the hospital director, Dr. Nadia Tariq, a young woman recently appointed by the Minister of Health. Dr. Tariq was also a resident physician who had not as yet completed her OB/GYN residency. While she was an earnest and enthusiastic woman whose intentions I am certain were genuine in terms of enhancing the quality of care at the hospital, her primary credential for this important role was rumored by the staff to be that she was the best friend of the wife of the president of Afghanistan, President Karzai.

Tribalism was evident throughout the hospital. Staff of the various Afghani tribes clustered and worked together and blatantly discriminated in providing (or not providing) care to women from tribes other than their own. We heard stories of pregnant women waiting in hospital hallways and then having to deliver their babies in the hall because midwives refused to assist or care for them because they were of a different tribe. The Hazara women seemed to bear the heaviest discrimination burden; there was clear evidence that Hazara women and infants had the poorest outcomes of care.

> Author's Note: In Afghan culture, boy babies are preferred. Hospital staff are bribed to switch a baby girl for a boy baby. Many "unwanted" girl babies were simply left at the hospital in hopes that some family might take them home.

Bribery was common at the hospital. Family members bribed the gatekeeper and other staff members to obtain entry into the hospital and be with their relative seeking care. There were stories of family members giving bribes to the surgeons who performed C-sections on women who, due to being under anesthesia, unknowingly delivered a girl and were given a baby boy to take home.

I tried to meet routinely with Dr. Tariq to assist her in developing organizational charts and accountability structures for the various functions of the hospital, and to help identify staff members to fill critical leadership roles. The hospital was severely short staffed, she said, and she constantly lamented the fact that the hospital experiences a no-show rate of 40 percent by the hospital staff including physicians. There is no incentive, she said, for staff to come to work since they are paid by the Ministry of Health regardless of whether they are present at work or not. Many of the hospital's attending physicians are also obstacles. Some refuse to see patients, take supplies and equipment from the hospital to stock their own offices, and even demand money/bribes from patients and families for their services.

Most of the staff physicians are also involved in the training of the OB/GYN residents, but the hospital director noted the medical staff provides unequal education and training and often conflicting information regarding patient-care protocols. Clinical training for residents was also largely based on a "who you know" basis. If residents didn't know or have pre-existing relationships with physician staff, they were largely left to their own devices to develop their clinical skills. Essentially, they were forced to employ a trial-and-error methodology in treating patients, hoping they were doing the right things and not inadvertently creating greater harm.

Dr. Tariq, as a resident herself, was trying to promote a more consistent and standardized medical curriculum for the residents that emphasized greater accountability, professionalism, and connectivity with senior medical staff at the hospital. All the while, she lamented the lack of good role models.

"We can teach clinical and patient management skills, but it is hard in this country to train moral skills without moral leaders or mentors," she said. Though she was young and inexperienced, I grew to admire Dr. Tariq for her dogged commitment to bring change to the dysfunctional culture of care that existed within the hospital. It was encouraging to see her perseverance in combatting corruption within the hospital and oppose efforts designed to discredit her abilities and plans. Facing seemingly insurmountable obstacles, hers was a voice for integrity and hope for the women of Kabul.

As disturbing and distressing these observations and stories were about how Afghani women were at risk due to insufficient staffing levels and inadequate clinical training for direct-care providers such as midwives and physicians, they paled in comparison to the horrific clinical-care situations we witnessed. These were inflicted on patients as a consequence of either societal culture or the prevailing culture of care at the hospital.

Donna Harris and Chris Gall from our Milwaukee team were both nurses seasoned by years of experience in practical nursing, including pregnancy and childbirth, and both were also specialists in pediatric and neonatal care. Donna and Chris were involved in basic nursing and midwifery education processes and daily engaged with trainees and staff in clinical activities. In our nightly debriefing, it was gut- and heart-wrenching to listen to them describe patient care incidents that they had observed. Donna diligently kept a diary, in which she painstakingly recorded her observations and shared with the team. Donna recorded the following entry describing an experience in the hospital's delivery room:

> I spent about 90 minutes in the delivery area. During my observation, a woman clearly in late labor walked into the delivery room, walked around, positioned herself on a delivery table, placed a towel under her perineal area, writhed in labor with contractions for 5 minutes and began to crown. Only then was she attended to. The baby was delivered but was not suctioned and did not breathe for about 45 seconds. An MD told the midwife to suction the baby. However, she could not find a suction bulb for another 15 seconds on so. She suctioned the baby. Apgars were about 3 at one minute ... 7-8 at 5 minutes. The baby was wiped with a rag-like cloth and placed on the scale and left for several minutes wrapped in the wet cloth with which

it was wiped. The baby was visibly cold. The temperature in the delivery room was probably in the 60s, since there is no source of heat. The baby was then placed on a pad, wet and stained with blood and meconium from previous infants, and was wrapped in an afghan-like blanket which looked like the same one used for a previous baby.

The baby was then wiped again, dressed, and swaddled with a blanket and sat (a traditional practice) and was placed in a "bin beside the table" beside 3 other babies. The bin was covered with a heavy quilt to keep the babies warm. However, no one observes or monitors the babies. I lifted the quilt and noted that one of the babies had nasal flaring and pointed this out. …

Babies are delivered into plastic garbage bags placed under the mother's perineum just before delivery and lay in the bloody drainage near the perineum while the cord is being tied off with string. Women deliver their babies with no privacy. There are no curtains between the delivery tables lined up side by side, 4 in a section. There is often only one midwife to attend to 7 women in the delivery room. There is no staff person routinely monitoring the babies, assuming the infants under the quilt are fine. There are no supplies for women who do not bring clothing or blankets for the infants with them. … Infants are not examined after delivery. An infant might be discharged with an imperforate anus after birth without this being identified.

Sadly, we saw many instances similar to that described by Donna in her diary reflection.

A daily ritual once we arrived at the hospital each morning is to attend and participate in what I'll refer to as "morning report," a time when "significant" patient issues that had occurred during the previous 24 hours are discussed. The meeting is attended by midwives and attending physicians and was typically led by an IMC physician and a hospital physician and midwife. These meetings highlighted for us so many of the clinical concerns that confront the hospital.

We learned that many women come to Rabia Balkhi in labor with preeclampsia (preeclampsia untreated can dramatically impact the health of the mother and infant). Daily, we heard of numerous fetal deaths of preterm infants. As we expressed amazement and concern over the number of reported daily deaths of women and infants, we were told that the death rates were actually declining. Even so, Donna at one point made the comment that through her observations in the delivery room and in the various patient-care units, she had witnessed many patient-care instances where she thought it was just pure luck that more women and infants had not died.

One evening, during our nightly dinner debrief at our compound, we discussed the fact that a set of triplets had been born that day. Chris reported that the infants all looked to be in good health and the mother also seemed to be doing well after the delivery. But what was disconcerting was that about three or four hours after delivery, the mother gathered up all three of her infants, wrapped them in blankets and quilts, and left to return to her home in a mountain village about a half-day's journey from Kabul!

Donna and Chris said that they and others had tried to prevent her from leaving, telling the mother that the infants and she should stay a day or two in the recovery areas of the hospital. They also shared their concerns with the mother about the extreme cold and how it might be harmful to the infants' health, particularly how the extreme cold might adversely affect their lungs.

Unfortunately, the mother refused to stay and left the hospital with a female relative helping her with the babies. Several days later, the mother returned to the hospital suffering from complications from the delivery. When asked how the three babies were faring, the mother responded that all three had died within a day of departing the hospital. The mother was despondent. She was treated and once again departed against the advice of medical personnel.

Having been initially involved in the delivery and care of the infants, our team was devastated by the news of their deaths, particularly after having pleaded with the mother to remain longer at the hospital for the good of both herself and her infants. However, we had grown to understand that this behavior was very typical of Afghani culture. Women delivered their babies and immediately returned to their homes and villages. It was common at Rabia Balkhi for women to arrive, deliver their babies and depart, all in the matter of hours. And oftentimes, women present at the hospital are not immediately attended to, and deliver their babies in the hallway with the assistance of a relative, or perhaps by the last-minute attendance of a midwife.

We learned that it was common for Afghan women, over the course of their reproductive years, to deliver as many as six to eight babies. Sadly, the infant death rate is so high that only one or two of the babies might survive to adulthood.

In her diary, Donna recorded a touching story of a woman who lost an infant:

> There was one woman in the post-surgical ward, quite isolated and without a baby as the other women were holding, feeding, caring for their babies. No one spoke to her. I approached the pediatrician and asked about her. She told me that this woman's baby had died prior to her C-section delivery. I approached the woman and just touched her hand, communicating my sorrow at the loss of her baby. She initially tried to hide her face but the tears began to flow down her cheeks. She looked at me with such sadness, with eyes of appreciation for support. Sadly, the OB physicians tell the staff not to give the women attention because they will demand even more. There is very little attention to emotional support and care, something the midwifery consultant is working hard to change......

Not a day went by that we weren't flabbergasted by events or occurrences in the hospital that either directly impacted patient care or reflected a cultural attitude of repression of or devaluation of women. We also heard of many issues that related to sanitary conditions around the hospital. Supplies and equipment were stored in the hospital's

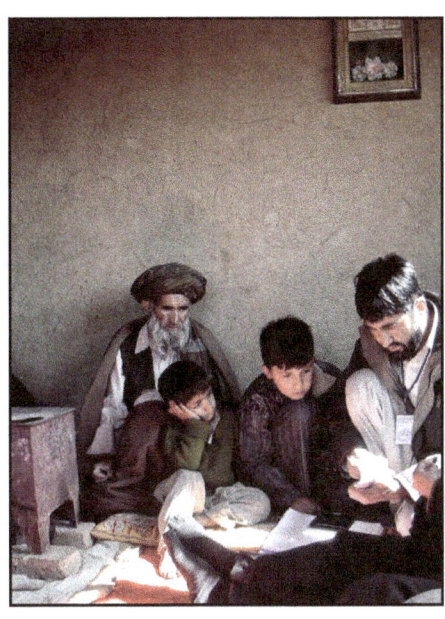

Sharing a meal with an Afghan family in rural Afghanistan

basement, but their dispensing was controlled by the head pharmacist, who routinely refused to provide requested supplies. One day, an obstetrician went to the basement to seek out Cesarean-section trays. To her dismay, she spied several cats eating dead birds in the basement, and was mortified when she saw several cats preparing to dine on placentas that were stored in one corner of the basement.

One morning, several of our team traveled with Suzanne Griffin from IMC and Dr. Greenfield from DHHS, to a village several hours outside of Kabul. The purpose of the field trip was to visit a basic Health Center and a small 20-bed village hospital. The conditions at both these facilities far exceeded those of Rabia Balkhi in terms of overall patient outcomes. Perhaps this was because of the cohesiveness of the village. Clearly there was not competition for care among different tribal units.

I'm sure the smaller scale of the facilities also permitted better training opportunities for the midwives and physicians as well. The training materials used were "talking books" that had been translated into Pastu, Dari, and English and covered a wide spectrum of clinical areas, including nutrition, prenatal care, infectious disease, breastfeeding, and so on. Candidly, this village experience reflected the best care for women that we had seen in Afghanistan.

At the conclusion of the visit, a village family invited the team for a meal. It was a feast of deliciously prepared traditional Afghani food and an incredible experience of hospitality. We all felt humbled by the fashion in which we, as strangers, were welcomed and fed. We knew too that the meal we shared with the family depleted their meager resources and was one they could hardly afford to share, yet their hospitality was unconditional.

The longer we worked in Rabia Balkhi, the more I began to understand the uncommon resiliency Afghan women displayed in the face of such overwhelming adversity. I was amazed by the courage they showed in spite of being forced to live lives in an environment of conflict and abhorrent conditions. I know I could never fully understand the context of their suffering as being the most vulnerable and lowliest regarded within their societies. Nevertheless, the steadfast perseverance I saw in them to go on in spite of their circumstances was their

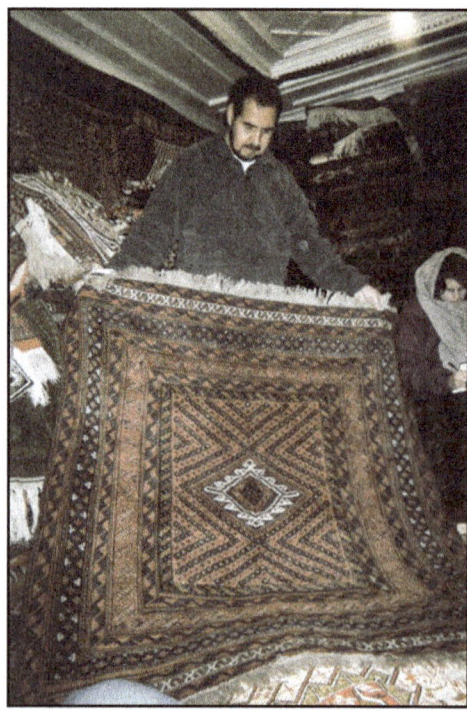

Carpet shopping on Kabul's famous Chicken Street

Welcome to Hell

witness and expression of hope for their future, and for the future of Afghanistan.

Despite the brutally cold weather, Donna, Chris, Suzanne from IMC, Dr. Greenfield, our driver Abdullah, and I on several occasions did venture into Kabul. Our first weekend in Kabul, we went for brunch at the International Hotel, which stands on the mountainside overlooking Kabul and provides a scenic view of the city and surrounding mountain ranges. By then, many of us were already suffering from colds, but we enjoyed being out and having the opportunity to see the city. The hotel served a wonderful buffet and had several small gift and craft shops where we shopped and found a few souvenirs, most of which were made by Afghani women. The hotel was also a routine target of shelling by remnants of the Taliban. In fact, just a couple of days earlier, it had suffered an attack, so we didn't loiter too long.

One afternoon, Abdullah took Donna, Chris, Doug, and me to Chicken Street in central Kabul. Chicken Street is Kabul's most famous shopping area for tourists who want to buy Afghan souvenirs. Abdullah told us that after the fall of the Taliban, many NGOs and occupying military arrived in Kabul and Chicken Street became the favorite site for tourists to shop. While apparently the street was named for a chicken shop that once stood in the area, it no longer existed and the street is lined with shops selling jewelry, oriental rugs, arts and crafts, antiques, knickknacks, and other Afghan exotica.

The street itself is a scruffy lane only a few blocks long and many of the shops are hole-in-the-walls.

The street's main attraction were the rug merchants, where we spent some time perusing the various carpets the merchants laid out for us as we drank tea. The carpets were beautiful, hand-woven rugs of varying colors and sizes. As specific carpets were laid out for our consideration, the merchant stated that each of his rugs had a small imperfection sown into the pattern, because he said, "Only God is perfect."

Bargaining is an art form in Afghanistan and I participated in the offer/counteroffer contest of skill for a small carpet. I knew I was in over my head immediately. I wanted to conclude the "deal" but the merchant was playing the long game, waiting me out to get his price. I walked away with the carpet, happy with my deal, but knowing I had been bested by the merchant in the bargaining game.

We returned to Chicken Street several times during our visit, never remaining long. US officials had issued an advisory cautioning against visiting the area, citing reports that areas proximate to Chicken Street had recently been targeted by suicide bombers. While the advisory did not restrict travel to the area, all NGO and US military personnel were advised to be extremely careful while visiting Chicken Street and surrounding locations. We were actually planning one last visit to the area prior to our departure, but another suicide bombing close to Chicken Street altered our plans.

Thirteen days after we touched down in Kabul, we departed for home. Our plan was to prepare a report of our trip for IMC and DHHS that included our educational and clinical observations and recommendations. A second trip by our team was already planned for June; our intent was to use the intervening months to develop additional training tools and materials for the midwives and physicians based upon our February findings.

Our departure was bittersweet. Despite the harsh weather conditions and the tragic conditions within Afghanistan's health delivery system that we had witnessed and experienced, we each felt that in some small measure, our visit had made a difference and our ongoing participation in the project could help save the lives of women and children. We also felt that we had developed a true kinship with the Afghani people and gained a profound sense of unity and purposefulness with them in their struggles to lay a foundation for something enduring particularly with respect to healthcare and medical education.

Twenty-one hours after departing Kabul, we landed in Milwaukee on February 28th. It was a bitterly cold day there, but after experiencing the brutal and vicious cold of Kabul, we felt we had landed in the midst of a heat wave.

Four months later, on June 24th, I landed again in Kabul airport, this time on a tattered and old Ariana Afghan Airlines airplane. For this trip, my team was a little different. Dr. Doug Laube was again part of

Welcome to Hell

the group; we were joined by newcomers Dr. Fritz Broekhuizen, an OB/GYN faculty member of the Medical College of Wisconsin, and Martty Berner, RN, a faculty member of the University of Wisconsin-Milwaukee' College of Nursing. Both Martty and Doug were veteran international volunteers—Doug previously in Afghanistan and Marrty in Africa. Both were affable and quick-witted. These two no-nonsense types were a delight!

Abdullah, the IMC employee and one of the drivers we had met on our February trip, picked us up at the airport and escorted us to our IMC guesthouse. Thankfully, this time our quarters were a little more appealing than our previous visit. We still were housed in a secure compound, but we were in a different location. Our guesthouse was known as Golf II, and Fritz, Doug, and I were in one section, while Martty was in a separate building known as Golf I, a guesthouse reserved exclusively for women. In our portion of the building, we actually had three "houseboys" who assisted with our basic needs of cooking, washing as necessary, and otherwise keeping the guesthouse clean. Our team were the only occupants of Golf I and Golf II while we were there. However, the guesthouses could easily accommodate a dozen or more people if need be.

Though we were in a different area of the city, the guesthouses still treated us to a magnificent view of the mountains. The building was tucked into an area of Kabul that felt more like a suburb. There were other compounds near us and we saw a great deal more pedestrian traffic than in our first visit. When we had visited in February, we were told that our visit coincided with the absolute coldest time of the year in Kabul. We learned that the current visit coincided with the absolute hottest time of the year.

Our rooms were more spacious in Golf I and II, and we actually had a nice common room and dining area, but there was no air conditioning. We had fans, some of which didn't work, but those that did rattled like airplane propellers and simply pushed warm air around the room, more like a heater than a cooler. The good news was while we lamented the cold showers we were forced to take in February, we reveled in them in June.

Through the Lens of Humanity

The evening of our arrival, our team had dinner with Dr. Mir Anwar, Head of Pediatrics at Rabia Balkhi and Suzannne Griffin of IMC, at the United Nations Club in downtown Kabul. Dr. Anwar, whom we had met in February along with Suzanne, brought us up to date on training since February. We were encouraged by their report and Martty especially looked forward to meeting with hospital staff to initiate the next wave of training for midwives and physicians alike.

As we drove into the hospital the next morning, Fritz and Martty, having not been to Rabia Balkhi before, were highly amused at the antics of the gatekeeper, who was still in residence at the front entrance with her ever-present entourage of "familiars" —the cats. Waiting for us inside the main entrance was Dr. Tariq, who had just returned from the United States and a fact-finding mission to visit several medical centers specializing in women's and children's healthcare. Part of her US visit was to attend training seminars on hospital and health administration. I was hopeful she would be able to put her learnings to good use, but given the enormity of the cultural challenges at the hospital, revamping the administrative structure of Rabia Balkhi would be a long and difficult struggle for even the most capable and experienced administrator, much less a novice administrator at the onset of a new administrative career.

We settled into a routine this trip much like our previous visit—up early with the *muezzin*'s call to worship, breakfast at the compound, then off to the hospital for training of midwifery staff by Martty, and physician training by doctors Laube and Broekhuizen. Occasionally, Fritz and Doug were able to have direct contact with patients so long as the patients were fully clothed and "chaperoned" by a family relative and Afghan female physician. In every instance, they were consulted, the patient thanked them profusely for their involvement, and most importantly, the Afghan physician "chaperone" had an unparalleled learning opportunity with a renowned OB/GYN educator.

For her part, Martty integrated herself nicely into the training regimen for midwives. She conducted daily workshops for approximately 20 midwives, and when she wasn't teaching, she was rounding with Afghan physicians and nurses and providing practical nursing experience instruction.

Suzanne Griffin and I spent many of our mornings attending Ministry of Public Health meetings at the ministry offices in downtown Kabul. The attendees of these meetings were an assortment of representatives from the various NGOs that were engaged with the Ministry in providing educational services or clinical care services throughout the Afghan healthcare system. US military personnel usually attended these sessions as well and provided security briefings relative to travel advisories within the city and the surrounding areas.

These meetings were useful for comparing notes and coordinating activities with other NGOs conducting similar projects. During our February visit, we had met Dr. Jeff Smith from JHPIEGO. JHPIEGO is an international NGO initially known as Johns Hopkins International Education in Gynecology and Obstetrics, renowned for its expertise in reproductive health, family planning, maternal, newborn and child health, and so on. Dr. Smith had been working in Afghanistan for some time and had developed a number of programs for Afghanistan's Ministry of Health along with the World Health Organization. During our visit, he was in Kabul working on the development of a national course for emergency OB care. Jeff was certainly familiar with the situation at Rabia Balkhi, and he agreed to have dinner with Fritz and me to discuss his work and how we might integrate it into our own.

Jeff suggested we meet at Flashman's Restaurant on Passport Lane. Flashman's was part of Gandamack Lodge, one of the more popular expatriate hangouts in Kabul. Gandamack Lodge had been described to us as a "resurrection of Victorian England in a walled compound bristling with security guards in an Afghan capital whose streets can quickly turn deadly."

Historically, the village of Gandamack in eastern Afghanistan was the site of an 1842 battle where the British suffered a humiliating defeat. The owner of Gandamack Lodge, Peter Juvenal, a British journalist and history buff, took the name of the lodge from this historic encounter between the British and Afghans. And, the name and decor of Flashman's restaurant/pub was inspired by the character of Brig.

Through the Lens of Humanity

General Sir Harry Paget Flashman, a fictional hero of English historical novels by George MacDonald Fraser. In one of his novels, Fraser describes Flashman as "a charming scoundrel and decorated coward" who survived the battle of Gandamack by "deceit and dastardly deeds".

Upon entering the lodge and the restaurant, one is confronted by several large 19th-century maps and faded photographs, antique calvary sabers, muskets, and other relics of faded glory. Adding to the Victorian motif are low ceilings, wooden beams, aging Afghan carpets, and several functional potbellied stoves . The clientele consists mainly of expatriates, diplomats, NATO and other military personnel, journalists and, reputedly spies. Enhancing the lodge's mystique was the fact that the building was once home to the fourth wife of al Qaida's Osama bin Laden.

An added attraction of Flashman's was that it was one of the few restaurants in Kabul where alcohol was served, and this, combined with a variety of superbly cooked Afghan dishes, made the restaurant a nice haven for us to adjourn to and have a nice dinner and discussion with Dr. Smith.

One of our other excursions during our stay was a visit to Bagram Air Force Base. The base itself is up on a mountainside and we were able to get a bird's-eye view of Kabul as we snaked up the mountain road. It was a bright, clear day and it seemed to me that the mountain views were even more spectacular from the vantage point of the base.

One of the physician military officers we coordinated with at the interagency NGO meetings accompanied us to the base and assisted in enabling us to get on the base. We were allowed to move freely around the base and had several chats with US servicemen, who inquired who we were and where in the States we were from. After lunch at a pizzeria on the base, we went to the Post Exchange (PX) and bought a few souvenirs, but one of our primary tasks at the PX was to purchase a few bottles of bourbon to enjoy in the evenings after we returned to Golf II from the hospital. Our mission complete, we returned to Kabul in the late afternoon.

It had become our practice—Doug's, Fritz's, and mine—to have a relaxing few fingers of bourbon at Golf II when we returned in the evening and prior to dinner. One evening, we poured our drinks, toasted each other, took our first sips, looked at each other, and started laughing. Our habit was to leave the bourbon in a cabinet in the dining room. As we each drank our drinks, we realized that the bourbon had been watered down.

By now, we knew Afghan Muslims weren't supposed to drink alcohol. What we suspected was happening was that our Afghan houseboys were helping themselves to a few shots of bourbon and were adding water to the bottle to make it appear that bourbon levels hadn't changed. We were greatly amused by what was going on and decided to discreetly let the houseboys know that it was okay with us if they wanted a shot of bourbon, we certainly weren't going to tell anyone, but please, we asked them, don't water down good bourbon!

While Martty spent the bulk of her days in the hospital teaching about two dozen midwives, a substantial portion of my time, along with Doug and Fritz's, was spent in meeting with Ministry of Public Health personnel discussing appropriate training curricula for the residency and midwifery programs. We also discussed the prospect of bringing clinical providers in the areas of anesthesiology, laboratory, and pharmacy in future trips. These were all disciplines that were sorely needed at Rabia Balkhi. It was clear to our team that the hospital wasn't going to achieve its goals of substantially reducing maternal and child death rates without a full complement of competent providers in these areas as well.

However, as our second trip drew to an end, we knew our ongoing participation in the project was at risk due to funding issues. Our funding was only for a year and it wasn't assured we'd receive funding for an additional period of time. We departed with the hope of returning again, but were prepared for the reality that this might our team's last visit. That said, we left with the knowledge that progress was being made in all the training areas in which we had been engaged. We knew too that the hospital staff had accepted members of our team not only as teaching professionals. In addition, many enduring friendships between our team and the Afghan healthcare providers had also been forged.

THROUGH THE LENS OF HUMANITY

Our trip reports from both our February and June visits reflected what we felt to be true: the strategic approach to improving the quality of care provided to Afghanistan's women and children and to reducing the country's maternal and infant mortality rates could not occur simply by training additional midwives and OB/GYN physicians. Certainly a chief obstacle to better health for women and children has been the lack of female health workers and female physicians. This training must be done recognizing the cultural pressures facing both patients and providers.

Long-term solutions to address the care of women and children in Afghanistan would require the elimination of many barriers that the men place upon women that preclude women from being integrated in meaningful ways in Afghan society. During our visits, we were aware that more and more Afghan leaders in the post-Taliban era wanted to incorporate women more fully into Afghan social and economic structures through education, employment, and participation in community and political entities as a means of rehabilitating and rebuilding Afghanistan. It was certainly our sense from our participation in the project that a more open and tolerant post-Taliban Afghan society in which women are afforded greater equality and self-worth would be paramount if the systemic changes necessary in the Afghan health system are to be achieved.

As we suspected, shortly after our June team's return from Kabul, we were notified that our participation in the project would be ending, at least for the time being. As I reflected on my experiences in Afghanistan, I was struck by the extremes of my life and that of the people of Afghanistan that we met. For a moment, I tried to put myself in their place. Would I want to be viewed as a person to be pitied due to the absence of material goods and resources? Would I be able to survive in an intolerant and repressive country? How would I adapt to not having access to quality healthcare for my family and myself? How would I emotionally and mentally deal with the deaths of family and friends from causes that were completely preventable? How would I handle being perceived as someone of less value than others? Just how would people from other countries and cultures view me—my humanity and my dignity?

As I reflected, I thought of some of our experiences in Afghanistan: a rural family welcoming us into their home and sharing their hospitality with us in ways I'm not so sure would have been as genuine and authentic if the tables were turned and we were opening our homes to them.

As I noted in earlier chapters, I have long been a fan of Rudyard Kipling's prose and poetry. His poem, "The Ballad of East and West," specifically the opening four lines, speaks to the topic of equality, the possibility of mutual understanding, and respect for polar opposites:

> Oh, East is East, and West is West, and never the twain shall meet,
> Till Earth and Sky stand presently at God's great Judgment Seat,
> But there is neither East nor West, Border, nor Breed, nor Birth,
> When two strong men stand face to face, though they come from the ends of the earth!

The story of the rest of the poem is that two men who are polar opposites, one an English officer and the other an Afghan horse thief, whose rivalry and animosity to each other in the end turns to great admiration and respect. The essence of the poem is that though the ends of the earth cannot meet, people cannot only transcend the boundaries of East and West, but also borders, birth, and breeding and appreciate each other's humanity, dignity, and rectitude.

In our travels to Afghanistan from Milwaukee, East did meet West, and I believe our team and the patients and providers we met are all better for it. Though our cultures were quite different, our common humanity enabled us to find mutual respect and admiration. It is only with this type of understanding can the hopes, dreams, and aspirations of the Afghan people for their future be realized.

Part Five

"Once a Hopie…"

CHAPTER 10

"Once a Hopie, Always a Hopie"

Beginning in 1987 and throughout the 1990s, I volunteered in international healthcare or Christian mission-oriented projects in India, in the Netherlands, Hungary and Germany in Eastern Europe, in Taiwan, in Chile, in the African countries of Malawi, Zambia and South Africa, and in China. Each journey had been an opportunity to reach out and share life and life experiences with other people and other cultures. Once I had a taste of such experiences, I couldn't get enough of them, and I knew that these journeys were my attempts to heal a few more of the world's wounds. And I knew these journeys were my own personal "hound of heaven," a steady, relentless pull towards a path of service commitment to the disenfranchised and disadvantaged abroad.

Therefore, I wasn't surprised when in June of 2000, I received the call that I knew one day would come, a call I knew I couldn't turn away from, a call to work full-time in the international arena. The call came from Project HOPE, a renowned international health education and training organization I knew and respected. The invitation to join the staff of Project HOPE was the culmination of an association with Project HOPE that had stretched over several years. Here's the story.

Growing up in the 1960s I often saw television commercials extolling the work of Project HOPE around the world. Like many others, I was captivated by photographs of the huge white hospital ship with the word HOPE emblazoned in black on its hull sailing out of New York Harbor with the Statue of Liberty in the foreground. As I grew older and learned the history and lore of the ship,

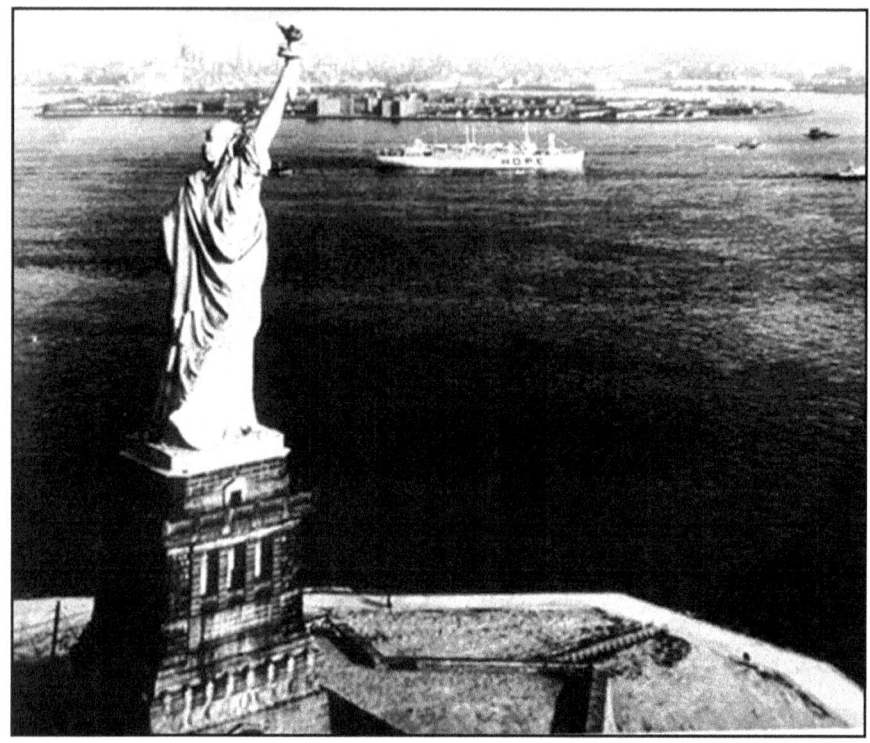

The *HOPE* sails out New York Harbor (Source: Project HOPE archives)

the SS *HOPE*, I became more intrigued by stories of its voyages to exotic locales to provide medical care and assistance to the most vulnerable people in every region of the world.

Project HOPE was founded by Dr. William B. Walsh, Sr. in 1958. Dr. Walsh, as the story goes, served in the US Navy on a destroyer during World War II, and was disturbed by the poor conditions he witnessed while serving in the Pacific.

Following the war, Dr. Walsh established a medical practice and became a noted Washington DC cardiologist. After President Dwight Eisenhower suffered a heart attack, Dr. Walsh was called in as a consultant. President Eisenhower and Dr. Walsh became fast and close friends, and Eisenhower, knowing of Dr. Walsh's interest in international healthcare, appointed Walsh co-chair of a committee whose purpose was to assist emerging nations with the development of medical and health professions.

Shortly thereafter, Dr. Walsh proposed the concept of a peacetime hospital ship to the president, and Dr. Walsh worked with Eisenhower to charter and lease a retired, mothballed Navy hospital ship, the USS *Consolation*, for one dollar per year. Dr. and Mrs. Walsh then raised $750,000 to transform the ship into the SS *HOPE*, a floating humanitarian vessel of healing and hope. Thus, Project HOPE was born.

The SS *HOPE* sailed out of San Francisco on its maiden voyage to Indonesia in September, 1960. Through the years, the ship sailed over 250,000 miles as part of 11 humanitarian voyages to various ports of call, where it provided health services to those in need, and health education and training to local healthcare professionals. In 1974, the SS *HOPE* was retired due to its age, rising maintenance costs, and increased requests to support land-based projects. With the ship's retirement, Project HOPE's humanitarian efforts were transitioned to land-based projects and programs, a transition that enabled Project HOPE to expand from a single-ship service provider to a global organization serving multiple countries via multiple projects and programs.

My first professional contact with Project HOPE occurred in the late 1980s. At that time, Project HOPE had initiated a partnership with the Shanghai municipal government and Shanghai's Jiao Tong University School of Medicine to help plan, develop, and construct a national children's medical center in Shanghai. Jiang Zemin, a future president of China, was then mayor of Shanghai (1984 to 1987), was supportive of the hospital project, and helped facilitate Project HOPE's involvement. Project HOPE was looking for someone with children's hospital administrative experience to live in Shanghai and essentially serve as Project HOPE's Project Director.

I was invited to Project HOPE's headquarters in Millwood, Virginia, to interview with Dr. Walsh, and his son, John Walsh, who was assigned to oversee Project HOPE's China initiatives. Project HOPE's headquarters were on a 200-acre site in Virginia's Shenandoah Valley, with the offices located in a building adjacent to Carter Hall, a classic Southern plantation mansion that had originally also been donated, and was presently owned by Project HOPE. Carter Hall was utilized as a conference center and guest house for conferees and visiting international dignitaries and delegations.

Dr. Walsh was charismatic and charming, and both he and John offered me the position. While I was tempted and flattered, at that point in my career, I wasn't ready to uproot myself and move to Shanghai for what clearly was going to be a project destined to take a number of years to complete in a very challenging and unpredictable environment.

Though I didn't accept this role, I was excited and gratified when Project HOPE asked me to participate as a consultant in several of their projects. One of the most fascinating was in Taipei, Taiwan, where the project was to evaluate whether an apartment building could be retrofitted as a hospital in an underserved and impoverished area of the city.

I was still able to contribute to the development of the national children's hospital, which became known as the Shanghai Children's Medical Center (SCMC). In my role as Executive Vice President of Children's Hospital of Wisconsin (CHW), I was able to help identify academic physicians from various pediatric subspecialties who could serve as consultants for the hospital as it developed its cadre of pediatric specialty services.

In January 1998, as the construction of the SCMC was being completed and plans for the facility's opening were being finalized, Jon Vice, Chief Executive Officer of CHW, and I traveled to Shanghai to consult with the Chinese academic and physician leaders charged with opening the hospital and to offer our recommendations and observations on how best to open the new facility. Six months later, on June 1, 1998, Shanghai's Vice Mayor Madame Zuo Huancheng and Hillary Clinton, then First Lady of the United States, presided over the inauguration ceremony for the Shanghai Children's Medical Center. The hospital's opening day, June 1, coincided with International Children's Day, certainly apropos for the collaboration between China and Project HOPE and other US partners.

"ONCE A HOPIE, ALWAYS A HOPIE"

In October 1999, I again traveled to Shanghai to speak at a Project HOPE-sponsored conference on hospital management, finance and fundraising that was held on the campus of Shanghai Children's Medical Center. Throughout 1998 and 1999, I assisted in bringing Chinese pediatric specialty physicians to Children's Hospital of Wisconsin as part of Project HOPE's Senior Technical Advisory Group (SENTAG) program, whose primary task was to recruit talented Chinese physicians for training as future Shanghai Children's Medical Center Medical Staff.

Over the years of working with Project HOPE senior staff, I had gotten to know them well, not only the staff at Project HOPE headquarters but also many in-country staff in nations around the world. In June 2000, when the offer to join Project HOPE on a full-time basis with responsibility for a portfolio of projects in Asia and the Middle East, including Shanghai Children's Medical Center, came along, it certainly piqued my interest.

The role I was offered was that of Senior Executive Director of Asia/Middle East Operations with responsibilities for existing projects in China, Indonesia, Thailand, Egypt, and Turkey. Project HOPE's intent was to expand operations in these countries and explore opportunities for expansion into other countries in these regions as well. The position would be based in HOPE headquarters in Millwood, Virginia, but I would be expected to routinely travel abroad to oversee the ongoing projects in the countries under my purview.

After a lot of soul-searching—I had been at Children's Hospital of Wisconsin 20 years—I decided to take the plunge and accepted the offer. While I could have stayed at Children's, I knew that I didn't want ten more years to pass and find myself looking back wishing I had taken another road, tried something different.

Leaving Children's Hospital and Milwaukee was difficult. Not only was I leaving professional colleagues and mentors I had known and worked with for years, I was upending my personal life as well. The move meant leaving behind friends, a church community that had fostered and supported my international interests, and a city that I had grown to know and love.

THROUGH THE LENS OF HUMANITY

My last day at Children's Hospital was Friday, September 29. The following day, I began a two-day drive from Milwaukee to Millwood, Virginia. When I resigned from Children's, I had begun house-hunting in the area surrounding Millwood and ultimately contracted to buy a town home in a development in Leesburg, Virginia, a fast-growing community about a 30-minute drive from Millwood. My townhouse wouldn't be available for occupancy for about six months, so Project HOPE had set aside a room for me in one of the guesthouses on the Carter Hall campus. My start date at Project HOPE was Tuesday October 2, 2000.

Two weeks later, I was on the road to Asia for a three-week trip that would include visits to Shanghai, Hangzhou, Beijing, Chengdu, and

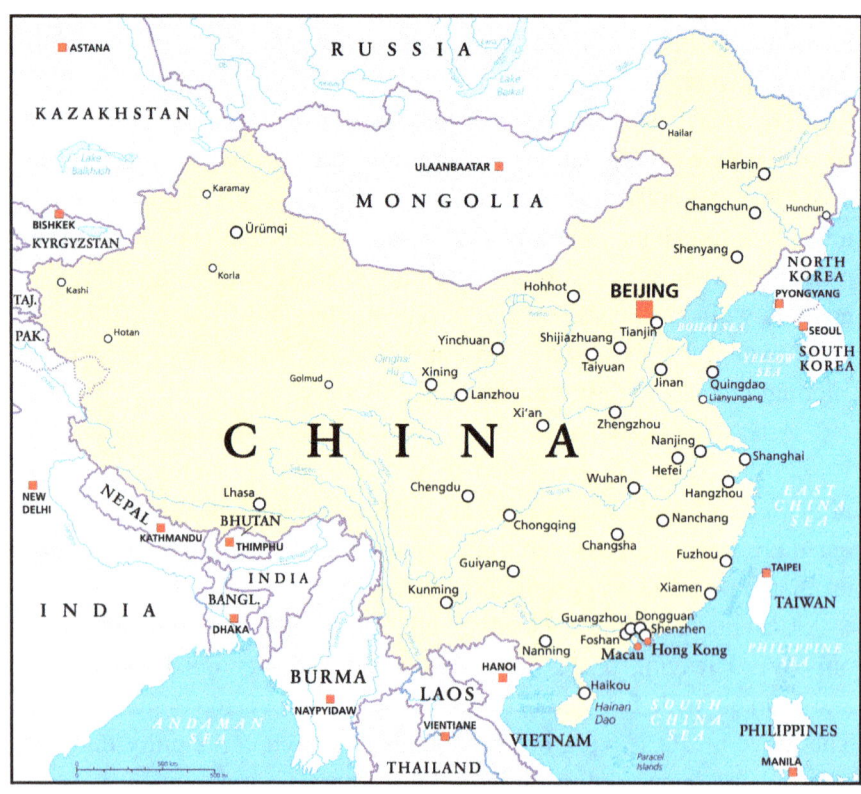

Destinations: Shanghai, Hangzhou, Beijing, Chendu, Xian, China; Hong Kong; Tokyo, Japan

"Once a Hopie, Always a Hopie"

Xian in China, as well as to Hong Kong and Tokyo, Japan. A major component of Project HOPE's mission was health education and training, so as HOPE moved into China, relationships were established with many of the major academic institutions in country, particularly those involved in medical education. The primary purpose of my first trip abroad as a HOPE employee was to meet my in-country Chinese staff in HOPE's Shanghai and Beijing offices, and to meet the leaders of the various Chinese academic institutions with which Project HOPE was aligned.

Bob Burastero, whom I was succeeding due to his retirement, accompanied me on my maiden voyage as a HOPE employee. Bob had worked for HOPE for years and was primarily responsible for setting up the relationships with the universities we were going to visit.

Our first stop was Shanghai. Dr. Frieda Law was the head of HOPE's operations in Shanghai; she and I had previously met during one of my consulting trips to Shanghai. We spent a day touring the Shanghai Children's Medical Center. I was amazed at how busy it had already become after only a year of operation. Shanghai Children's constituted HOPE's primary focus in Shanghai.

Bob also introduced me to the presidents of Shanghai Second Medical University and Jiao Tong University and together, we strategized about ongoing physician training programs that HOPE coordinated between their universities and US-based medical schools.

While in Shanghai, I was fascinated to learn that the city had been growing so rapidly since the 1990s that more than half the building cranes in the world were in Shanghai! I believed it—everywhere you looked, you saw dozens and dozens of cranes.

The Bund in Shanghai is a rich cultural asset of historic Shanghai. It is a waterfront area of the Huangpu River and faces the many splendid skyscrapers in the Pudong area of Shanghai. One of the Bund's great tourist attractions is the Peace Hotel, where President Nixon stayed during his historic visit to China in the early 1970s. A popular attraction in the Peace Hotel is the downtown bar where the "Old Jazz Band" plays. The band's name is correct—it is composed of elderly musicians who have played in the bar for decades. They might not hit every note correctly anymore, but a visit to the Peace Hotel bar is truly an enjoyable experience!

Next stop on our agenda was the city of Hangzhou, one of seven cities that had once been capitals of ancient China. A two-and-a-half-hour train ride from Shanghai brought us to Hangzhou, one of the largest cities in China with, at that time, over twenty million people. Project HOPE was conducting a diabetes training conference and our arrival coincided with the opening ceremony of the program. Dr. Shell Xue, Project HOPE's Beijing Director, was in Hangzhou facilitating the training conference, so it was an ideal opportunity to meet her and see her Beijing-based staff in action. Shell was an impressive young woman. She described herself as a "daughter of China" and she certainly had a missionary zeal to accomplish good things for her country.

Diabetes is a significant health issue in China and HOPE's diabetes program encompassed training components for patients and families, as well as health providers such as nurses and physicians. Funding for the program was provided through a collaborative partnership with three pharmaceutical companies: Eli Lilly, Roche, and Becton-Dickensen. The program HOPE had developed was national in scope and well-received by Chinese universities, even the Chinese Ministry of Health. The pharmaceutical companies were excited by the program because it gave them an opportunity to introduce their products into China in a way that was endorsed and supported by the Chinese government.

Project HOPE's academic partner in Hangzhou was Zhejiang Medical School. We met with former President Zheng Shu, who, in 1982, had met with Dr. Walsh and subsequently facilitated meetings between Dr. Walsh and numerous Chinese medical schools presidents. Through his relationship with Dr. Walsh, Dr. Shu in many ways had helped lay the groundwork for Project HOPE to establish a foothold in China.

We returned to Shanghai from Hangzhou, again by train, in order to attend a Project HOPE conference on Gaucher disease, an inherited genetic disorder that causes bone and organ abnormalities, and neurological problems. Project HOPE provided medicine in China for

"Once a Hopie, Always a Hopie"

Gaucher through a grant from Genzyme Corporation. This afforded me an opportunity to spend time getting to know the Shanghai HOPE staff. I also was able to spend time with Dr. Shen Xiao Ming, who had recently been appointed President of Shanghai Children's Medical Center. Dr. Shen was a rising star within China's medical landscape; he clearly was being groomed for higher positions within the Chinese governmental structure. Dr. Shen and I had become fast and good friends and he was always fascinating to talk with given his insights into the way China's healthcare system was evolving.

> Author's note: Dr. Shen's meteoric rise has continued over the years. He has served as President of Shanghai Children's Hospital, President of Shanghai Second Medical University, Executive Vice President of Shanghai Jiao Tong University, Vice Mayor of Shanghai for Health and Education, Party Secretary of Pudong, and Administrator of the Shanghai Free-Trade Zone. I saw Dr. Shen last in September of 2019 when we had dinner together in Haiku, Hainan Province, where since 2017, Dr. Shen has been Governor of the Province.

Chengdu, the capital city of Sichuan Province in western China was next on our tour itinerary and a three-hour flight west of Shanghai. Its population at that time was approximately nine million people. Project HOPE's partner in Chengdu was West China University of Medical Science, a relationship that had existed since the early 1980s. As we were being transported to our hotel by our West China University hosts, we were informed that the government had decided to merge the university into the larger Sichuan University over the next year or so. That would actually be advantageous to Project HOPE, given that Sichuan University was a larger and more prestigious organization.

Dentistry and diabetic programs were the staple of HOPE's programs within West China University. We were encouraged to learn that West China's president was eager to expand its collaboration to include cardiovascular care, hospital and healthcare management, as well as HIV/AIDS and tuberculosis programs.

Through the Lens of Humanity

Chengdu is famous for being the home habitat for the giant panda bear, another national treasure of China. And as the capital of Sichuan, it is renowned for its food, and notorious for its hot and spicy hotspots dishes!

The ancient city of Xian is an hour by air from Chengdu. Massive walls and gates surround this majestic old city, which is home to thousands of terra cotta warrior sculptures. Emperor Qin She Huang, had the terra cotta warriors buried with him to protect him in the afterlife. Though one of the oldest cities in China, Xian is presently a bustling city of approximately six million people. We visited Xian Medical University, which had just merged into Xian Jiaotong University. The Xian Medical University was collaborating with Project HOPE's diabetes training program and also eager to partner in Project HOPE's cardiovascular training programs.

From Xian, we flew to Hong Kong. In 1987, I had flown into Hong Kong's old airport, where it seemed like one was flying over the bay literally between the city's buildings. This time, I flew into the new airport, recently completed and one of the largest airports in the world. Our mission in Hong Kong was to meet with several prospective donors and encourage funding for new HOPE programs in the areas of cardiovascular care and healthcare management.

Next, I flew from Hong Kong to Beijing to meet with Beijing staff and pharmaceutical donors who were funding HOPE's diabetes program. While in Beijing, I traveled to visit perhaps China's greatest icon, the Great Wall of China. When one views this structure, one not only sees the extravagance and creativity of Chinese architecture, but one also understands that this structure is one of the greatest feats of engineering history. This wall was not just a wall; it was an integrated military defensive system spanning hundreds of miles of Chinese borders.

The final stop in my inaugural journey as a Project HOPE employee was Tokyo, Japan, to attend a Project HOPE Japan board meeting. It was my first visit to Japan, and more than any other place I'd visited, the pace and press of people in Tokyo was palpable. One could literally feel the rush of people as they passed—their kinetic energy if you will.

Bob Burastero and I had landed in Narita Airport and then taken a shuttle bus downtown to the Washington Hotel in Tokyo's Shinjuku District. We had dinner in the hotel's bar/restaurant, and as we dined, we watched US presidential election news coverage. It was Wednesday night, November 9, 2000, in Tokyo and Al Gore and George W. Bush were deadlocked in the presidential election. The presidency, intoned the newscasters, would hinge on a recount of Florida ballots. As we sat and ate, we noticed the waiters and other patrons watching the news as well, and looking, nodding, and smiling at us with friendly and sympathetic glances. Little did anyone realize at the time that it would be another month before the election was decided!

Our agenda in Tokyo was to meet with officials from Project HOPE Japan, an affiliate of Project HOPE, which funded HOPE projects in Asia. Thailand and Indonesia were two Asian countries under my jurisdiction, and each country's HOPE program directors were young Japanese women. Project HOPE Japan also provided limited funding support for Shanghai Children's Medical Center.

Project HOPE Japan leased space in an industrial complex outside of Tokyo proper. Bob and I were met in the hotel lobby by a senior staffer of HOPE Japan who was to guide us to HOPE Japan's offices. This necessitated taking the subway/railway. As we were entering the subway station, several trains pulled in. I have never seen such a mass of humanity scurrying and surging through the station like human tidal waves. This was one of the few times in my life I felt claustrophobic as I was squeezed against the crowd pushed and pulled along. My goal was to not get crushed or lose sight of Bob or the HOPE Japan official; literally thousands of people poured and gushed through the station's corridors like water out of a firehose. We were pushed aboard the subway and stood shoulder to shoulder as the train rocketed out of the station. When we disembarked at our stop, Bob and I looked at each other, shook our heads, and laughed, both thankful we had survived the subway without injury!

Through the Lens of Humanity

A full day of program and budget meetings ended with a wonderful Japanese banquet at a restaurant near our hotel.

Twenty-three days after departing the US on my inaugural Project HOPE trip, I returned to my new temporary home at Carter Hall. The journey had been quite an education, not only in terms of meeting my Asia-based staff and learning of HOPE's current programs and future opportunities in Asia, but more specifically and more enjoyably, in learning more about the customs and culture of the Asian people.

I would be remiss if I didn't say a few words about the practices and symbolism of Chinese and banquets. The Chinese certainly share a key concept with the rest of the world, which is that fine food and good drink, shared in the company of good friends and colleagues, certainly constitutes one of the great pleasures in life. However, I learned that many aspects and values of Chinese banquets and dining are approached very differently from those common in the West.

During our travel within China, each day culminated with an elaborate banquet. The Chinese banquet is a layered experience, a staged drama rivaling the best dramatic screenplays. Our experience was that round tables were typically set for eight up to twelve people. As the guests of honor at the banquet, Bob and I were seated in the best seats and then surrounded by our Chinese hosts according to their social hierarchy and professional position.

Then the festivities started, usually with a welcoming toast by the senior Chinese host. This is followed by a parade of courses, typically as many as eight cold-dish and eight hot-dish servings, each served one at a time. Major cooked items such as a whole fish, chicken, suckling pig, or cuts of beef are placed in the middle of the banquet table to be shared by all. The variety of food texture and colors serves Chinese aesthetic purposes, while the ritual of dish sharing conveys friendship and relationship. Depending on the section of the China you're visiting, the cuisine can be very different.

Our banquet dinner dishes were never dull, commonly challenging, and always interesting. I tried to be a good sport and at least taste everything I was served. Since our journey spanned a great deal of China, we experienced a wide array of Chinese cuisine (Cantonese,

"Once a Hopie, Always a Hopie"

Shandong, Szechuan, Anhui). I can say that I've tasted and eaten among other things: duck blood soup, bird's nest soup, chicken soup, stinky tofu, pig brains, frog legs, fried cicada, pigeon-on-a-stick (this in a local market), Peking duck (including the webbed feet and tongue), bamboo rice, chili chicken, spring rolls, spicy peri-peri chicken satay, shrimp, sucking pig, turtle soup (turtle included), glazed fish, sweet-and-sour pork, braised beef, fried scorpion, dumplings, and all manner of rice (steamed rice, fried rice, vegetable rice), and much more. Given the number of dishes served, Chinese banquets are notoriously long. The final dish served is fruit, most often watermelon. I can't describe how happy I was at times to see the watermelon arrive!

Long before the watermelon arrives, the toasting begins. *Gan bei* in Chinese means "dry the cup," or "bottoms up." The senior host starts the *gan-bei*-ing sometime during the dinner, usually specifically offering the toast to an individual. The recipient responds to the host with the top of his glass lower than that of the person offering the toast, as a sign of respect. I was told that rather than simply taking a sip, the custom is for both parties to drink up—"dry the cup"—at one time. At the banquets I've attended, the waiters seem far too attentive to filling all the glasses up with wine, so as you finish a *gan bei* with one person, another is likely on the horizon. The culture behind *gan bei* is the more you drink, the more respect you show. Trust me, it is quickly easy to be highly respectful and highly drunk at a Chinese banquet. Many were the nights after our banquets that I *gan bei*-ed Pepto Bismal to counteract all the food and drink!!

After my inaugural trip with HOPE, I took some time that November to help celebrate my parents' 50th wedding anniversary and to enjoy Thanksgiving Day. And, like millions of my fellow Americans, I watched the ongoing and unfolding constitutional drama and suspense of the 2000 Presidential election. "Hanging chads" entered the public lexicon and the month of November ended with people throughout the US anxious for this national nightmare to end.

In early December, I began another three-week sprint across the world to visit countries within my area of responsibility. This time, my travel encompassed China, Turkey, and Egypt. China was becoming old hat, but I had never visited Turkey before and it had been several years since I had been to Cairo.

Project HOPE's office in Turkey was located in Istanbul, formerly known as Byzantium and Constantinople. Having never been to Istanbul, I was delighted to get the opportunity to tour this exotic city straddling Eastern and Western cultures. HOPE's programs in Turkey revolved around rehabilitation projects and ongoing humanitarian support for survivors of the 7.4 magnitude earthquake that had devastated the Marmara region of Turkey in 1999 and left over 17,000 dead. Project HOPE's Turkey director toured me through the epicenter of the earthquake. We discussed with Turkish Ministry of Health officials how HOPE, via an airlift, could assist in providing relief supplies for the ravaged areas. We agreed that HOPE would also bring "visiting physicians" from the US to the region to assist in providing complex trauma and injury care to residents still recovering from the aftermath of the earthquake.

Didem, HOPE's country director, also provided a first-rate tour of Istanbul, including the Topkapi Palace, Taksim Square, the Sultan Ahmed Mosque—a.k.a. the Blue Mosque—Hagia Sophia, the Dolmabahce Palace, and of course, the famous Istanbul bazaar. I learned the fine art of negotiation from Didem in the bazaar as I bargained over several Turkish rugs. Over dinner during my last night in Istanbul came the breaking news that the US Supreme Court had decided in Bush's favor and that he would become the 43rd President of the United States, thus ending a weeks-long drama that had captivated people worldwide.

I traveled next to Cairo, and felt like I was in a 1940's Hollywood adventure film, going from the mystique and mystery of Istanbul to the mystique and mystery of ancient Cairo. I always feel like I'm putting on the cloak of history when I'm in a city like Cairo and walking the thousand-year old streets and alleyways. One of the treats of this trip was touring the museums in Cairo with HOPE Egypt staff and seeing the antiquities housed there.

My visit to Cairo coincided with Ramadan, which, in the Islamic calendar, is the ninth lunar month and commemorates the Prophet

Muhammad's first revelation. Ramadan is celebrated with 30 days of fasting, during which time Muslims go without food or drink from sunrise until sunset. Hoda Zaki, HOPE's Egypt country director, and her staff were all Muslims and observed the fast during the day, but after sunset, they were able to break their fast. We had some wonderful meals at restaurants along the Nile, and one even on a night cruise on the Nile, which included entertainment by belly dancers and whirling dervish dancers.

Project HOPE had been working in Egypt since 1975, and one of the most promising initiatives was a collaboration between Egypt's Ministry of Health, Pfizer pharmaceutical company, and Project HOPE to develop and implement a national training institute in Cairo to provide training for healthcare professionals from Egypt and other countries in the Middle East. HOPE's role in the partnership was to help manage the institute and assist in the development of multi-disciplinary training courses for the health professionals. Several of my meetings in Cairo were relative to this initiative, including with the Minister of Health and Population, Dr. Mohammed Awad-Taj Eddin.

While in Cairo, word came that we would be able to meet with First Lady Suzanne Mubarak. The First Lady's background was in sociology and she had actively championed causes in Egypt that focused on improving the welfare of women and children. The First Lady was aware of Project HOPE's participation in the development of the Shanghai Children's Medical Center in China, and she had expressed interest in creating a similar national children's medical center in Egypt. Given my background as a pediatric hospital administrator, this was certainly an appealing idea to me. Unfortunately, her schedule prevented a meeting on this trip. Nevertheless, over the course of several visits to Cairo, we met with representatives of the First Lady's staff and Dr. Awad Taj Eddin to discuss child healthcare in Egypt and ways in which Project HOPE could assist efforts to improve women's and children's health in the country.

Through the Lens of Humanity

> Author's note: The concept of a children's hospital remained an interest and priority of the First Lady's, but unfortunately her dream did not materialize during her years in that position.

I returned home just before Christmas and reflected on the fact that as I was concluding my first 90 days with Project HOPE, I had already spent 46 of those 90 days out of the country. I was living in guest housing on the Project HOPE campus while my townhouse was being built in Leesburg, Virginia, so in some ways, I felt it was just as well that I was out on the road.

The grueling travel pace wasn't about to slow down. In January, 2001, I traveled to Beijing, Hong Kong, Shanghai, and Cairo over a 14-day stretch to visit the country offices, attend HOPE-sponsored training sessions in the various cities. We were also to meet with sponsoring programmatic donors and prospective donors, as well as with in-country academic partners and in-country governmental employees, many of whom were senior Ministry of Health officials. Much of my time was spent with HOPE in-country staff identifying potential new programs proposals, and responding to US governmental funding opportunities specific to the HOPE's Asia/Middle East Region.

In February, I visited Indonesia and Thailand, the two remaining countries under my administrative umbrella that I had not visited. After flying first to Japan to meet with prospective donors and the Project HOPE Japan Advisory Board, which provided funding for the projects in Indonesia and Thailand, I flew to Jakarta, Indonesia, and then onward to Denpasar, Bali Province, Indonesia to meet with Mika Ito and HOPE's Indonesia staff.

Denpasar is the capital of Bali Province and its center of commerce and tourism. Its population is a mix of cultures and religions with over 60 percent of the population Hindu, perhaps 25 percent Muslim, and the remaining population split between Christianity, Buddhism, and other religions. HOPE's projects were concentrated around oral and dental health, primarily emphasizing children. Mika and I toured several clinics and hospitals and met with many local governmental and health officials. Indonesia was the SS *HOPE* ship's first port of call in the

"Once a Hopie, Always a Hopie"

1960s and there remained much good will and enthusiasm for HOPE and its work. I departed Indonesia for Thailand with the grateful thanks of the Indonesian people for HOPE's ongoing support—and with a severe sunburn from the country's tropical climate!

Chiang Mai is the headquarters for HOPE's Thailand offices and projects. A former capital of the ancient Lanna Kingdom, Chiang Mai is located in northern Thailand approximately 430 miles from Bangkok. It is surrounded by misty mountains and is renowned for its ancient and colorful temples. During the day, Akiko Otani, HOPE country director, escorted and toured me through HOPE's Thai projects: a treatment and educational center for those suffering with HIV/AIDS, a cervical cancer detection and treatment program, and a pediatric cardiovascular program. In addition to surveying HOPE's medical services, I also partook of Thailand's medical services myself. My sunburn from Indonesia was so severe and created so much discomfort that a local doctor Akiko knew recommended that I go to a hospital emergency room to get ointments and salves to better treat the burn and swelling.

The ointment wasn't a miracle cure, but it did diminish my discomfort to the point that I was able to tour several of the city's many cultural and historic sites, such as the Old City with its ancient walls and perfectly square moat. The night bazaar we visited was bustling and chaotic and vibrant. As Akiko laughed at my negotiation efforts, I did manage to secure a couple of nice silk carpets that I arranged to have shipped to the United States.

With this trip under my belt, I had, over a five-month period, traveled to all five of the countries within my regional purview—some of them several times—logging tens of thousands of miles in the process! When I returned to the States, it felt good to have visited all the countries and to now personally know all my staff both abroad and at HOPE's Millwood headquarters.

My routine over the succeeding months became one of spending several weeks at HOPE Center in Millwood, and then several weeks abroad to attend various HOPE-sponsored training sessions, stay in touch with in-country governmental officials, and work toward creating new programs and projects.

Through the Lens of Humanity

A major organizational shift occurred in May 2001, when Dr. John Howe became the new president and CEO of Project HOPE. For forty years, the Walsh family had been synonymous with Project HOPE. With the death of founder Dr. William Walsh in 1996, gradually the family ties with HOPE faded for varieties of reasons, even though William Walsh Jr. had served as president and CEO for several years. The Board selected Dr. Howe, a cardiologist by training, to lead Project HOPE. As is common with new leadership, Dr. Howe's arrival created some anxiety as to what organizational changes he might make and how current staff would be affected. During my tenure at HOPE, I had reported to Dr. Leslie Mancuso, the Chief Operating Officer. Speculation was rampant that changes structurally would be made within the organization so the rumor mill was ripe with all sorts of intrigue and gossip!

Throughout the summer, while Dr. Howe settled in at Millwood, I continued my travel regimen to the various countries under my supervision. While in China in August, with staff from both Shanghai and Beijing offices, we planned two national nursing conferences, the first to be held September 4th though 7th in Shanghai, followed by the second, September 9th and 10th in Beijing. At that time, basic nursing training in China was inconsistent, and there was minimal ongoing research relative to formalizing standardized Chinese nursing practices.

Project HOPE would host both conferences, develop the conference agenda and training segments, and secure Chinese as well as international nursing leaders to be faculty and presenters for the conferences. Nurses from China's major hospitals and universitys would be invited to participate. We anticipated that several hundred nurses would attend the conferences.

I invited Nancy Korom, Chief Nursing Officer at Children's Hospital of Wisconsin (CHW) during my tenure as Executive Vice President, to be one of the guest presenters, and afterwards, she and her husband John would travel to Beijing as tourists before heading back to the United States. Also participating in the Shanghai conference were two physician colleagues from CHW, a husband-and-wife team, Dr. Stu Berger, a pediatric cardiologist, and Dr. Julie Biller, a pediatric pulmonologist. Doctors Berger and Biller would be conducting mentoring sessions for physician staff at Shanghai Children's Medical Center while in Shanghai.

My intention with the conference was also a means of bringing my entire regional leadership together, so my HOPE country directors from Turkey, Egypt, Thailand, and Indonesia were all scheduled to attend. Each of the country directors was to share how HOPE was assisting with nursing education in their countries.

My trip itinerary included not only Shanghai and Beijing, but after the conclusion of the conference in Beijing, I would be flying on to Tokyo for several days of discussions about initiating programmatic activities in Cambodia. Project HOPE Japan had explored several program possibilities with health officials in Cambodia and I was certainly eager to learn HOPE Japan's assessment of the possible prospects and opportunities.

I flew out of Dulles Airport on September 2, 2001 with Dr. Leslie Mancuso. Leslie, who describes herself as first and foremost a nurse, was going to be addressing the nursing conferences in both Shanghai and Beijing. We flew first to San Francisco, where we met Nancy and John Korom. Nancy, Children's Hospital of Wisconsin's VP of Nursing, was to be the featured speaker at the Shanghai and Beijing conferences, and her husband John, a professional photographer, had arrived in San Francisco earlier in the day from Milwaukee. Nancy, John, Leslie, and I traveled together from San Francisco to Shanghai. We arrived the evening of September 3rd and were met by HOPE Shanghai staff, who transported us to the Grand YouYou Hotel.

The Shanghai conference was held in the auditorium/lecture hall of Shanghai Children's Medical Center. It was gratifying to see every seat taken and standing-room-only crowds of young Chinese nurses over the next four days. The conference proceeded with nary a hitch, a memorable highlight being the recognition of Madame Lin, the acknowledged matriarch of

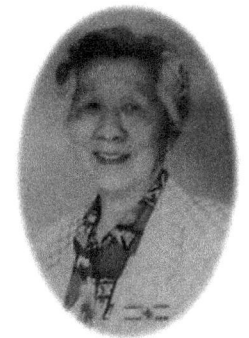

Madame Lin Ju-Ying (Laureate 2001)

nursing in China. As she was recognized with the Princess Srinagarindra Award and her accomplishments noted, the Chinese nurses and nursing students gave her a standing ovation that went on for several minutes. It was a truly exceptional tribute to a remarkable woman whose entire life had been spent in service of others and in raising the standards of nursing care within China!

By all accounts, the nursing conference was a success, and on the evening of September 7th, Project HOPE hosted the closing banquet at the Grand YouYou Hotel. I enjoyed watching Nancy and John Korom's faces as course after course of food was brought to the tables—and then came the toasts. Shouts of *gan bei* were heard throughout the banquet hall.

Many of us were flying to Beijing early the following day, so we tried to keep the *gan beis* to a minimum. Though the Koroms and doctors Berger and Biller were heading to Beijing as well, I bid them thanks and adieu that evening as they were departing later in the day and would be on holiday in Beijing for several days.

Leslie and I caught an early flight to Beijing the next morning, September 8th. All systems were go with the Beijing conference preparations, and over the next several days, the Beijing nursing conference was a successful repeat of the Shanghai conference. The Beijing conference was held in the Beijing Continental Grand Hotel with approximately 150 nurses in attendance. On the final day of the conference, Madame Lin was again honored and received another heartfelt expression of thanks and love from the gathered nurses.

Dinner that evening was a smaller crowd, comprised of Leslie, my in-country directors, and myself. It was a more casual and informal dinner. Most of the group were returning the next day to their homes and usual roles. Leslie was heading back to the United States. I was traveling to Tokyo for my meetings with Project HOPE Japan regarding Cambodia.

Leslie and I arrived at the Beijing International Airport at 7:15 a.m. on Tuesday, September 11, 2001. We both immediately discovered that our respective flights were delayed due to a typhoon off the coast of China. Leslie rescheduled her flight route with a new departure time for the States at approximately noon. My flight to Tokyo was delayed until almost 1 p.m., and with the hour time differential between Beijing and Tokyo—Tokyo is an hour ahead of Beijing—I arrived in Tokyo's Narita airport at about 5:30 p.m. I caught the bus shuttle to downtown Tokyo and arrived at the Shinjuku Washington Hotel about 7:30 p.m.

I had dinner in the hotel restaurant and then took a walk around the area surrounding the hotel. The crowds were massive and music filled the air. Bright lights and spotlights caromed off high-tech advertising boards, advertising God knows what, and after a short time, suffering from sensory overload, I went back to my room and flipped on CNN International News.

It was 11 p.m. Tokyo time, 10 a.m. in New York City. From 6,750 miles away, I watched in horror the replay of two commercial airplanes striking the Twin Towers and I knew the world would never be the same again.

The magnitude of the 9/11 attack expanded as news came of the plane crashing into the Pentagon and then of the plane crashing into the field near Shanksville, Pennsylvania. There were unimaginable visuals of people jumping to their deaths from Twin Tower windows hundreds of feet above the ground. Suddenly, live television showed the visual of first one tower, then the second, seemingly in slow motion, collapsing in upon themselves, sending plumes of smoke, dirt and debris high into the sky.

Over the next several hours, I watched horrified at the unfolding drama in New York. I also made several phone calls to the States. One call was to my parents to let them know where I was and that I was safe. Another call went to HOPE Center to confirm my location and to determine where other HOPE staff and our consultants were.

News reports had already acknowledged that all air traffic within the United States was being instructed to land immediately. All international flights heading into the United States were being diverted and instructed to land as well.

As evening became morning in Tokyo, the folks at HOPE Center had notified me that they were attempting to arrange for all US-based HOPE personnel to return to the United States immediately. The dilemma was not knowing how long the flight restriction mandate would be in place or when foreign air carriers might resume service to the United States.

My meeting with Project HOPE Japan staff was not until Thursday morning the 13th, and it was clear the United States' no-fly order wouldn't be lifted before then, so I decided to keep the meeting as planned.

I had agreed to meet the Project HOPE Japan staff in the lobby of my hotel on Thursday morning, and as I got off the elevator, Mr. Watanabe, an elderly and distinguished Japanese man I had gotten to know, and who was a consultant with Project HOPE Japan, approached me and bowed deeply and with tears in his eyes and in a voice quivering with emotion and sadness said, "Sixty years ago, my country attacked yours without warning. Yesterday, your country was again attacked in such a terrible way. I had hoped to never again see such treachery in my life. My heart is with you and your country."

I was momentarily speechless and filled with emotion myself. Then I bowed and thanked him for his kind words. This is one of my most poignant and touching memories of the tragedy of September 11, 2001.

Later that day, HOPE Center advised me that the no-fly restriction in the States might be lifted on Friday, and we agreed that the best course of action for me would be to book a hotel room near Narita so that I could be available should a flight become available. No flights to the US departed Narita on Friday, but HOPE Center said they did have me booked on an early flight out of Narita on Saturday morning. They advised that I should get to the airport early, anticipating that many people who had been stranded in Tokyo would be eager to return to the US.

I'm someone who typically arrives everywhere early anyway, and Saturday was no exception. I got to Narita fully expecting a madhouse of stranded travelers seeking to get home. I was booked on a Japan Airlines (JAL) direct flight to Dulles Airport and was the first person checked in for the flight. HOPE Center had procured a business class seat for me and after check-in, I waited for the flight in JAL's lounge, hoping the flight wouldn't be cancelled at the last moment. Several other Americans were in the lounge waiting for the Dulles flight as well, and when the flight was called for boarding, we were all stunned. Only 28 passengers were booked on a plane that normally carried 300+ people. It seems many were leery of being the first to fly again in the United States.

The flight attendants moved everyone into first and business class seats. When we landed and taxied to our gate, I saw an enormous American flag hanging at the international arrival gate. It was good to be home.

Over the next several months, I continued my travel routine: a few weeks out of the country, a few weeks in the States. One of these "out of the country" trips was to Phnom Penh, Cambodia, to explore establishing education and training programs in nursing and in HIV/AIDS prevention and treatment. Our assessment team entourage included Adriana Mikullu, my Millwood-based regional analyst, Akiko Otani, whose HIV/AIDS program in Thailand had garnered good reviews and donor support, Dr. Marcia Petrini, a long-time nursing consultant of Project HOPE's, Ms. Yokoo, a representative of Project HOPE Japan, the potential donor for any projects that might emerge, and myself. We met with Ministry of Health (MOH) officials from Cambodia, and began serious discussions regarding both programs. Given the enthusiasm of the Cambodian MOH officials, upon her return, Ms. Yokoo recommended to the Project HOPE Japan Advisory Committee that they fund both projects within the next budget cycle.

Things shifted dramatically for me in May 2002, when Leslie Mancuso left to assume the CEO role at Johns Hopkins Program for International Education in Gynecology and Obstetrics (now simply known as JHPIEGO). With Leslie's departure, I was named Interim Vice President of International Affairs. In this role, I retained my day-to-day responsibility for the Asia/Middle East region, but also assumed oversight for all other regions as well. The most immediate impact: more travel!!

And though the travel pace was demanding, I enjoyed the exposure to other regions, and, as attested by my frequent flyer miles over a six-month period, I had flown more than 175,000 miles. This included multiple visits to my own region, as well as to Malawi and Ghana in Africa, Kazakhstan and Armenia in Central Asia, and the Dominican Republic in the Caribbean.

However, by the end of the year, I also was being recruited for a CEO role in another organization, known at the time as the Milwaukee International Health Training Center (MIHTC), which later became the Center for International Health (CIH). CIH was located in Milwaukee and afforded me the opportunity to not only return to a city and friendships I loved and missed, but also gave me the opportunity to grow and expand an organization devoted to improving the health status of people around the globe.

Similar to Project HOPE, CIH's mission was to provide health education and training to health professionals around the world, particularly in emerging and developing nations, where there is a paucity of healthcare services and integrated health systems to provide care to vulnerable peoples. CIH was organized as a consortium of distinguished and eminent academic and health institutions and provided a ready-made platform for identifying resources and faculty to address the challenges of underdeveloped health systems abroad.

I announced my resignation from Project HOPE on January 6, 2003, with my last day being February 7th. I had one last trip scheduled with Project HOPE to Beijing, China from January 10th to 17th, and from there to Cairo from January 18th to 23rd.

The Beijing trip had been on the books for a number of weeks. Dr. Charles Sanders, Chair of the Board of Project HOPE and Dr. Howe, Project HOPE President and CEO, were conducting a series of meetings in association with the Center for Strategic and International al Studies (CSIS), of which Dr. Sanders was a board member. CSIS is a bipartisan think tank "dedicated to advancing practical ideas to address the world's greatest challenges." The CSIS meetings in China were primarily dealing with the impact of HIV/AIDS in China and throughout Asia. Dr. Louis Sullivan, Former Secretary of Health and Human Services under President George H.W. Bush, Dr. Randy Wykoff, who had assumed the role of Chief Operating Officer for Project HOPE, and I were accompanying doctors Sanders and Howe.

Another priority of the trip was a scheduled meeting with President Jiang Zemin of China to discuss/celebrate Project HOPE's activities over the years in China. The meeting had been months in the making and Dr. Shen Xiao Ming, President of Shanghai Children's Medical Center, was largely responsible for arranging the meeting. The meeting with President Jiang Zemin was scheduled for Friday, January 17th, at his Beijing office.

Randy and I arrived in Beijing on January 11th and doctors Sanders, Howe, and Sullivan arrived on 12th. The CSIS meetings were held all day Monday the 13th at the Shangri-La Hotel, and were well attended by senior Chinese government and academic leaders. The gathering received widespread coverage by Chinese media outlets and governmental agencies. The requisite closing banquet was a long and very scripted affair as protocol required recognition of all senior Chinese leadership in attendance.

On Thursday evening, our delegation met with Zou Xiao Ning, a foreign affairs liaison officer for Shanghai Second Medical University who had worked and interfaced for years with Project HOPE's staff in Shanghai, and who had come to Beijing to assist with our meeting with President Jiang Zemin.

Mr. Zou went through Chinese meeting Protocol 101 for such meetings with very senior Chinese leaders. He described the meeting venue and how seating would be set up. President Jiang Zemin and Project HOPE's senior-most leader, who in this meeting was Dr. Sanders as Chair of the Board, would be seated adjacent to each other at one end of the room, with their respective entourages seated in descending order of rank on either side of the leaders. A translator would be seated behind and between the two senior leaders. The conversation would be carried on between the two senior leaders. It was not protocol nor customary for members other than the most senior leaders of the delegation to speak.

Mr. Zou mentioned that at the conclusion of the meeting, several group photographs would be taken.

Through the Lens of Humanity

The next morning, our delegation was picked up in several vans to transport us to the meeting. We arrived at a nondescript, single-story building in central Beijing enclosed by a thick surrounding wall. The vans pulled into a driveway and dropped us at a door, where several Chinese security officers dressed in dark blue suits met us and escorted us into the building and on to the meeting venue. The room was large with walnut or mahogany wood-covered walls. It was brightly lit by an enormous chandelier and decorated with lively Chinese paintings. The seats were set up in the style that Mr. Zou had described and were huge and luxurious. Ornate wooden side tables were between each chair.

We milled about the room for a few moments, and then Mr. Zou asked us to stand in front of our seats. Dr. Sanders stood at the seat adjacent to where President Jiang Zemin would sit, then down our side were Dr. Howe, Dr. Sullivan, Randy Wykoff, myself, and Shell Xue, Project HOPE's country director.

President Jiang Zemin entered the room with his entourage and moved to his seat. Once his staff had reached their seats, we all sat down. Utilizing the translator, Dr. Shen Xiao Ming made a few introductory comments about the long-term relationship between Project HOPE and China, and made some very brief introductions of the delegations in the room.

President Jiang Zemin then initiated a conversation with Dr. Sanders and Dr. Howe for about 15 minutes that discussed various projects that had taken place over the years with the leaders, thanking each other for their commitment to raising the standard of care for the people of China. Occasionally during their discourse, President Jiang Zemin spoke in English, but primarily he spoke in Chinese and allowed the translator to interpret his message.

After about 20 minutes or so, President Jiang Zemin paused and looked at our delegation. Then he started asking each member of our delegation in English if he or she had anything to say. As he went down the row of our delegation, no one spoke. Based on Mr. Zou's instructions that only senior leaders speak, none of our delegation wanted to break "protocol".

"Once a Hopie, Always a Hopie"

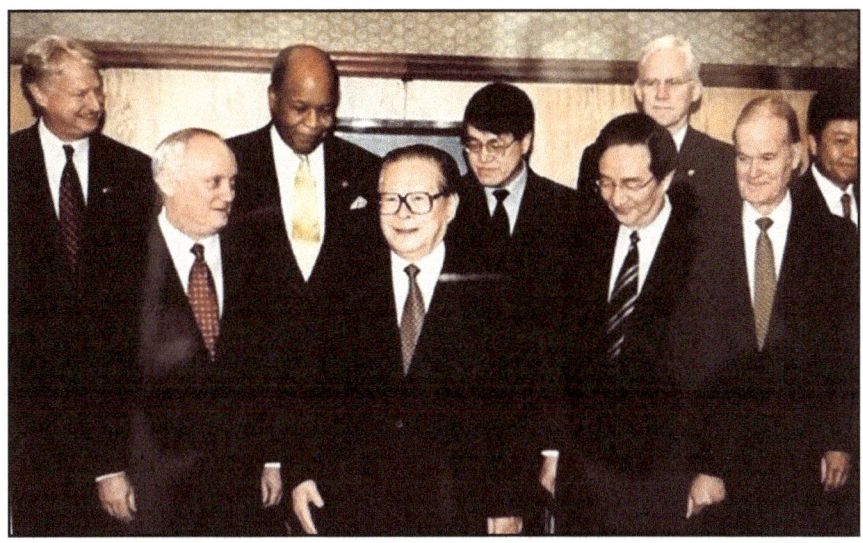

Project HOPE Delegation with Chinese President Jiang Zemin
Back Row from Left: Mark Anderson, Dr. Lewis Sullivan (Former US Secretary of Health and Human Services), City of Shanghai Party Secretary, Dr. Randy Wycoff (Project HOPE). Front Row from Left: Dr. John Howe (President of Project HOPE), Chinese President Jiang Zemin, Shanghai Mayor, Dr. Charles Sanders (HOPE Chair of the Board), Dr. Shen Xiao Ming (Shanghai Second Medical University President).
(January 17, 2003))

When he came to me, I figured that since he was directly asking me a question, I'd respond. So I replied that I knew of his initial support for the development of the Shanghai Children's Medical Center and thanked him for his vision for helping children with a hospital dedicated to their specific needs. I noticed I drew a few surprised looks from my delegation, but President Jiang Zemin quickly said he was very pleased with the hospital and he talked about how it had first been discussed when he was mayor. He asked if I had worked on the project, and I told him I had and also on other projects in Shanghai and Beijing. He nodded and then thanked me for working in China.

The president then spoke in Chinese to Shell Xue, who was sitting next to me. She too responded, saying that she was responsible for HOPE's programs in Beijing and she specifically mentioned the diabetes and cardiovascular care programs. Speaking in English, President Jiang Zemin said that his youngest son had diabetes and he remembered when his son was very little, he used to give his son shots. It was an unexpectedly intimate and very personal moment from a major world leader not known for unscripted or unguarded speech and whose life was mainly cloaked in mystery.

President Jiang Zemin then wrapped up the meeting, praising the relationship that had been created between China and Project HOPE. A photographer then directed us to a small stage and took several pictures of the combined delegations. He then departed and we were ushered back out to our waiting vehicles.

Afterwards, in the van. I asked Zou Xiao Ning if I was wrong for answering President Jiang Zemin.

"It's okay, it's okay," he said. "He asked you a direct question. You should have responded."

Immediately after our meeting with President Jiang Zemin, I departed for Cairo for several days of discussions regarding the national training institute. Knowing that it would be my last visit to Cairo as a HOPE employee, Hoda Zaki, HOPE's Egypt Country Director, the entire Egypt office staff, and I, took a leisurely dinner river cruise on the Nile. It was a very special and rewarding way to end my travel days with HOPE, at the place of one of the world's oldest civilizations!

I have always looked back with fondness on my tenure with Project HOPE. On the Project HOPE website, there is a wonderful statement and acknowledgment of the work of HOPE staff and volunteers:

> Anyone who has ever been involved with Project HOPE understands the adage, "Once a HOPIE always a HOPIE" .....
> HOPIES, are an extraordinary group of individuals because their bond is one of giving…of themselves, their time and their treasure …to improve the health of people around the world.

I am and always will be proud to say that I am "Once a HOPIE, always a HOPIE"

Part Six

Through the Lens of Humanity

CHAPTER 11

Through the Lens of Humanity

When I reflect on my mission and humanitarian trips abroad, I close my eyes and in my mind's eye, thousands of images burst upon the canvas of my consciousness. Images from the streets, alleyways, markets and slums of big cities and small towns like Miraj, Calcutta, Mumbai, Varanasi, Agra, Kathmandu, Cairo, Sarajevo, Kabul, Cape Town, Mwandi, Embangweni, Phnom Penh, Shanghai, Beijing, and so many others I've visited. Among the most vivid, vibrant and evocative images are those of the people I walked among, those I worked with, shared meals and hospitality with, shared joys and sorrows with, shared laughter and tears with. Particularly potent are the images of these and other people in their unguarded moments, when, as renowned photographer Steve McCurry says, "Their essential soul peeks through," and I glimpsed what it was like in that time and place, to be that person in the human conditions and challenges they confronted.

Photographer Steve McCurry for decades has been the source of incredible pictorial images that have become iconic photographic classics. From the iconic "Afghan Girl" taken in 1984 at the Nasir Bagh refugee camp in Pakistan to literally thousands of magical and powerful photographs taken all over the world, his photography has enabled McCurry to "write" pictorial stories through his remarkable ability to bring a spectacular confluence of light, color, and cultural context to his photographs. In this manner, he says, he captures the true "sacredness" of the moment.

In 2008, through the convergence of efforts of numerous individuals, an extraordinary opportunity unfolded—the possibility of a collaboration between Steve McCurry, arguably the best photographer in the world, and Johan Stengard, a unique and soulful saxophonist with his own world-class reputation.

The opportunity? Create a multi-movement orchestra composition whose musical score is synchronized with thousands of McCurry's most vibrant and iconic photos. The idea captured our imaginations, and so over several months, utilizing Stengard's musical and orchestral connections, coupled with McCurry's consultation and collaboration in the selection of literally thousands of photographs, slowly this creative idea became an artistic reality. *Human Reflection: The Photo Symphony* was born.

And with its inception came the notion that the world premier performance would be a charitable event hosted by the Center for International Health and proceeds would benefit the Center's efforts to raise the standard of care available to peoples worldwide.

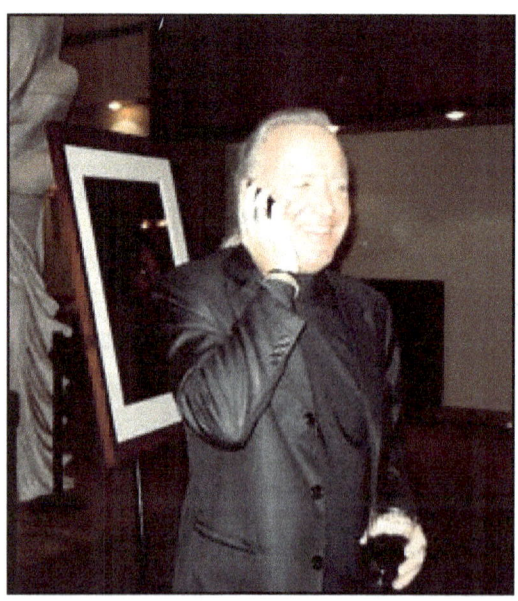

Renowned saxophonist Johan Stengard relaxing after his *Human Reflection* performance

Through the Lens of Humanity

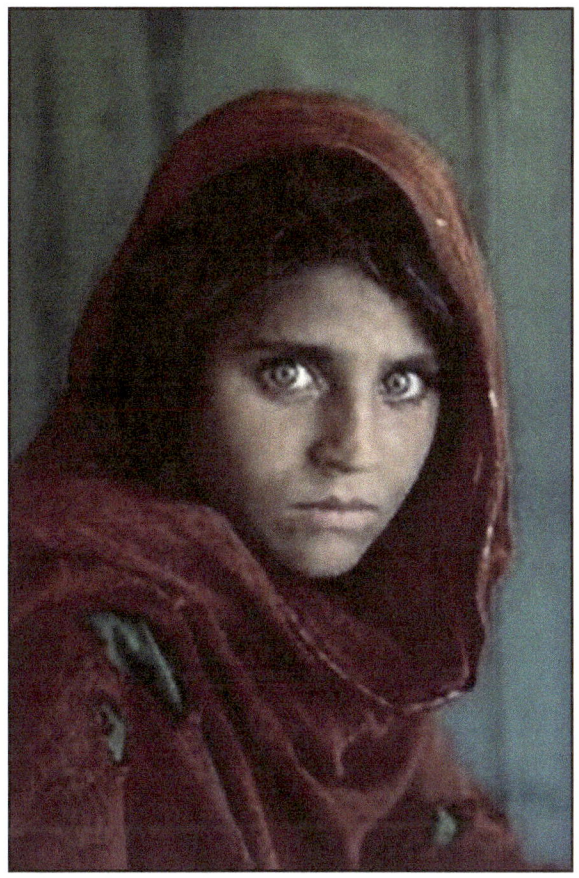

Afghan Girl, at Nasir Bagh refugee camp near Peshawar, Pakistan, 1984. Photograph by Steve McCurry

    As *Human Reflection: The Photo Symphony* moved toward fruition, various efforts were made to advertise the symphony. One of these was an article entitled, "Through the Lens of Humanity" published in Milwaukee magazine *Exclusively Yours*. With permission of *Exclusively Yours*, the article is reprinted here. The original *Exclusively Yours* article featured five McCurry photographs that were interspersed within the article. I have included the same McCurry photographs in the reprint.

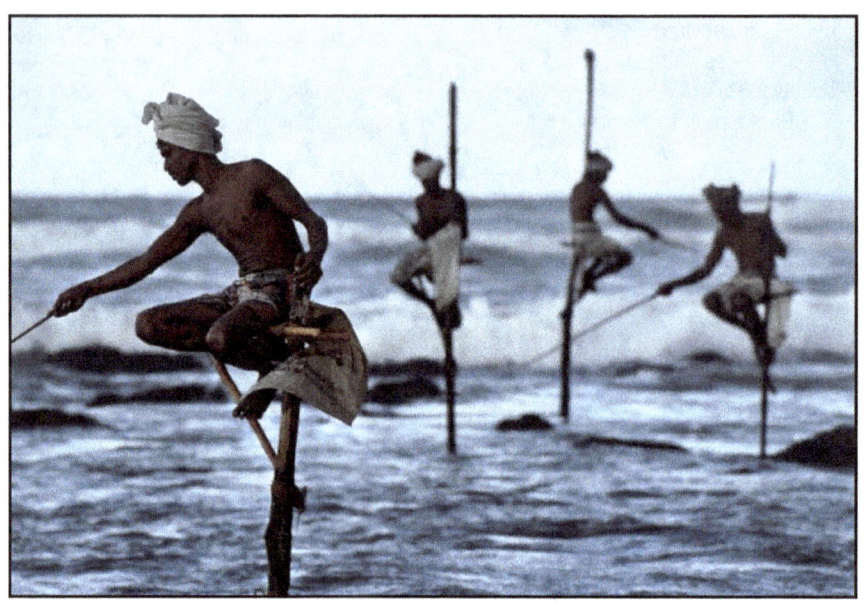

Fishermen, Weligama, South Coast, Sri Lanka, 1995.
Photograph by Steve McCurry

THROUGH THE LENS OF HUMANITY
(Reprinted with permission from *Exclusively Yours* magazine)

Upon first hearing the music joined with a widescreen projection of photographs deeply evocative of powerful human experience and emotion, you might for a moment mistake the sound of a saxophone for a human voice moved to the edge where vocal expression cannot be contained.

Human Reflection: The Photo Symphony has been billed as a "symphonic journey through the lens of humanity." It features the work of documentary photographer Steve McCurry, best known for his striking portraits of real people caught in extraordinary moments of color and light amidst their everyday lives, accompanied by Jorge Calendrelli, Andreas Landegren, and Jay Chattaway, and performed by Sweden's premier tenor and soprano sax player, Johan Stengard, with

THROUGH THE LENS OF HUMANITY

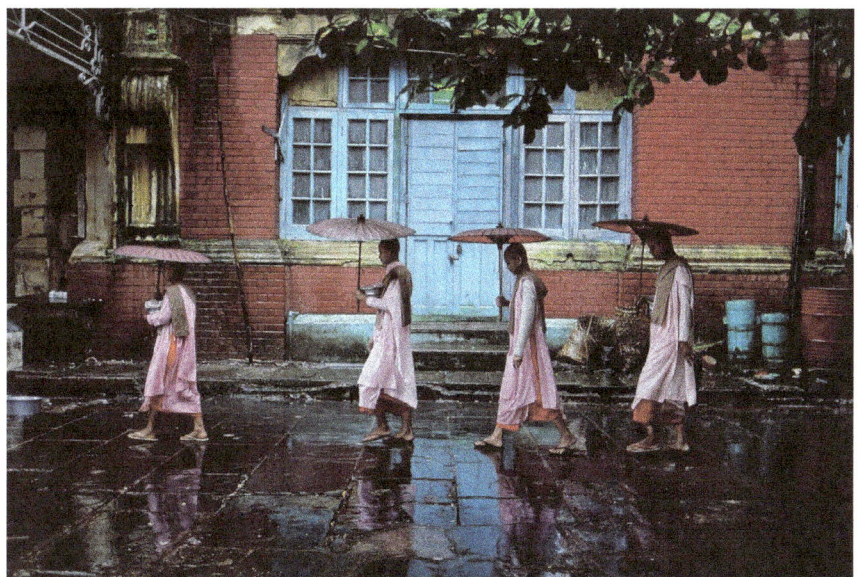

Procession of nuns, Rangoon, Myanmar (Burma), 1994.
Photograph by Steve McCurry

symphonic accompaniment under the direction of Frank Zuback of New York.

Frank Zuback is well known for his work with such renowned artists as Tony Bennett, Frank Sinatra, Maureen McGovern, Aretha Franklin, Ray Charles, Stevie Wonder, and more. As a musical contractor, he has been involved in television specials (such as the Tony Awards, Bi-Centennial Closing Ceremonies, the U.S. Olympic Festival and the Grand Opening of Ellis Island), films (such as *Tron*, *The Shining*, and *All That Jazz*), and Broadway shows (such as *Joseph and the Amazing Technicolor Dreamcoat*, *The Three Musketeers*, and *Mowgli*). As a music director and/or conductor, Zuback's recent engagements have included NBC pilots for *Swing It Again*, MGM/UA world premieres for *Tomorrow Never Dies*, and *Golden Eye*, the Pepsi Cola 100th Anniversary Gala, and the Radio City Music Hall Amway Celebration.

THROUGH THE LENS OF HUMANITY

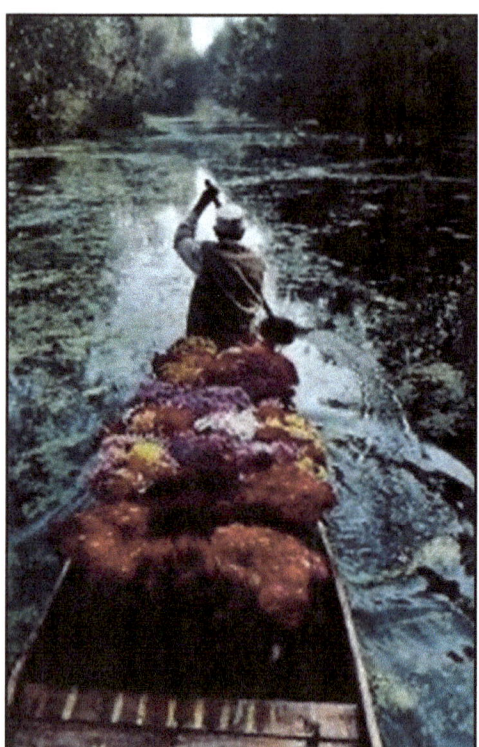

Srinagar, Kashmir, India, 1996
Photograph by: Steve McCurry

Johan Stengard has earned a world-class reputation as an unique and soulful musician known for his 15 completed solo albums, more than thousand solo performances, and hundreds of recordings as an orchestra musician with noted artists such as Michael Bolton, ABBA, Woody Herman, Celine Dion, Pete Cetera, Nelson Riddle, Tommy Steele, Mel Lewis, Clark Terry, Lena Horne and Sammy Davis, Jr. Played on both the tenor and soprano saxophones, his performances entail a mix of pop favorites, jazz standards and original compositions, turning songs like "Somewhere Over the Rainbow" into a smoldering salute to the yellow brick road and leaving his audiences breathless with his blues version of "Amazing Grace."

Though touring mainly in Europe and the United States, Stengard is the King and Queen of Sweden's musician when on official state visits and has been formally invited by the Thailand government to perform during official ceremonies. As he integrates stories about his history and world travels between songs, the performances of Johan Stengard carry a warm and spiritual, yet riveting, appeal right to the heart of the audience.

Another world traveler, Steve McCurry is best known as the eye behind the famous "Afghan Girl" *National Geographic* magazine cover, known as the Mona Lisa of photography. McCurry's career was launched when, disguised in native garb, he crossed the Pakistan border in rebel-controlled Afghanistan just before the Russian invasion. Smuggling his film out of the country by sewing it into the folds of his jacket, McCurry's images of the conflict were among the first seen by the global community. His coverage won the Robert Caps Gold Medal for Best Photographic Reporting from Abroad, an award dedicated to photographers exhibiting exceptional courage and enterprise.

Since then, McCurry has covered many areas of international and civil conflict, including Beirut, Cambodia, the Philippines, the Gulf War, Afghanistan, Tibet, and the former Yugoslavia. His work focuses

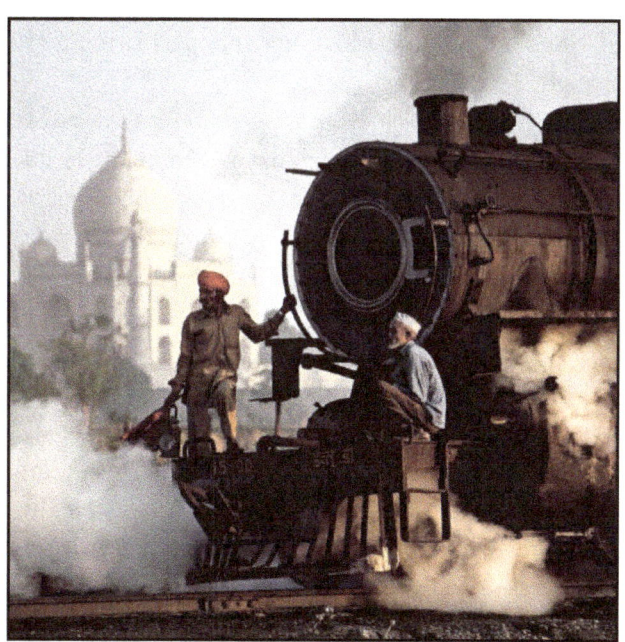

Uttar Paradesh, India,1983
Photo by Steve McCurry

on the human consequences of war, not only showing what war impresses on the landscape, but rather, on the human face.

Though featured in every major magazine in the world, McCurry's photos most often appear in *National Geographic* magazine, with recent articles on Tibet, Afghanistan, Iraq, Yemen, and the temples of Angkor Wat, Cambodia. McCurry is driven by an innate curiosity and sense of wonder around the world, paired with an uncanny ability to cross boundaries of language and culture to capture stories of human experience.

He has been recognized universally as one of the world's finest image-makers and has won nearly all of photography's top awards, including Magazine Photographer of the Year, awarded by the National Press Photographers Association, four first prizes in the World Press Photo Contest, and two Olivier Reboot Memorial Awards.

A high point in his career was the rediscovery of the previously unidentified "Afghan Girl," which many have described as the most recognizable photograph in the world today. When McCurry finally located Sharbat Gula after almost two decades, he said "her skin is weathered, there are wrinkles now, but she is as striking as she was all those years ago."

Human Reflection: The Photo Symphony showcases McCurry's unforgettable photos, many of which have become modern icons. "Most of my images are grounded in people. I look for the unguarded moment, the essential soul peeking out, experience etched on a person's face. I try to convey what it is like to be that person, a person caught in a broader landscape, that you could call the human condition," said McCurry.

Human Reflection: The Photo Symphony will be held on Wednesday, October 1 at the Sharon Lynne Wilson Center for the Arts. Proceeds from this incredible evening of photographic art and music will benefit Milwaukee's Center for International Health (CIH), an internationally recognized 501(c)(3) organization that offers food aid, medical training, technical assistance, material resources, and health systems development techniques to strengthen communities, their healthcare systems and the capabilities of their health professionals in emerging and developing countries.

CIH serves as the lead agency of an area-wide consortium that comprises Children's Hospital of Wisconsin, Froedtert Memorial Hospital, the Medical College of Wisconsin, the Blood Center of Wisconsin, the University of Wisconsin–Milwaukee, Marquette University, Milwaukee County government, and GE Healthcare.

Based on the belief that, despite dramatic divisions of geography and politics, every person in the world should share the same basic human right to health, including adequate healthcare, education and nutrition, CIH and its consortium member institutions have participated

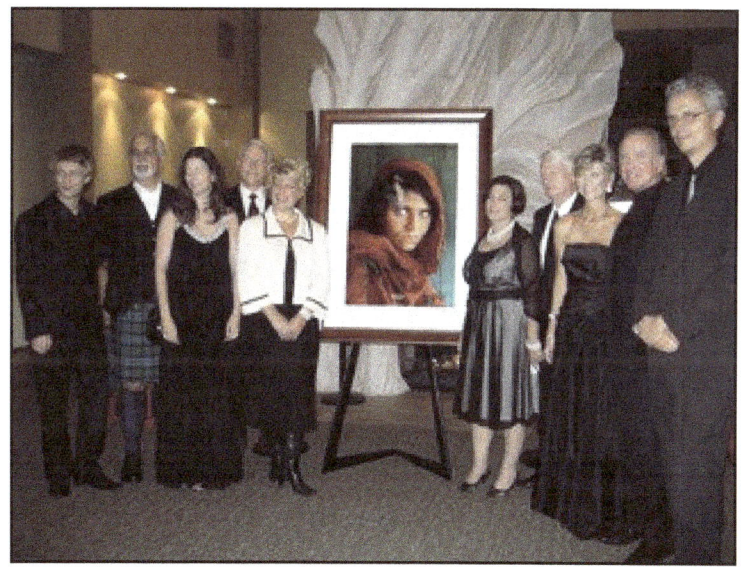

Human Reflection Event Committee beside "Afghan Girl"

in over 50 International health partnerships and projects focused on HIV/AIDS, nutrition, health professions education, disease prevention and management, and health systems development.

Enjoyment of the right to health is vital to all aspects of a person's life and well-being and is crucial to the realization of many other fundamental human rights and freedoms. As *Human Reflection: The Photo Symphony* brings your attention to the difficult and sometimes startling realities in other parts of the world, your very presence will help to generate the funds needed to create change.

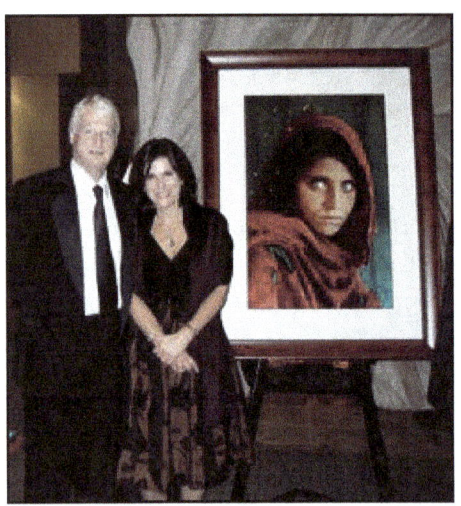

The author and Kathleen Spini alongside the iconic "Afghan Girl"

[**Author's Note**: On October 1, 2008 hundreds attended the concert at the Sharon Lynne Wilson Center in Milwaukee. The performance was universally heralded in the press locally, nationally, and internationally. Most importantly, through the generosity of those in attendance and of a specific donor in particular, more than $2.5 million was pledged to enhance the health status of those in need throughout the world!

POSTSCRIPT

Tempus Fugit — Time Flies

Fifty years have elapsed since I boarded the aircraft that would take me on my first journey abroad. Hundreds of thousands of miles and a million memories later, I marvel at what I experienced and learned from so many "teachers" along the path of my many journeys. As I walked among the people I met on my travels, so many shared with me their life's challenges and their hopes and dreams and aspirations for their and their children's futures. I learned the stories of the poor and poverty-stricken. I learned from those who had been marginalized and ostracized; I learned the tortured histories of those ravaged by decades of war and oppression. And I learned from the saints living among us who "go where they are needed" and who along the way sow seeds of hope, justice and peace.

Much has changed over five decades, though sadly, too much is the same. Afghanistan remains one of the most dangerous places on the planet, and new conflict zones such as Ukraine, Iran, and Iraq have emerged. COVID 19 wrought terrible costs throughout the world, not just in terms of lives lost, but in emotional, economic, and social costs and trauma. And the world lost a number of ethical and moral giants with the passing of Mother Teresa, Margrietha van der Kreek, Archbishop Desmond Tutu, and so many others. Now more than ever the challenges facing the world community compel us to understand as Archbishop Tutu reminded us, "We all belong in the bundle of life, my humanity is caught up and is inextricably bound up in yours, we all belong to a greater whole."

I have been blessed in all my journeys with "traveling mercies" and was fortunate to have experienced a vision of a greater sense of wholeness and human connectiveness that I truly believe beckons us all.

ACKNOWLEDGMENTS

"*Come see me after class. I think you should be one of Lee High School's exchange students to Barranquilla, Columbia.*"

Those words from my high school Latin teacher, Kay Grilliot, altered my life in spring 1972. She helped ignite my wanderlust bug and I will forever be in her debt. God bless her!

While Mrs. Grilliot ignited the fire, so many other stoked my wanderlust flames. First and foremost, my parents, Audie and Mary Anderson, who wholeheartedly encouraged and supported my high school exchange trip. In addition, my grandfather, Reverend George S. Jarman, challenged me to be conscious not only of my own, but the life stories and experiences of others as well.

As I grew older and began my travels in earnest, church friend and travel agent Ed Eisendrath booked dozens of my journeys over the years. Through his experience and guidance, I was remarkably free of travel mishaps and always appreciated his recommendations of where else to visit "while I was in the neighborhood" on my journeys

Constant supporters too were Milwaukee's Immanuel Presbyterian clergy—The Reverend Doctor Deborah Block and The Reverend Doctor William Johnstone—and the entire church congregation, who aided and abetted my travels, not only with prayers of support, but often with financial support for medical supplies, field ambulances, and ongoing financial support for mission hospitals and sites abroad, particularly in India and Africa.

To Jon Vice, President and Chief Executive Officer Emeritus of Children's Hospital Health System, friend and mentor. Thanks for creating a culture of care and excellence at Milwaukee's Children's Hospital that recognized and encouraged individuals to pursue their passions, both professionally and personally. Thank you for indulging and encouraging my pursuits

Thanks to Linda Galecke, a Special Assistant and special person who kept my work life afloat while I was off on one journey or another.

I am indebted to Dr. Fred Tavill and the late Dr. John R. Petersen, whose gentle cajoling enticed me to explore global health as a full-time professional endeavor and for their wisdom and guidance along the way.

Thanks to the leadership and staff of Project Hope for their concern, care, and commitment to health professionals and their patients around the world. To my friends and colleagues at Project Hope, with you I say, "Once a HOPIE, always a HOPIE!

Presbyterian missionaries Salvador and Irma de la Torre, Paul and Judy Jewett, and Cherian and Kalindi Thomas were sources of inspiration and awe for their unconditional commitment to their patients and those they served on the mission field, often at the expense of their own health and well-being. Blessed indeed are these peacemakers.

To Kira Henschel, thanks for guiding me through the process of bringing my story to others. I am grateful for your keen insights, helpful spirit, and guiding hand.

Finally, to Kathy Spini, life partner and fellow wanderlust soul. Thanks for your support, prodding, and partnership in making my dream of sharing my experiences a reality! My true joy now is looking forward to our next adventures and the extraordinary memories we'll share.

About the Author

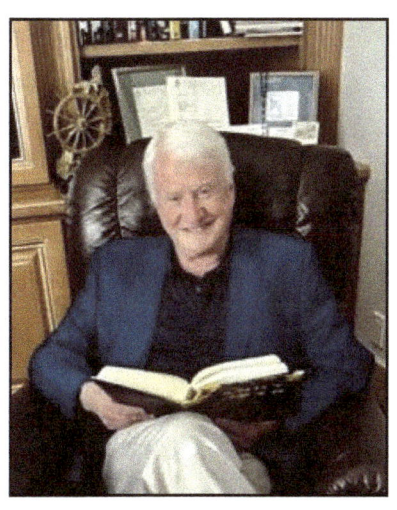

Dr. Mark Anderson is a health administrator whose career has encompassed senior executive roles in prominent hospitals, academic health centers, and renowned global health and health education organizations. He holds master's and doctorate degrees in Health Administration from the University of Alabama at Birmingham and a master's degree in Theology from McCormick Theological Seminary in Chicago. His many travels have provided him with a bird's-eye view of life for those living in remote, developing, and war-torn countries, and has brought him face to face with several of the leading humanitarians of our day. His debut memoir, *Through the Lens of Humanity*, recounts both his halcyon and harried journeys as he pursued his lifelong wanderlust. It reflects on who we are and who we can be as human for ourselves and others. Dr. Anderson was born in Alabama and lives in Illinois and Arizona.

Email: meamander@gmail.com

www.ingramcontent.com/pod-product-compliance
Lightning Source LLC
Chambersburg PA
CBHW050201240426
43671CB00013B/2209